AF663905

Common Drug Plants and Ayurvedic Remedies

By

Dr. Anil Kumar Dhiman

Ph. D.(Botany). FES, FUWAI

APSI Young Scientist and Gold Medal Awardee 1999

Information Scientist

Gurukul Kangri University

Haridwar -249 404 (India)

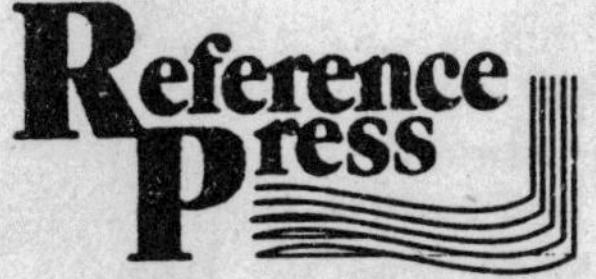

4831/24, Ansari Road
Darya Ganj
New Delhi-110 002
Phone : 23260807
Fax : 23274173
E-mail: essess@del3vsnl.net.in

First Published 2004

ISBN : 81-88583-51-0

Price : Rs. 1325/-

Published by :

Reference Press

4831/24, Ansari Road, Darya Ganj,
New Delhi - 110 002
Phone : 23260807
Fax : 23274173

Laser Typesetting:

Mukesh Graphics

L-2/8. DDA Market.
Mangolepuri, New Delhi
Ph. : 27924405

Printed at :

Print Line

DEDICATED

To

My Parents

Shri Ramlal Dhiman & Shrimati Kamla Devi

And

My beloved wife

Shrimati Yashoda Rani

DISCLAIMER

This book is a reference book not meant for treatment, diagnose or prescription. The material contained in this book is in no way to be considered as a substitute for consultation with a duly licensed medical professional.

Contents

Preface

Today, we are living in the fast culture and have no time to cure ourselves. We are forced to live in a very special yet very dangerous time, wherein a new global culture is painfully struggling to be born. It is the challenge of the time to integrate human culture and knowledge to evolve a balanced system for healing.

The modern system of medicine has made a tremendous progress and synthetic drugs and antibiotics have revolutionized the complete scenario. But their toxic side effects are also being realized which has attracted the attention of whole world towards natural system of medicine, i.e., the ayurveda. Ayurveda, the system of life, is based on the herbs. This is an eternal system that has already integrated eight limbs of healing within itself, from herbs to surgery to psychology. It is seen that during last two decades, the people's attention of whole European countries and American sub-continents has increased many times and in USA alone, 25 percent health prescription is found to contain natural plant products. Day by Day, more and more people are switching over to plant drugs, herbal health foods and herbal tea in western world.

This book '*Common Drug Plants and Ayurvedic Remedies*' aims to provide a bird's eye view on common drug plants met with in Indian subcontinent. This is divided into three parts; the first part is introductory, the second part contains information about common plants of the country and the third parts deals with the ayurvedic remedies for common ailments. Its first part starts with the introduction, then the history of Indian medicine system i.e., ayurveda, energetics and therapeutics of herbs and various types of herbal preparations etc are given. In its part second, the plants are arranged with their common names, followed by theirs' Latin names and families. The main identification characters of the plants are given besides, the parts used and medicinal uses. The third part of the book gives a list of various recipes for common ailments for the general users, which are based on the standard works like that of Nadkarni (1954) and Chopra et al., (1958) and mainly of Miller (2002). Though, the utmost care has been taken in providing the remedies for common ailments yet the readers are advised to consult the doctors in case of seriousness.

In preparing this monograph, the works of various authors has been consulted, for which author is grateful of them. As far as the personal help is concerned, the author is thankful to Dr. P. Kaushik, Professor of Botany, Department of Botany and Microbiology, Gurukul Kangri University, Haridwar (U.A.); Dr. S.K. Gupta, Secretary, APSI, and Former Head of Botany Department, DAV (PG) College, Muzaffarnagar (U.P.) for their suggestions. The author is also thankful to Mr. S.C. Sinha, Ex – Library Officer, Central Building Research Institute, Roorkee (U.A.) and of Mr. S.K. Sharma, Central Library, Indian Institute of Technology, Roorkee (U.A.) for their help in various ways. The author also feels grateful to Mrs. Sheel Sethi and Mr. Sumit Sethi, the owners of Reference Press, New Delhi for publishing this work in a attractive form on time.

The author is indebted to his parents Mr. Ramlal Dhiman, and Mrs. Kamla Devi for their blessings and moral encouragement and to his sister Ms. Alka Rani for her help in writing of the manuscript. The author is also thankful to his son Aman, to whom he could not pay much attention, which he deserved while writing the book. In the last but not least, my sincere thanks are due to my wife Mrs. Yashoda Rani, who has been a source of inspiration to enable me to complete this work.

This is hoped that this book will serve not only as a practical guide to cure the diseases but also produce the faith in ayurvedic system of medicine.

Dr. Anil Kumar Dhiman

Dated : January, 2004

Information Scientist
Gurukul Kangri University
Haridwar -249 404 (U.A.)

Other books of the author

* Citation Analysis of the Research Field and Information Technology Development. Ess Ess Publications, New Delhi. 2001.
* Prolegomena to Universe of Knowledge. Ess Ess Publications. New Delhi, 2002.
* Research Methodology. 2 Vols. Ess Ess Publications, New Delhi, 2002.
* Special Libraries: Technical and Research Libraries. Ess Ess Publications, New Delhi, 2002.
* Academic Libraries. Ess Ess Publications, New Delhi, 2002.
* Basics of Information Technology for Librarians and Information Scientists. 2 Vols. Ess Ess Publications, New Delhi, 2003.
* Cataloguing of Non Book Materials. Ess Ess Publications, New Delhi, 2004.
* Medicinal Plants and Raw Drugs of India. Bishen Singh Mahendra Pal Singh, Dehradun, 2000.
* Medicinal Plants of Uttaranchal State. Chowkhamba Sanskrit Series Office, Varanasi, 2003 (In Press).
* Sacred Plants and their Medicinal Uses. Daya Publishing House, New Delhi, 2003.
* Wild Medicinal Plants of India. Bishen Singh Mahendra Pal Singh, Dehradun, 2003 (In Press).

Part I
Introductory Part

1
Introduction

Ayurveda is one of the great gifts of the sages of ancient India to mankind. It is one of the oldest scientific medical systems in the world, with a long record of clinical experience. However, it is not only a system of medicine in the conventional sense of curing disease but also a way of life that teaches us how to maintain and protect health. It shows us both how to cure disease and how to promote longevity. Ayurveda treats man as a "whole" - which is a combination of body, mind, and soul. Therefore it is a truly holistic and integral medical system.

The "Ayu" means all aspects of life from birth to death and "Veda" means knowledge or learning. Hence Ayurveda indicates the science by which life in its totality is understood. It is a way of life that describes the diet, medicine, and behavior that are beneficial or harmful for life. The roots of Ayurveda can be traced to the beginning of cosmic creation. Indian philosophers state that Ayurveda originated from Brahma, the creator of the universe. Brahma is not a mere individual but the unmanifest form of the Divine Lord, from whom the whole manifest world comes into being. The desire to maintain fitness, health, and longevity is one of the basic instincts of all creatures. Ayurveda in this respect sets the pattern for other systems of medicine. It is a tradition with an antiquity comparable to that of life itself:

AYURVEDA AND THE VEDAS

The Vedas are regarded as the oldest and most sacred written record of knowledge. The Vedas state that the Supreme

Being who created the Universe, out of love and concern for humanity, gave the Divine Vedas to all mankind through the Rishis or seers of wisdom. The words of the Vedas were carefully memorized according to metrical chants and transmitted from generation to generation. Thus the four Vedas – *Rig, Yajur, Sam* and *Atharva* – have come down to us through several thousands of years of oral transmission before finally being recorded in writing.

The *Rig Veda,* the oldest repositories of human knowledge were written about 4500-1600 B.C., described about 99 medicinal plants. *Yajur Veda* listed 82 plants and *Sam Veda,* described various medicinal plants already mentioned in *Rig Veda,* particularly, the Soma plant. *Atharva Veda,* dealt with 288 plants almost all with medicinal ingredients which were used to cure deadly diseases. Though all the Vedas contain references to Ayurvedic concepts, the *Atharva Veda* contains more of these, so much so that Ayurveda is considered to be an Upaveda or a subsidiary teaching of the *Atharva.* In the *Atharva* we find references to anatomical and physiological factors, the disease process, treatment of specific diseases, and other systematic knowledge about Ayurveda.

In fact Ayurveda, is the foundation of the ancient medical science of life and art of healing. The eight divisions of Ayurveda were followed by the comprehensive works of Charaka (1500 B.C.) and of Sushruta (1500 B.C.), which gave a detailed description of the materia medica as it was known to ancient Vaidyas. Charak samhita, the first recorded treatise on Ayurveda was an edited version of an old scientific treatise by Agnivesha, who wrote on Ayurvedic medicine based on teaching of Ayurveda from his preceptor, Atreya, the great sage. This work dealt primarily with medicine and its seventh chapter was devoted entirely to the consideration of purgatives and emetics. There were six pupil of Acharya Punarvasu; Agnivesha, Jatukarana, Parashara, Kshreepani, Bhel and Harit around 1500 B.C. Each of them described his own thoughts in the form of Samhitas. Bhel presented his own thoughts in '*Bhel Samhita*' which now-a-days, is available only in scattered form. The other pupil of Punarvasu, Harit also wrote '*Harit Samhita*' that is available today also. But the present '*Harit Samhita*' is not the original one because the pattern of its description does not resemble with other samhitas of that time. Although, some learned researchers considered this work as much older as were the other Samhitas. The other Samhitas; '*Agnivesha Samhita*' of Agnivesha, '*Jatukaran Samhita*' of Jatukaran, '*Parashar Samhita*' of Parashar and '*Ksheerpani Samhita*' of Ksheerpani are not available now. '*Kashyap Samhita*' or '*Vrahad Jivakiya Tantra*' was also written nearly of Charak's time but it is also available only in scattered form.

CHARAKA

The *charaka Samhita* is the oldest of the three and was probably first compiled around 1500 BC. It is considered the prime work on the basis concepts of Ayurveda. Charaka represents the Atreya school of physicians. It is a systematic work divided into eight Sthanas or sections, which are further divided into 120 chapters. The first section of the *Charaka Samhita* describes the fundamental principles of Ayurveda. Then it elaborates the physiological and anatomical structure of the human body, various etiological agents, along with their role in pathogenesis, symptoms and signs of various diseases, the methodology for examination of patients, treatment, and prognosis. The preventive aspects of treatment include daily and seasonal regimens, as well as dietetics and social behavior conducive to mental health. The chapter on dietetics is a vast store of information. The section on curative treatments includes detailed descriptions of medicinal plants and their properties, various herbal preparations, and therapeutic procedures such as elimination therapy. The chapters on rejuvenation therapy and prevention of the aging process are today considered as good sources for modern research work. The *Charaka Samhita* is written in prose as well as in beautiful poetry, comparable to any Sanskrit classic. Its combined medico-social and medico-philosophical approach is a source of inspiration to anyone who studies the original text.

Acharya Charka has divided the drugs into 50 Vargas (groups) as follows :

1. **Jeevaneeyam (Promoting Life)** : Jivaka, Rishabhaka, Meda, Mahaamedaa, Kaakoli, Ksheerakaakoli, Maashaparni, Mudgapami, Jeevanti and Yastimadhu.
2. **Brimhaneeyam (Promoting Growth)** : Ksheerini, Raajakshavaka, Bala, Kaakoli, Ksheerakaakoli, Vatyaayani, Bhadroudani, Bhaaradwaaji, Payasyaa and Rishyagandhaa.
3. **Lekhaniyam (Reducing Growth)** ; Mustaa, Kushta, Haridraa, Vachaa, Daaruharidraa, Ativishaa, Katukarohini, Chitraka, Karanja and Haimavati.
4. **Bhedaneeyam (Proroting Evacuation)** : Trivrit, Arka, Eranda, Agnimukhi, Danti, Chitramula, Chirbilwa, Sankhini, Katukarohini and Brahmadandi.
5. **Sandhaaneeyam (Promoting Union)** : Yastimadhu, Guduchi, Prisnipami, Ambashtaa, Samangaa, Mocharasa, Dhaataki, Lodhra, Priyangu and Katphala.
6. **Deepaneeyam (Promoting Appetite)** : Pippali, Pippalimoola, Chavya, Chitraka, Sunthi, Amiavetasa, Maricha, Ajamodaa, Bhallathakaasthi and Hingu.
7. **Balyam (Promoting Strength)** : Indravaaruni, Vrishabha, Sataavari, Maashaparni, Vidaari, Aswagandhaa, Sthiraa, Rohini, Balaa and Atibalaa.
8. **Varnyam (Promoting Complexion)** : Chandana, Tunga, Padmaka, Useera, Yashtimadhu, Manjistaa, Saaribaa, Ksheera-kaakoli, Sitaa and Lataa.
9. **Kanthyam (Promting Voice)** : Saaribaa, Ikshumoola, Yastimadhu, Pippali, Draakshaa, Vidaari, Kaayaphala, Hansapadi, Brihati and Khantakaari.

10. **Hridyam (Promoting Happy feeling)** : Aamra, Aamraataka, Lakucha, Karamarda, Vrikshaamla, Amiavetasa, Kuvala, Badara, Daadima and Maatulunga.

11. **Triptighanam (Destl-oying Satisfaction)** : Sunthi, Chitramoola, Chavya. Vidanga, Murva, Guduchi, Vachaa, Musta, Pippali and Patola.

12. **Arsoghnam (Destroying Piles)** : Kutaja, Bilwa, Chitraka, Sunthi, Ativisha, Haritaki, Dhanvayaasaka, Daaruharidra, Vachaa and Chavya.

13. **Kustaghnam (Destroying Skin Diseases)** : Khadira, Haritaki, Aamalaki, Haridraa, Bhallaataka, Saptaparna, Aaragwadha, Karaveera, Vidanga and Jaathi Pravaala.

14. **Kandughnam (Destroying Itching)** : Chandana, Jataamaansi, Aaragwadha, Naktamaala, Nimba, Kutaja, Sarshapa, Yastimadhu, Daaruharidra and Mustaa.

15. **Krimighnam (Destroying Parasites)** : Sigru, Maricha, Gandira, Kebuka, Vidanga, Nirgundi, Kinihi, Gokshura, Bhaarangi and Aakhuparnika.

16. **Vishaghnam (Destroying Poison)** : Haridraa, Manjistaa, Raasnaa, Sukshmaila, Syaamaa, Chandana, Kathaka, Sireesha, Sindhuvaara and Sleshmaataka.

17. **Sthanyajananam (Producing Milk)** : Virana, Saali, Shastika, Ikshumoola, Kusamoola, Darbhamoola, Kaasamoola, Gundra, Utkatamoola and Katrinamoola.

18. **Sthanyasodhanam (Purifying Milk)** : Paathaa, Sunthi, Devadaaru, Mustaa, Murvaa, Guduchi, Kutajabeeja, Bhunimba, Katukarohini and Saaribaa.

19. **Sukrajananam (Producing Sperm)** : Jivaka, Rishabhaka, Kaakoli, Ksheerakaakoli, Mudgaparni, Maashapami, Medaa, Sataavari, Jataamansi and Karkatakasringi.

20. **Sukrasodhanam (Purifying Sperm)** : Kushta Elavaaluka, Katphala, Samudraphena, Kadambaniryaasa Ikshukanda, Ikshuraka, Vasuka and Useera.

21. **Smehopagam (Promoting lubrication)** : Draakshaa, Yastimadhu, Guduchi, Medaa, Vidaari, Kaakoli, Ksheerakaakoli, Jivaka, Jivanti and Saalaparni.

22. **Sedopagam (Promoting Sweet)** : Sigru, Erandamula, Arka, Vrischira, Punarnava, Yava, Tila, Kuluttha and Maasha.

23. **Vamanopagam (Promoting Vomiting)** : Madhu, Yastimadhu, Kovidaara, Karbudaara, Neepa, Vidula, Bimbi, Sanapushpi, Arka and Pratyakpushpi.

24. **Virechanopagam (Promoting Purgation)** : Draakshaa, Kaasmari, Parushaka, Abhayaa, Aamalaki, Vibheetaki; Kuvela, Badara, Karkandhu and Pilu.

25. **Aasthaapanopagam (Useful for Non-oily Enemata):** Trivrit, Bilwa, Pippali, Kushta, Sarshapa, Vachaa, Kutajabeeja, Satapushpaa, Yastimadhu and Madanaphala.

26. **Anuvaasanopagam (Useful for Oily Enemata)** : Raasnaa, Devadaaru, Bilwa, Madanaphala, Satapushpaa, Punarnavaa, Vrischeera, Gokshura, Agnimantha and Syonaka.

27. **Sirovirechaniyam (Purging Doshas in the Head)** : Jyotishmati, Kshavaka, Maricha, Pippali, Vidanga, Sigru, Sarshapa, Apaamaarga, Sweta and Mahaaswetaa.

28. **Chardinigrahanam (Controlling Vomitting)** : Jambu, Aamrapallava, Maadiphala, Badara, Daadima, Yava, Yastimadhu, Useera, Mrith and Laaja.

29. **Trishnaanigrahaanam (Controlling Thirst)** : Sunthi, Dhanvayaasa, Mustaa, Parpataka, Chandana, Bhunimba, Guduchi, Useera, Dhaanyaka and Patola.

30. **Hiccaanigrahanam (Checking Hiccough)** : Sati, Pushkaramoola, Badarabeeeja, Kantakaari, Brihati, Vriksharuha, Haritaki, Pippali, Duraalabhaa and Karkatakasringi.

31. **PurishaSangrahaneeyam (Reducing Faecal Matter):** Priyangu, Ananthaa, Aamraasthi, Katwanga, Lodhra, Mocharasa, Samangaa, Dhaataki, Bhaarangi and Padmakesara.

32. **Purisha Virajaneeyam (Pruifying Faecal Matter) :** Jambu, Sallakitwak, Kachchura, Yastimadhu, Mocharasa, Devadaaru-niryaasa, Bhrustamrit, Payasyaa, Utpala and Tilakana.

33. **Mootra S angrahaneeyam (Reducing U rine) :** Jambu, Aamra, Plaksha, Vata, Kapitana, Udumbara, Aswattha, Bhallataka, Asmantaka and Somavalka.

34. **Mootra Virajaneeyam (Purifying Urine) :** Padma, Dtpala, Nalina, Kumuda, Sougandhika, Pundareeka, Satapatra, Madhuka, Priyangu and Dhaathaki-pushpa.

35. **Mootra Virechneeyam (Increasing Urine) :** Vrikshaadani, Swadamstra, Vasuka, Suryaavarta, Paashaanabhedi, Darbha, Kusa, Kaassa, Mustaa and Utkatamoola.

36. **Kaasahara (Relieving Cough) :** Draakshaa, Haritaki, Aamalaki, Pippali, Duraalabhaa, Karkatasringi, Kantakaari, Punamavaa, Taamalaki and Vruschira.

37. **Swaasahara (Relieving Dyspepsia) :** Sati, Pushkaramula, Amiavetasa, Elaa, Hingu, Agaru, Surasaa, Taamalaki, Jeevanti and Chandana.

38. **Swayathuhara (Relieving Swelling) :** Paatala, Agnimandha, Syonaka, Bilwa, Kassmari, Kantakaari, Brihati, Saalaparni, Prisniparni, Gokshura and Dasamoola.

39. **Jwaraharam (Relieving Fever) :** Saaribaa, Sarkaraa, Paathaa, Manjistaa, Draakshaa, Peelu, Parushaka, Haritaki, Aamalaki and Vibheetaki.

40. **Sramaharam (Relieving Exhaustion) :** Draakshaa, Kharjura, Piyaala, Badara, Daadima, Phalgu, Parushaka, Ikshu, Yava and Shastika.

41. **Daahaprasamanam (Relieving burning Sensation):** Laaja, Chandana, Kaasmari, Madhuka, Sarkaraa, Neelotpala, Useera, Saaribaa, Guduchi and Hribera.
42. **Seethaprasamanam (Relieving Cold) :** Tagara, Agaru, Dhaanyaka, Sringabera, Ajmadaa, Vachaa, Kantakaari, Agnimandha, Syonaaka and Pippali.
43. **Udardaprasamanam (Relieving Rashes) :** Tinduka, Piyaala, Badara, Khadira, Kadara, Saptaparna, Aswakarna, Arjuna, Asana and Irimeda.
44. **Angamardaprasamanam (Releiving Body Pains) :** Vidaarigandhaa, Prisniparni, Brihati, Kantakaari, Eranda, Kaakoli, Chandana, Useera, Elaa and Madhuka.
45. **Sulaprasamanam (Releiving Colic) :** Pippali, Pippalmoola, Chavya, Chitraka, Sunthi, Maricha, Ajamodaa, Ajagandha, Jeeraka and Gandeera.
46. **Sonitaasthaapanam (Restoring Blood) :** Madhu, Madhuka, Kunkuma, Mocharasa, Loshta, Lodhra, Gairika, Prenkhana, Sarkaraa and Laaja.
47. **Vedanaasthaapana (Relieving Sufferings) :** Arjuna, Katphala, Kadamba, Padmaa, Kumuda, Mocharasa, Sirisha, Vanjula, Elaavaluka and Asoka.
48. **Samgnaasthaapana (Restoring Consciousness) :** Hingu, Katphala, Irimeda, Vachaa, Sati, Braahmi, Golomi, Jataamaansi, Guggulu and Katurohini.
49. **Prajaasthaapana (Fixing Pregnancy) :** Indravaaruni, Braahmi, Durvaa, Swetadurva, Paatali, Aamalaki, Haritaki, Katurohini, Balaa and Prenkhana.
50. **Vayasthaapana (Fixing Youthfulness) :** Guduchi, Haritaki, Aamalaki, Raasna, Swetaa, Jeevanti, Sataavari, Braahmi, Sthiraa and Punaravaa.

SUSHRUTA

Sushruta represents the Dhanvantari school of surgeons, and is considered in Ayurveda to be the father of surgery. In the

Sushruta Samhita there are sophisticated descriptions of surgical instruments. Its classifications of fractures, wounds, abscesses, and burns as well as its elaboration of procedures for plastic surgery and anal-rectal surgery have all stood the test of time. He has also described the original concepts of pathogenesis. Sushruta describes a procedure for dissection of the human body by the maceration method. The knowledge of anatomy — bones, joints, nerves, heart, blood vessels, and circulation — is surprising and praiseworthy. The descriptions of the "marmas," vital points in the body, is comparable to the system of acupuncture points used in traditional Chinese medicine. He clearly states the importance of both theoretical and practical knowledge and describes ways and means to develop the surgical skill.

Acharya Susruta has divided the plants into 38 ganas (groups) as follows.

1. **Vidaarigandhaadigana** : Vidaarigandhaa (Saalapamee), Vidaaree, Viswadevaa (Gangerukee), Sahadeva (a variety of Balaa), Swedamshtraa (Gokshura), Prithaakpamee (Prisniparnee), Sataavaree, Saaribaa, Krishna saaribaa, Jeevaka and Rishabhaka, Mahaasahaa (Maashaparnee), Kshudasahaa (Mudgaparnee), Brihatee, Kantakaaree, Punarnavaa, Eranda, Hansapaadi, Vrischikaalee and Rishabhee.

   TheVidaarigandhaadigana counteracts Vaata and Pitta.It is useful in Sosha (emaciation) Gulma (tumour), Angamarda (body soreness), Oordhwaswaasa (a kind of Swassa) and Kaasa (Cough).

2. **Aaragwadhaadigana** : Aaragwadha, Madana, Gopaghonta (Karkotee), Kantakee (Vikarnkata), Kutaja, Paathaa, Paatalaa, Moorvaa, Indrayava, Saptaparna, Nimba, Kurantaka, Daaseekurantaka, Gudoochee, Chitraka, Saarngeshtaa (Kaakajanghaa), Karanja and Vitapakaranja, Pgtola, Kiraatatiktaka and Sushavee (Kaaravella).

TheAaragwadhaadigana checks Kapha and poison. It is also used in Prameha, Kushta, Jwara, Vami (Vomitting) and Kandu (Itching) and to purify Vrana (Dushta).

3. **Varunaadigana** : Varuna, Aartagala (Kakubha), Sigru, Madhusigru, Tarkaaree, Meshasringee (Karkatasringee), Pooteeka (Chiribilwa), Naktamaala (Brihat Karanja), Morata (Ankolapushpa), Agnimantha, two kinds of Saireyaka (red and blue flowers), Bimbee, Vasuka (Buka), Vasira (Markatapippalee), Chitraka, Sataavari, Bilwa, Ajasringee (Chagalavishanikaa), Darbha (Kusa), Brihatee and Kantakaari.

   The Varunaadigana checks Kapha and Medas. It is also useful in hèadache, Gulma, and Aabhyantara vidradhi (internal abscess).

4. **Veeratarwaadigana** : Veerataru (Savara), two kinds of Sahachara, Darbha, Vrikshaadanee, Gundraa (Paadaraka bhedah), Nala, Kusa, Kaasa, Asmabhedaka, Agnimandha, Morataa (Ankola-pushpa), Vasuka, Vasira, Bhallooka, Kurantaka, Indeevara, kapotavankaa, and Swadamshtra (Gokshura).

   The Veerataraadigana checks vaata diseases. It is useful in Asmaree (Stone), Sarkaraa (Sand in urine etc.),Mootrakrichra (painful passage of urine),Mootraaghaata (retention of urine etc.) and Ruja (a kind of pain connected with passing of urine).

5. **Saalasaaraadigana** : Saalasaara, Ajakarna (Sarja), Khadira, Kadara (Swetasaara), Kaalaskandha, Krarnuka (Pooga), Bhoorja, Meshasringa (Karkatasringi), Tinisa (Syandana), Chandana, Kuchandana, Simsapaa, Sireesha, Asana (Beejaka), Dhava (Sakata), Arjuna (Kakubha) Taala, Saaka, Naktamaala, Pooteeka, Aswakama, Agaru and Kaaleeyakam (Daaru-haridraa).

   The Saalasaaraadigana is very helpful in Kushta. It also acts as a curative in Prameha and Paandu (anaemia) and lessens Kapha and Medas.

6. **Rodhraadigana** : Rodhra, Saavaralodhra, Palasa, Kutannata, Asoka, Phanjee (Bhaarangee), Katphala, Elavaalukarn, Sallakee, Jinginee, Kadamba, Saala and Kadalee.

   The Rodhraadigana lessens Medas and Kapha. It is curative ofYoni Dosha (Disorders of Yoni), astringent (Stambhee), develops complextion (Varnya) and mitigates the poisons (Vishvinaasana).

7. **Arkaadigana** : Arka, Alarka (Sweta Arka), Karanja, Vitapakaranja, Naagadantee, Mayooraka (Apaamaarga), Bhaargee, Raasnaa, Indrapushpee, Kshudra Swetaa (Sephanda), Mahaaswetaa, Vrischikaalee, Alavanaa (Jyotishmaee) and Taapasa Vriksha (Inguda).

   The Arkaadigana checks kapha, aredas and visha. It is helful Krimi and Kustha and is a purificator of Vranas (Viseshaat Vrana Sodhanah).

8. **Surasaadigana** : Surasaa (Krishna Tulasee), Sweeta Surasaa (Sweta Tulasee), Phanijjaka (Maruvaka), Arjaka (Swetakutheraka), Bhoosthrina (Angudaaka), Sugandhaka (Dronapushpa), Surnkha (Raajikaa), Kaalamaala (Krishnamallikaa), Kaasamarda, Kshavaka (Chinkini), Kharapushpaa (Kshavakabhedah), Vidanga, Katphala, Surasee (Bilwanasee), Nirgundee, Kulaahala (Mundikaa), Undurukarnika (Mooshikakarnikaa), Phanjee (Bhaargee), Praacheebala (Matsyaakshaka), Kaakamaachee and Vishnumustika.

   The Suraasadigana checks Kapha and destroys Krimees (parasites). It is also useful in cold, loss of appetite, hardbreathing and cough and it also purifies Vrana.

9. **Mushkakaadigana** : Mushkaka (Kshaaravriksha), Palaasa (Kinsuka), Dhava, Chitraka, Madana, Vrikshaka (Kutaja), Simsapaa, Vajravriksha and Thriphala (Hareetaki, Vibheetaki and Aamalaki).

   The Mushkaadigana reduces Medas and useful in

Sukradosha (impurity of Semen). It also acts as a curative in Prameha, Árass, Paanduroga and Sarkara.

10. **Pippalyaadigana** : Pippalee, Pippaleemoola, Chavya, Chitraka, Sringabera (Sunthee), Maricha, Hastipipalee (Gajapippalee), Harenuka, Elaa, Ajamodaa, Indrayava, Paathaa, Jeeraka, Sarshapa, Mahaanimbaphala, Hingu, Bhaarangee, Madhu-rassa (Moorvaa), Ativisha, Vachaaa, Vidangaa and Katurohinee.

The Pippalyaadigana reduces Kapha Dosha, P ratisyaaya (cold), Vaata, anorexia, Gulma, and soola (pain). It creates appetite (deepana) and digests (resolves) Aama-Dosha (Aama paachana).

11. **Elaadigana** : Ela, Tagara, Kushta, Maamsee, Dhyaamaka (Mattrina) Twak, Patra (Patrakarn), Naagapushpa (Naagakesara), Priyangu, Harenuka, Vyaaghranakha, Sukti (Vyaaghrana-khabheda), Chandana, Sthouneyaka (Thuneraka), Sreeveshtaka (Saraladruma), Chocha, Choraka, Vaaluka, Guggulu, Sarjarasa, Turushka (Sihiaka), Kunduraka (Sallakee Chopa), Agaru, Sprukkaa, Useera, Bhadrudaaru, Kunkumam and Punnaagakesara.

The Elaadigana checks Vaata and Kapha and Visha (Poison). It creates lustre of the skin (Varna Prassaada) and destroys itching (Kantoo), Pidakaa (Diseases with elevated skin on account of an abscess etc.) and Kotha (eruption on skin).

12. **Vachaadigana** : Vachaa, Mustaa, Ativishaa, Abhayaa, Bhadradaru and Naagakesara.

The Vachaadigana purify the breast-milk and acts as amelioratives (Samana) in amaateesaara. This is especially digestives of the Doshaas (Viseshaat Doshapaachanou).

13. **Haridraadigana** : Haridraa, Daaruharidraa, Kalasee (Prisnipamee), Kutajabeej and Yastimadhu.

The Haridraadigana purify the breast-milk and acts as ameliorative (Samana) in Aamaateesaara. This is especially digestives of the Doshaas (Viseshaat Doshapaachanou).

14. **Syaamaadigana** : Syaama (Sweta Trivrut), Mahaasyaama (Vriddha-daaraka). Trivrut (having red root), Dantee, Sankhinee (Yavatiktabhedah), Tilvaka (Rodhra), Kampilaka (Rochanikaa), Ramyaka (Mahaanimba), Krarnuka, Putresrenee, Gavakshee, Raajavriksha, Karaanja, Vitapakaranja, Gudoochi, Saptala (Snuheebheda), Chagalaantree (Vriddhadaarakabheda), Sudhaa (Sehunda) and Suvarnaksheeri.

    The Syaamaadigana, checks Gulma and Visha (poison), Aanaaha (Distension of abdomen), Udara and Udaavarta. It causes free evacuation of the bowels.

15. **Brihatyaadigana** : Brihatee, Kantakaarika, Kutajaphala, Paathaa and Madhukarn (Yasthimadhu).

    The Brihatyaadigana is a digestive (Paachaneeya) and it checks Vaata and Pitta. It is also beneficial in Arochaka (Anorexia) due to Kapha, Hridroga and Mootrakrichra (Dysuria).

16. **Patolaadigana** : Patola, Chandana, Kuchandana (Raktachandana), Moorvaa, Gudoochi, Paathaa and Katurohinee.

    The Patolaadigana cures Pitta, Kapha and Arochaka (Anorexia). 11 a Hays j wara a nd c ures vomitting, itching and Visha (Poison) and is also beneficial in Vranas.

17. **Kaakolaadigana** : Kaakolee, Ksheerakaakolee, Jeevaka, Rishabhaka, Mudgaparnee, Maashaparni, Medaa, Mahaamedaa, Chinnaruhaa (Gudoochi), Karkatasringi, Tugaaksheeree (Vamsa-lochanaa), Padmaka, Papoundareeka, Riddhi, Vriddhi, Mridweeka (Draakshaa), Jeewantee and Madhukarn.

    The Kaakolyaadigana cures Pittasonita (Rakta vitiated by Pitta; or Pitta and Sonita) and Vaayu. It is Jeevana (increases vitality), Brimhana (promotes body growth) and Vrishya (increases semen) and increases breast-milk and Kapha.

18. **Ooshakaadigana** : Ooshaka (Kshaaramrittika), Saindhavalavana, Silaajathu, Kaaseesadwaya (Vaalukaaseesam and Pushpakaaseesam), Hingu and Tuththaka.

The Ooshakaadigana allays Kapha and diminishes Medas. 11 acts as curative in Asmaree (stone), Sarkaraa (sand in urine), Mootrakrichchra and Gulma.

19. **Saaribaadigana** : Saaribaa, Madhuka (Yashtimadhu), Chandana, Kuchandana (Rakhtachandana), Padmaka, Kaasmareephala, Madhookapuspha and Useeram.

The Saaribaadigana allays thirst and Raktapitta. It is beneficial in Pittajwara and cures daaha (burning sensation).

20. **Anjanaadigana** : Anjana (Souveeraanjanam), Rasaanjanam, Naaga-puspha (Naagakesaram), Priyangu, Neelotpala, Nalada (Maamsee), Nalinakesa (Padmakesara) and Madhukarn.

The Anjanaadigana cures Raktapitta and is beneficial in Visha (poisoning). It also allays internal burning sensation.

21. **Parooshakaadigana** : Parooshakaa, Draakshaa, Katphala, Daadima, Raajaadana (Ksheerika), Katakaphala and Saakaphalas (fruits of Saaka tree).

The Parooshakaadigana cures Vaata and disorders urine. It is pleasant to take (Hridya) and allays thirst and creates appetite.

22. **Priyangwaadigana** : Priyaangu, Samangaa (Anjali-Kaarikaa of Lajjalu), Dhaatakee, Punnaaga (Tunga), Naagapusphpam, Chandanam, Kuchandanam, Mocharasa (Saalimali chupa), Rasaanjana, Kumbheeka, Srontonjana Padmakesara, Yojanavalli (Manjishta) and Deerghamoolaa (Duraalabhaa).

The Priyangwaadigana is useful in Pakswaateesara and causes Sandhaana (union of bones etc.). This is also beneficial in Pitta and healing the ulcers (Vranaanam chaapi Ropanou).

23. **Ambashtaadigana** : Ambashtaa (Machikaa), Dhaatakikussuma, Samangaa (Lajjaalu), Katvanga (Araluka), madhuka, Bilwapesikaa (Baala Bhilwagirah), Saavaraprodhra (Lodhra), Palaasa, Nandeevriksha (Kaasmaree) and Padmakesaram.

The Ambashtaadigana is useful in Pakswaateesara and causes Sandhaana (union of bones etc.). This is also beneficial in Pitta and healing the ulcers (Vranaanam chaapi Ropanou).

24. **Nyagrodhaadigana** : Nyagrodha (Vata), Udumbara, Aswattha, Plaksha, Madhuka, Kapeethana (Aamraataka), Kakubha, Aamra, Kosaamra, Chorakapatra (Laakshaavrikshaa), Jamboodwaya (Raajajamboo and Kaakajamboo), Piyaala (Saaradruma), Madhooka (Gudapushpa), Rohinee (Katphala), Vanjula (Vetasa), Kadamba, Badaree, Tindukee (Tinduka Vriksha), Sallakee, Rodhra, Saavararodhra, Bhallaataka, Palaasa and Nandeevriksha.

The Nyagrodhaadigana is beneficial in the treatment of Vranas (Vranyah). It is astringent (Sangraahee) and is useful in fractures (Bhagna Sandhaana). Fruther, it allays Raktapitta (haemorrhage) and Daaha (burning sensation) and reduces Medas (Obesity) and it is useful in Yonidosha (Yonivyaapat) also.

25. **Gudoochyaadigana** : Gudoochi, Nimba, Kustumburu (Dhaanyakarn), Chandanam and Padmakarn.

The Gudcochyaadigana checks all jwars (fevers) and increases appetite (Deepana). It allays Hrillaasa (nausea accompanied with hawking of mucuos etc. from the mouth), Arochaka (Anorexia), Vami (Vomiting), thrist and burning sensation.

26. **Utpalaadigana** : Utpala (Neelotpala), Raktopala, Kumuda (Swetot-pala), Sougandhika (a sweet-scented blue lily different from Neelotpala), Kuvalaya (Utpala having blue-

white colour), Pundareeka (White lotus) and Madhukarn (Yashtimadhu).

The Utpalaadigana allays daaha (burning sensation), Pitta and Rakta, Thirst, Visha (Poisoning), Hridroga, Chardi (Vomiting) and Moorchaa (Syncope).

27. **Mustraadigana** : Mustaa, Haridraa, Daaruharidraa, Hareetakee, Aamalaka, Vibheetakea, Kushta, Haimavatee (Vachaa), Paathaa, Katurohinee, Saarngeshtaa (Yavatikaa), Ativishaa, Draavidee (Elaa) Bhallaataka and Chitraka.

The Mustakadigana reduces Kaphaand is digestive (Paachana). It also cures Yoni-dosha and purifies breast-milk.

28. **Triphalaa** : Hareetakee, Aamalaka and Vibheetaka.

The Thriphala reduces Kapha and Pitta. It is useful in Prameha and Kushta and is also beneficial to eyes. It creates appetite and is used in Vishamajwara.

29. **Trikatukam** : Pippalee, Marichaa and Sringabera (Sunthee).

The Trikatukam is also called Tryooshanam and Vyosha. It reduces Kapha and Medas and is useful in Prameha, Kushta, Twagaamaya (skin diseases) and creates appetite. It is also useful in Gulma, Peenasa and Agnyalpataa (poor digestion).

30. **Aamalakyaadigana** : Aamalakee, Hareetakee, Pippalee and Chitraka.

The Aamatakyaadigana is useful in all jwaras (fevers), beneficial to eyes and also used as an aphrodisiac. It also cures Kaphaa-rochaka (Anorexia due to Kapha).

31. **Trapwaadigana** : Trapu (Vangam-Tin), Seesa (Lead), Taamra (Copper), Rajata (Silver), Krishaloha (Steel), Suvarna (Gold) and Lohamala (Mandoor).

The Trapwaadigana is useful in gara (poisoning usually through worms (Krimi), thirst, Visha, Hridroga, Paandu, and Prameha.

32. **Laakshaadigana :** Laakshana, Aarevata, (Kiramaalaka), Kutaja, Aswa-maaraka (Karaveera), Kathphala, Haridraa, Daaru-haridraa, Nimba, Saptachchada, Maalatee and Traayamaanaa.

The Laakshaadigana is Kashaaya (astringent), bitter and sweet in taste and it reduces ailments due to Kapha and Pitta. It is also useful in Kushta and Krimi (worms) and purifies Dushta Vranas.

33. **Kaneeyahpanchamoola (Hraswapanchamoolam or Laghupanchmool) :** Trikantaka (Gokshura), Brihatee, Kantakaari, Pithakparnee and Vidaarigandhaa (Saalaparni).

The Kaneeyahpanchamoola is Kaashaaya, Tikta and Madhura in Rasa (taste) and it reduces Vaata and ameliorates Pitta. It is Brimhana (tissue builder) and increases strength (Balavardhanah).

34. **Mahaapachmoola (Brihat Panchamoola) :** Bilwa, Agnimandha, Tuntuka (Syonaaka), Paatala and Kaasmaree.

The Mahaapanchamoolam is bitter (tikta) and checks Kapha and Vaata. It is Laghu in Paaka and promotes appetite with slightly sweet in Rasa (taste).

35. **Dasamoola :** Kaneeyahpanchamoola and Mahaapahchamoola collectively are called Dasamoola.

The Dasamoola gana reduces swaasa (hard breathing) and checks Kapha, Pitta and Vaayu. It digest Aama-dosha and is curative of all type of jwaras (fevers).

36. **Valleepanchamoola :** Vidaaree, Saaribaa, Rajanee (Haridraa), Gudoochee and Ajasringi.

The Valleepanchamoola is beneficial in Raktapitta and is used in three-kinds of Sopha (Aama, Pachyamaana and Pakwa), Prameha and Sukra.

37. **Kantakapanchamoola :** Karmarda, Trikantaka (Gokshura), Saireeyaka, Sataavaree and Gridhranakee.

The Kantakapanchamoola is beneficial in Raktapitta

and is used in three-kinds of Sopha (Aama, Pachyamaana and Pakwa), Prameha and Sukra.

38. **Trinapanchamoola** : Kusa, Kaasa, Nala, Darbha and Kaandekshuka.

    The Trinapanchmoola cures disorders of urine (Mootra Dosha), Raktapitta when it is used especially with milk. Laghupanchamoola and Mahaapanchamoola usually reduce Vaata Trínapanchamoola reduces Pitta; the other two, namely, Valleepanchamoola and kantaka Pachaa-moola, reduce Kapha. It should be understood that the substances in the groups (Ganas) may be altered or individually used and variously combined according to the Doshaas or Dooshyas etc. existing individually or in various combinations in a person.

VAGBHATTA

The next important authority in Ayurveda after Charaka and Sushruta is Vagbhatta of Sind, who flourished about the seventh century AD. His treatise called *Ashtanga Hridaya* presented a summary of Charaka and Sushruta with gleanings from other Ayurvedic writers like Agnivesha, Bhela, and Harita, and again brought the subject up-to-date. He introduced a number of new herbs and made valuable modifications and additions in surgery. He did all this in spite of strong opposition from the orthodox school. *Ashtanga Hridaya* is classified in six sections and contains 7,444 verses in 120 chapters.

Vagbhatta has divided the drug plants into 32 ganas (groups) as follows :

1. **Vamanaoushadhaga :** Madana, Madhuka (Yastimadhu), Lambaa (Tumbee), Nimba, Bimbee, Vissalaa (Indravarunee), Trapusa, Kutaja, Moorva, Devadaalee, Krimighna (Vidangam), Vidula (Jalavetasa), Dahana (Chitraka), Chitraa (Mooshikarparm\nee), Kosavatyou (Ghantalikaa and Dhamargava), Karanja, Kanaa (Pippalli), Lavana (Saindhavalavana), Vacha, Elaa and Sarshapa.

2. **Virechanaoushdhagana** : Nikumbha (Dantee), Kumbha (Trivruth), Thriphala, Gavakshee (Visalaa), Snuk, Sankhinee (Yavatiktaa), Neelinee, Tilwaka (Rodhra), Samyaka (Aaragwasdha), Kampillaka, Hemadugdhaa (Swarnakheeree), Dugdham (Milk) and Mootram (the urine of cow etc.).

3. **Niroohana Dravyagana** : Madanaphala, Kutaja (twak), Kushtam, Devadalee, Madhukarn, Vachaa, Dashamula, Daaru (Devadaaru), Rasana, Yava, Misi (Satapushpa), Kritavedhanam (Dhaamaargava), Kulmuttha (Madhu), Lavanam (Saindhavarn) and Trivruth.

4. **Seershavirechaneeyagana** : Vella (Vidanga), Apamarga, Vyosha (Trikatutam), Daarvee (Daruharidra), Suraalaa (Sreshta Sarjrasa), Saireeshabeeja, Baarhatabeeja (Brihatibeeja), Saigravam-beejam (Sigru beeja), Maadhooka Saara (Madhupushpasaara), Saindhavarn, Taarkshysailam (Sushkarasanjanam), Trutyou (Sookshma elaa and Sthoola elaa), and Prithveeka (Hinupatree).

5. **Vaataharaganas** : Bhadradaaru, Natam (Tagaram), Kushtam, Dasamoolaam and Baladwaya (Bala and Atibala).

6. **Pittaharaganas** (To check Pitta) : Doorwaa, Anantaa (Yavassa), Nimba, Vassa, Aatmaguptaa (Kapikachhu), Gundraa (Padayerakah), Abheeru (Sataavaree), Seetapaakee (Kaakanantikaabheda), and Priyangu. Besides, Nayagrodhaadi gana, Padmakadi gana and dwe sthire (Salparnee and Prishnipamee), Padam (Lotus), Vanyam (Kutannatam) and Saaribaaadi gana are also knowm to ameliorate pitta.

7. **Kapharaganas** : Aragwhaadhigana, Arkaadigana, Mushakaadigana, Surasaadigana, Mustaadigana and Vatsakaadigana.

8. **Jeevaneeyaadigana** : Jeevantee, Kaakolee, Ksheerakaakolee, Medaa, Mahamedaa, Mudgapamee,

Maashaaparnee, Rishabhaka, Jeevaka and Madhuka.

9. **Vidaayaadigana** : Vidaree, Pandhcaangula (Eranda), Vrischikaalee (Meshasringee), Vrischeeva (Kshudravarshaabhoo), Devaahvaya (Devdaaru)< Soorpaparbee (Mudga pamee and Masha pamee), Kandookaree (Kapikachoo), Jeevana Panchamoolam (Abheeru, Veeraajeevantee, Jeevaka and Rishsabhaka), Haraswapanchamoolam (Brihatee, Kanatakaaree, Saalaparnee, Prishniparnee and Gokshuraka), Gopasutaa (Sariba) and Tripaadee (Hamsapadee).

10. **Saaribadigana** : Saaribaa, Useeram, Kaasmarya, Madhooka, Sisiradwayam (Chandanam and Raktachandam), Yashtee (Yastimadhu) and Pai-ooshakam.

11. **Padmaakadigana** : Padmaakam, Pundr (Prapoundareekarn), Vridhi (Sraavanee), Tunga (Vamsalaochanna), Rodhi (Mahaasraavanee), Sringee (Karkatasringee), Amritaa (Gududchi) and the drugs constituting Jeewantyaadigana.

12. **Parooshakadigana** : Parooshakarn, Varaa (Triphala), Draakshaa, Katphalam, Katakaphalam, Raajaahavam (Aargwadha), Daadimam and Saakam.

13. **Anjanaadigana** : Anjanam (Srotonjanam), Phatinee (Priyangu), Maamsee (Krishnajataa), Padarnam (Lotus), Utpalam (Lily), Rasaanaganam, Elaa, Madhukarn (Yastimadhu) and Naagaahavam (Nagakesaram).

14. **Patolaaadiagana** : Patola, Katurohinee, Chandanam, Madhusravaa (Surangee), Gudoochee and Paathaa.

15. **Guduochyaadigana** : Guduchee, Padmaka, Arista (Nimba), Dhanakaa and Raktachandanam.

16. **Aaragwadhaadigana** : Aragwadha, Indryava, Paatali (Vasantha Dootee), Kaakatiktaa (Saarangeshtaa), Nimba, Amritaa (Guduchi), Madhurasaa (Moorva), Sruva Vriksha (Vikarnkata), Paathaa (Ambashtaa), Bhoonimba, Sairyaka (Sahachara, Patola, Karanjayugma (Pooteekaranja) and

Naktamalaa, Saptachchada (Saptaparna), Agni (Chitraka), Sushavee (Kaaravee), Phala (Madanphala), Baana (Sahachara) and Ghonta (Poogavisesha).

17. **Asanaadigana** : Asana (Peeta Saala), Tinisha (Syadana), Bhoorjt. Swetavaaha (Arjuna), Prakeerya (Pootikaranja), Khadira, Kadara (Swetasaara), Bhandee (Sireesha), Sinsapaa (Mandala - patrika), Meshasringee, Trih (Chandanam, Rakta - chandanam and Daaruharidraa), Tala, Palaa (Kinsuka), Jongaka (Aguru), Saakan (Varadaaru), Saala, Krarnuka (Poos), Dhava (Sakata), Kulinga (Sakrayava), Chaagakama and Aswakarna.

18. **Varanaadigana** : Varuna, Sairyakayugma (Kuravaka and Kurantaka), Sataavaree, Dahana (Chitraka), Morata (Moorva), Bilwa, Vishaanikaa (Ajasringee), Dwibrihatee (Brihatee and Kantakaari), Dwikaranja (Pootikaranja and Naktamala), Jayaadwayam (Tarkaaree and Hareethakee), Bahalapallava (Shobaanjana), Darbha (Kusha), and Ruiaakara (Hitaalu).

19. **Ooshakaadigana** : Ooshaka (Kallara), Thuththakarn (Kitiha), Hingu, Kaaseesadwaya Pushapakaaseesam and Paansukaaseesam), Saindhavarn and Silaajatu.

20. **Veerataraadigana** : Vellaantara (Veeratara of Useera), Aranika (Agnimantha), Booka (Easwara mallika), Vrisha (Vaasa), Asmabheda (Pashanbheda), Gokantaka (Gokshuru), Itkataa, Schaachara.Baana, Kaasa, Vrikshaadanee, Nala, Kusadwaya (Sthoola Darbha and Sookshma Darbha), Gunthaa (Vrintartrina), Gumdraa (Pada Eraka), Bhallooka (Syonaka), Morata, Kuranta (Stivaaraka), Karambha (Uttamaarain) and Paartha (Suvarchalaa).

21. **Rodhraadigana** : Rodhra, Saavarka Rodhra, Palaasa (Sathee), Jinginee (Krishnasaalmalee), Sarala (Devadaru), Katphalam, Kutsitaamba (Kadamba), Kadalee, Gatasoka (Asoka), Elavaalu, PAripelavarn (Kutannatam) and Mocha.

22. **Arkaadiagana** : Arka, Alarka, Naagadanti Visalyaa (Langalee), Bhaargee, Rasana, Vrischikalee (Ushtradhoomaka), Prakeeryaa (Karanjaka), Pretyakpushpee (Apamarga), Peetataila (Kakaadanee), Udkeerya (Karanjaka), Swetaa Yugmarn (Kinhi and PAtlindee) and Taapasavrisksha (Ingudee).

23. **Surasaadigana** : Sursayugma(Krishna Tuisi and SwetaTulsi), Phanijjam(Mareechaka), Kaalamaalaa (Krishnaarjaka), Vidngam, Kharebuse (Maruvaka), Vrishakarnee (Mooshikakamee), Katphalam, Kaasamarda, Kshavaka, Sarasee (Tumbarapatkrikaa), Bhaargee (Angaaravalee), Kaamukaa (Raktamanjaree), Kaakamachee, Kulahala (Alambusa), Vishamushti (Kuchilaa), Bhoostrina (Atichatra) and Bhootakesee (Maamsee Putrachaaraa).

24. **Mushkaakaadigana** : Mushakaka (Mokshaka), Snuk (Gudaa), Varaa (Triphala), Dweepi (Chitraka), Palaasa, Dhava and Sinsapaa.

25. **Vatsakaadigana** : Vatsaka (Vanatiktaka), Moorva, Bhaargee, Katukaa (Katurohinee), Maricham, Ghunapriyaa (Ativishaa), Gandeeram (Snuhee), Elaa, Paatha, Ajaajee (Jeerakam),Karvangaphalam (Aralukaphalam), Ajmoda (Deepyaka), Siddhaartha (Goura Sarshapa), Vachaa, Jeeraka, Hingu, Vidangam, Pasugandhaa (Ajagandhaa) and Panchkolakarn (Pipalee, Pippaleemoola, Chavya, Chitraka and Sunthee).

26. **Vachaadigana** : Vschaa, Jalada (Musta), Devaashwa (Kilimarn), Naagaram (Sunthee), Ativihsa and Abhayaa.

27. **Privangawaadigana** : Priyangu (Syaama), Pushpaanjanam (Reetipushpam), Anjanayugmam (Srotoanjaman and Souveeranajanam), Padmaa (Padmachaarinee), Padmakesaram), Yopjanavalee (Manjishtaa), Anantaa (Yavaasa), Maanadruma (Salmalee), Mochasrasa (Saalmalee Niryasaa), Samangaa

(Namaskaaree), Punnaaga (Tunga), Seetham (Chandanam) and Makaneeyahetuh (Dhaatukee).

28. **Ambashtaadigana** : Ambaashtaa (Mayoorashikaa), MAdhukarn (Yashti - madhu), Namaskaree (Samangaa), Nandeevriksha (Prarohee), Palaasa, Kachchuraa (Dhanvayaasa), Rodhram, Dhaatakee, Bilwapesika, Kstwanga (Syonaka) and Kalodhbhavan Rajah (Padmakesaram).

29. **Mustaadigana** : Mustaa, Vachaa, Agni (Chitrak), Swinisaa (Haridraa and Daarunharidraa), Dwitikta (Katurohinee and Kaakatikta), Bhallaataka, Paathaa, Triphala, Vishaakhyaa (Sukiakandaa), Kushtam, Trutee (Elaa) and Haimavatee (Swetavachaa).

30. **Nyagrodhaadigana** : Nyagrodha (Vata), Pipplaa (Aswattha), Sadaaphala (Udumbara), Rodhrayugman (Rodhra and Saavara Rodhra), Jaboodwaya (Raajajamboo and Kaakajamboo), Arjuna, Kapeetana (Vaaneera), Somavalka (Sitasaarakhadira), Plaksha, Aamra, Vanjul (Vetasa), Piyaala, Palaasa, Nandee (Jayavriksha), Kolee (Bedaree), Kakamba, Viralaa (Tindukee), Madhukarn (Yasti - madhu) and Madhookarn.

31. **Elaadigana** : Elaayugmam (Sookshmaa Elaa and Sthoola Elaa), Turushka, Kushtam, Phalinee (Gandha Priyangu), Maamsee (Naladam), Jalam (Hreeberam), Dhyaamakam (Devedaghakarn), Sprikkaa (Devee), Chouraka (Grandhiparne), Chocha (Twak), Patram (Gandhapatram), Tagaram (Chakram), Sthouneyam (Tailapeetakarn), Jeateerasa (Bola), Sukti (Nakha), Vyaaghranakha, Amaraahwam (Devadaaru), Aguru, Sreevaasakam, Kurnkurnam, Chandana, Guggulu, Devadhoop (Sarjarasa), Khapura (Kunduruka), Punnaga (Raktakesara) and Naagaahwayam.

32. **Syaamaadigana** : Syaamaa (Syaamaa Trivrit), Dantee (Chitraa), Dravantee (Indurukamikaa), Kramuka

(Pattikaalodhra), Kutaranee (Sukiaa), Sankhinee (Yavatiktaa), Charmasaahwaa (Saatalaa), Swarnaksheeree, Gavaakshee, Sikhari (Apamaarga), Rajanaka, Karanja, Bastaantree (Vrishagandhaa), Vyaadhighaata (Kritamaala), Bahalabahurasa (Ikshu) and Teekshnabrikshaphala.

LATER AYURVEDIC WRITERS

Coming nearer to our times, we meet with the name of Madhava or Madhavacharya, who in the twelfth century wrote several works embracing almost all branches of Hindu learning. In his medical work named *Madhava Nidana* he dwells exclusively on the diagnosis of diseases. It contains 1,552 verses in 69 chapters. During the Muslim period, up to the sixteenth century, activity in Ayurveda was mainly focused on Rasakriya or alchemical preparations. Systematic works were written on the subject by Chakrapani and Vrinda. Narhari Pandita and Madanpal wrote two masterpieces on medicinal herbs. *Raja Nighantu* and *Madanpala Nighantu,* Sharangdhara, the son of Damodara, in the fourteenth century systematized various materia medicas and his is still a most popular and reliable treatise on the subject. His book contains 2,500 verses, is divided into three parts and has 32 chapters. The *Sharangdhara Samhita*, *Madhava Nidana,* and *Bhava Prakasha* are regarded as the Laghu Tray a or Junior Triad of Ayurvedic classics.

The next celebrated writer on Ayurveda is Bhavamishra, the author of *Bhava Prakasha*. This physician lived in the sixteenth century and was considered to be the best scholar of his time in northwest India. His treatise contains 10,831 verses and is divided into three sections. In the time of Bhavamishra, India began to come into contact with the European nations, notably the Portuguese, who were attracted by trade. A syphilitic disease, in which hands and feet were affected, was then common among the Portuguese. Bhavamishra deals with this at length under the name of *Firanga Roga*, Foreigner's disease.

During this time the main Ayurvedic texts were translated into Arabic. The Unani system of medicine, which the Arabs developed out of the older Greek medicine, was to a great extent founded on Ayurvedic knowledge from India. The Indian Unani system, which grew up under Muslim rule in India, never lost touch with its parental source.

The Muslim invasion of India, which began in earnest in the eleventh century and resulted in a series of wars lasting into the eighteenth century, caused a decline in Ayurveda. The violence of the conquest and its anti-Hindu and anti-Buddhist crusades weakened the older culture as a whole and made it difficult to maintain the arts and sciences at their highest level.

BRITISH INFLUENCE ON AYURVEDA AND MODERN TIMES

The advent of the British was another big landmark in the decline of Ayurveda. The British not only denied state patronage to Ayurveda, but also took a negative attitude toward the system. The East India Company closed down existing schools of Ayurveda and started a medical school of their own at Calcutta in 1833. In spite of suppression and the lack of patronage, Ayurveda remained popular with the masses and still served about 80% of the population of the country. The tremendous national awakening around 1920, with the establishment of national schools and universities, encouraged the revival of Ayurveda. Different state governments were compelled to start regular teaching of Ayurveda and thus established state boards, faculties and councils of Indian medicine. The government of India also appointed a committee under the chairmanship of Sir R. N. Chopra in 1946, which made several recommendations for teaching and research in Ayurveda. After independence, the government of India, and the state governments took more interest in Ayurveda. Over fifty universities in India now have faculties of Ayurveda and over one-hundred Ayurvedic colleges are affiliated with these universities.

Presently the government of India has initiated a more open policy and allows the founding of more private Ayurvedic institutions on a non-grant basis. Therefore many new Ayurvedic schools are arising all over India today. In the next decade the scope of Ayurvedic education in India would expand greatly. Ayurveda in the twenty-first century looks to inherit its old glory of ancient times and will be one of the most important forms of naturopathic medicine practice in the world.

Today, it is especially important for the presentation of Ayurveda to be updated so that it may best continue to stand the test of time. It should be studied rationally using modem experimental methods from various disciplines of science and technology. This does not mean Ayurveda should accommodate itself to allopathic medicine and its standards, which are not appropriate for it, but that it has to be presented in a clear, modern and rational language, and subject itself to proof through observation and clinical experience.

BASIC CONCEPTS OF AYURVEDIC SYSTEM OF MEDICINE

Encyclopaedia Britanica has defined ayurvedic medicine as "an example of well - organized system of traditional health care, both preventive and curative. It is still a form of health care in large parts of the Eastern world specially in India, where a large percentage of population use this system exclusively or combined with modern medicines". It is the science which imparts knowledge of Ayus (life), provides longevity, contains relevant informations and discussed all allied topics and the objective of this system of medicines are that the persons should remain full of health endowed with strength and vigour and well protected from disorders and the sick should be treated for alleviation of diseases.

The medical knowledge of ayurveda is divided in to eight parts which are known as *Astanga Ayurveda* of the ayurveda. These include the following :

EIGHT BRANCHES OF AYURVEDA (ASHTANGA AYURVEDA)

1. Internal Medicine (Kayachikitsa)

Ayurveda treats man as a whole, comprising body, mind, and soul. Mind and body both affect each other and together form the seat of disease. The approach of Ayurveda from the very beginning is psychosomatic. Ayurveda groups all human beings into seven different types of constitutions (Prakriti) according to the predominance of biological humors (Doshas), and similarly groups them into seven psychological constitutions according to the predominance of mental humors. These factors are always taken into account in diagnosis, prognosis and treatment of disease. Diseases are caused by imbalance of the humors, the three energy principles, which in turn damage various tissues and systems. Pathologically, diseases have six different stages of treatment.

A number of infectious diseases are described in Ayurveda but great importance is not given to pathogens as their cause. Ayurveda emphasizes internal factors, the condition of the host, behind all diseases, even those appearing to come from the outside. It is well-known that if the soil remains sterile, the seed will not grow. In the same way, if the internal energies are benefited, disease has no field in which to act.

In the course of treatment, the Ayurvedic physician takes note of the aggravation of humors (Dosha), the tissues damaged (Dushya), environmental influences, the patient's vitality, digestive power, constitution, age, psychological factors, personal inclinations and diet.

Ayurvedic medicines *are* derived from the mineral, vegetable, and animal kingdoms. More than 20,000 species of medicinal plants and herbs are found in India, out of which 2,000 are in use in Ayurveda. Six or seven hundred are commonly used in Ayurvedic preparations. A number of minerals and metals are used, but they are subject to various and complex processes of purification and oxidation before becoming suitable for internal usage. The special therapy of Pancha Karma, the five purification practices, is also used in treatment. These five are the use of emetics, purgatives, nasal medications, and medicated enemas with or without oil. Pancha Karma utilizes certain preliminary practices of Snehana (oleation internal and external) and Swedana (different kinds of fomentation or sweating therapies), and related follow-up practices like Rasayana or rejuvenation.

2. Surgery (Shalyatantra)

Surgery is not just an invention of modern medicine. It was already highly advanced in several ancient cultures, including India, Greece and Egypt. Its low condition in Europe in the Middle Ages was a period of decline, a temporary dark age, and was not at all indicative of its condition in ancient and Oriental cultures.

In Ayurveda, Sushruta describes surgery as the first and foremost specialty of the system. He describes various surgical procedures including abdominal operations like those for intestinal obstruction and stones in the bladder, and also delineates specialized surgery like plastic surgery. He was the first person to advocate knowledge of anatomy through the dissection of the dead body as essential for a good surgeon. Later in Indian history, the philosophical emphasis on non-violence came in the way of development of this branch of medicine. Even today, the *Sushruta Samhita* contains a great deal of useful material for research work.

3. Shalakya Tantra

This is the Ayurvedic branch of Ophthalmology and Otorhinolaryngology, concerned with diseases of the eyes and head. Around seventy-two eye diseases are described by Sushruta along with surgical operations for such conditions as cataract and pterygium. Special techniques are also described for many diseases of the ear, nose and throat.

4. Pediatrics (Kaumarabhritya)

This branch deals with prenatal and postnatal baby care and with the care of the mother before conception and during pregnancy. Ayurveda describes methods for conceiving a child of the desired sex, intelligence, and constitution. Various diseases of children and their treatment come under this branch.

5. Toxicology (Agadatantra)

This branch deals with the toxins of the vegetable, mineral, and animal kingdoms. Most interesting to note is that the concept of pollution of air and water in particular times and places has been given due consideration. Such pollution is said to be the cause of various epidemics and the collapse of civilizations.

6. Psychiatry (Bhutavidya)

Ayurveda is equally concerned with mental diseases and their treatment. Treatment methods include not only diet and herbs, but also the yogic methods for improving the condition of the mind. There is ample material for further research on this branch in the *Atharva Veda* and other Ayurveda Samhitas.

7. Science of Rejuvenation (Rasayana)

This therapy is used to prevent diseases and for promotion and prolongation of a healthy life. As mentioned earlier, Pancha Karma therapy is an essential prerequisite for Rasayana. A code of right conduct in life has also to be observed as part of the rejuvenation process. Details of regimen in terms of dietetics have also been described.

8. Science of Aphrodisiacs (Vajikarana)

This branch deals with the means of increasing sexual vitality and efficiency. For achieving good progeny, the therapy of Rasayana and Vajikarana are closely interrelated. Vajikarana medicines also act as rejuvenatives.

PANCH MAHABHUTAS OR THE FIVE GREAT ELEMENTS

The basic material constituents which exist in the universe and in man are called the "five great elements" (Pancha Mahabhutas) of ether, air, fire, water, and earth. The original substance of this group pervades the universe and is not completely observable, hence it is called the "great element" (Mahabhuta). These elements refer to the etheric, gaseous, radiant, fluid, and solid states of matter and their respective principles of space, movement, light, cohesion, and density. Hence they are far more subtle and comprehensive than their visible counterparts on earth. According to the Sankhya-Yoga system they evolve from the mind.

Each of these primal elements possesses its characteristic quality (either essential or auxiliary). The essential qualities of sound (ether), touch (air), light and colour (fire), taste (water), and smell (earth) are grasped by the corresponding five sense organs of the ear, skin, eye, tongue, and nose. When these are not perceived, the alternative five auxiliary characteristics are observed indirectly through the skin. They are non-resistance (ether), vibrations (air), change of temperature (fire), fluidity (water), and shape (earth).

Characteristics of Five Elements

Elements	*Essential*	*Auxiliary*	*Related to*
Ether AKASHA	Sound	Non-resistance	Rarefaction
Air VAYU	Touch	Vibration	Propulsion
Fire TEJAS	Appearance	Heat & Color	Conversion
Water APAS	Taste	Fluidity	Degree of Liquidity
Earth PRITHIVI	Smell	Solidity	Density of Particles

TRIDOSHA THEORY: THE THREE BIOLOGICAL HUMORS

The scientists of old explained all body functions relative to the happenings in the universe. They found certain phenomena common to both man and nature. There are three main causative factors in the external universe: the sun, moon and wind. The sun is the energy of conversion represented as fire; the moon is the agency of cooling represented by the combination of earth and water and the wind is the principle of movement or propulsion represented by the combination of air and ether.

All activities in the universe or in the human being are grouped into the three basic functions of creation, preservation, and destruction. These are the functions of three main Hindu Gods of Brahma, Vishnu, and Shiva. The Tridosha theory relates these three functions to the three biological humors or Doshas. Vata, the energetic humor, controls destruction, Pitta, the thermogenic humor, organizes body activities after transformation. Kapha, the cohesive humor, is responsible for maintaining the creation.

Relation of Five Elements to Three Energy Principles in the Universe

Structure of Universe			***Function of Universe***
Ether	Space	WIND	Principle of propulsion, movement
Air	Motion		
Fire	Energy	SUN	Principle of conversion, transformation
Water	Cohesion	MOON	Principle of cooling
Earth	Mass		cohesion or preservation

Universal Function	***Man***
Principle of propulsion	Vata Dosha
Principle of Conversion	Pitta Dosha
Principle of Preservation	Kapha Dosha

Relationship of Five Elements, Three Gunas and Tridosha

Elements	***Gunas***	***Humours***	***Gunas***
Ether	Sattva		
		VATA	Sattva 1 + Rajas 1
Air	Rajas		
Fire	Sattva + Rajas	PITTA	Sattva 1 + Rajas 1
Water	Sattva + Tamas		
		KAPHA	Sattva 1 + Tamas 2
Earth	Tamas		

All the natural happenings observable in the universe are caused by one of the three energies:

* Agency of propulsion
* Agency of interchanging
* Agency of cohesion

This energy of propulsion causes the change in position of all things in the universe — like dust, smoke and clouds — in the direction in which the wind or force of propulsion is moving. In human beings, functions like respiration, heart beat, and the expulsion of waste products all are manifestations of change in position.

The energy inside the body is termed as Vata, which is

similar to wind. But it must be remembered that Vata should not be simply equated with wind. Vata is any propulsive force and the principle of movement generally on the level of the life-force (Prana). The lower part of the large intestine is the seat of this humor. The functions manifested here (drying of the waste matter by removing the liquid portion) resemble those of the wind in nature.

When any substance comes in contact with the heat of the sun, it changes its temperature, form, appearance, or taste. In the human body the same type of thermogenic energy causes the food taken in to be changed into tissues and waste products. It is responsible for the complexion and temperature of the body. Hence it is named Pitta, that which is thermogenic in nature. Sweat, which is increased by heat, and blood, which is red in colour, thus having properties common to fire, are the main seats of Pitta.

The effects of these two energies are inhibited by the third energy, the agency of cold and cohesion or, in nature, the rainfall. This is responsible for new growth. Hence it is named Kapha, or that which gets activated by water. The nutrient fluid pool, secretions, muscular tissues, bony structures, the nervous system, and the reproductive system are the chief sites of this humor.

HUMOURS, TISSUES, AND WASTE MATERIALS: DOSHA, DHATU, AND MALA

Ayurvedic scientists have classified all bodily constituents into three categories. They are Dosha, Dhatu, and Mala — the humors, tissues, and waste materials.

Mala or the waste products are the constituents that are constantly eliminated from the body. Their physical appearance varies from gaseous, liquid, semi-solid to solid form. The gross waste products (sthula) are urine, feces, and sweat The subtle waste products (sukshma malas or kleda) are exudations eliminated from the epithelial linings of the eyes, nose, mouth, ears, and smegma. Similarly, the many minute waste products that are formed in the body during tissue formation from food are also included in subtle waste materials. Health is maintained when these waste products are eliminated properly. When they accumulate in excess, various diseases are produced.

Dhatus or tissues are the constituents which do not get eliminated from the body (except the reproductive) and they are maintained within a particular limit. This limit is the skin from the outside and the internal linings (of the gastrointestinal tract, bladder, joints, and cerebral linings) from within the body. As bodily strength grows these tissues continue to develop. They are seven in number, with their characters and functions as follows:

Name	Character	Function
Rasa Dhatu PLASMA	Circulating nutrient fluid	Nutrition
Rakta Dhatu BLOOD	Hemoglobin portion of the blood	Oxygenation
Mamsa Dhatu MUSCLE	Muscular tissue	Movement
Meda Dhatu FAT	Lubricating fat deposits	Lubrication
Asthi Dhatu BONE	Supporting and Accommodating bony structure	Support
Majja Dhatu NERVE	Nerve tissues	To promote understanding
Shukra Dhatu REPRODUCTIVE	Reproductive Tissue	Reproduction

The most important function of this group is to give maximum support and strength to the body. The body cannot afford to eliminate the tissues in this group like the waste materials. If they cross the limit of the skin or the internal linings, then the disease condition becomes very serious, as essential substances are being lost.

The humors (Doshas) play a dual role. They do not continue developing like the tissues, nor are they completely eliminated from the body like the waste materials. Vata has no physical form. It is understood by the various movements it sets in motion. Pitta and Kapha are of a fluid character, Pitta consisting of lighter fluids and Kapha of heavier fluids.

Formation of Vata

The movements of breathing and swallowing trigger the cycle leading to absorption of external food. This movement also depends upon previously absorbed food. Thus Indian scientists have understood a relationship between energy and food absorption. Hence Vata is described as the ejectable product of food. Anna Mala, the waste material from food = Vata Dosha. This energy is then utilized by the body for essential movements like breathing, heart beat, passage of food, excretion of waste products, and so on. These movements cannot be measured or weighed. Thus Vata is perceived by the totality of its functions.

Formation of Pitta and Kapha

The movements that appear in the upper part of the gastro-intestinal tract disappear during the process of absorption of food. Saliva and mucous secretions (Kapha) and other digestive secretions including various enzymes and hormones (Pitta) appear in the proximal part and then re-enter in the distal part with absorbed food.

Kapha, when it appears in the mouth, gastro-intestinal tract, lungs, or cerebral circulation is the ejectable product from Rasa Dhatu, the plasma or the nutrient body fluid. Such Kapha Dosha looses certain characteristics of Rasa Dhatu. Hence Rasa Mala, the waste product of the Rasa or plasma = Kapha.

When it leaves the circulating channels this nutrient fluid forms various tissues according to need: it may change into muscle tissue, provide its lubricating material for adipose tissue, or help in the formation of bones, nerves, or reproductive fluids. The channeled nutrient fluid is Kapha Dosha because it helps in the cohesion of various tissues.

Pitta is the product of the breakdown of the blood (Rakta Dhatu). Rakta Mala, the waste product of the blood = Pitta Dosha. This Pitta Dosha appears as coloured secretions in the middle portion of the gastro-intestinal tract and is thus responsible for the central conversion function.. The blood (Rakta) does not combine with any other constituent in the body, hence it is different from other tissues. Pitta Dosha, however, which is a breakdown product of hemoglobin, helps in various conversions; in the eye for vision, in the skin for complexion, and in the liver for formation of various tissues.

PROPERTIES OF THE THREE HUMORS

Vata is recognized by its qualities as dry, cool, rough, less nourishing, propulsive, and subtle. It possesses an astringent taste. When the living body comes into contact with substances of such qualities, it loses bodily constituents. Even though these qualities are harmful to existing tissues in the body, they are essential for body functions. If subtleness in the structure of a tissue is nullified, there can be no movement in it at all.

Pitta is slightly oily in character, has a sharp odour, secretary and vasodilating properties, is penetrating and hot, and is pungent and sour in taste. In the process of digestion it appears as an easily flowing fluid. All colours except white, dusky or violet denote the existence of Pitta. Kapha is oily, cool, smooth, soft, heavy, nourishing, slimy, compact in arrangement, white in colour, and is sweet and salty by taste.

Functions of Vata

As the principle of propulsion, Vata carries out many diverse functions in the human body. It controls cell arrangement and division, the formation of different tissue layers, and the differentiation of organs and systems. It conducts impulses like those from the sense organs to the brain and from the brain to the motor organs. Vata controls the expulsion of feces, urine, sweat, menstrual fluid, semen, and the fetus. It controls respiratory, cardiac and gastro-intestinal movements, as well as all higher functions in the brain and spinal cord. It also controls the mind and gives the energy to perform all bodily and mental activities.

Functions of Pitta

Pitta is responsible for the formation of tissues, waste products, arid energy from the food, water, and air that we take in from the outside. It controls metabolic activities and is responsible for all the secretions in the gastro-intestinal tract, and the enzymes and hormones from ductless glands into the blood stream. It controls body temperature, hunger, thirst, fear, anxiety, anger, and sexual desire. It is also responsible for courage and will power, and assimilation of knowledge from the outside world.

Functions of Kapha

Kapha increases the deposits in the cell mass as well as being essential for the interlinking of cells, tissues, and organs. It is thus responsible for the growth of the body. It prevents destruction of tissues from wear and tear — due to friction and movement by Vata — by maintaining the strength and immunity of the body. Capacities for reproduction, happiness, and correct retention of knowledge depend upon the proper functioning of Kapha.

Ayurveda attributes great importance to the equilibrium of the three humors or Tridosha. Although they are in a constant state of flux, due to the impact of internal and external factors, their equilibrium is usually maintained. When this equilibrium gets disturbed, the disease process starts. According to the Indian system of medicine, all diseases are caused by aggravated humors

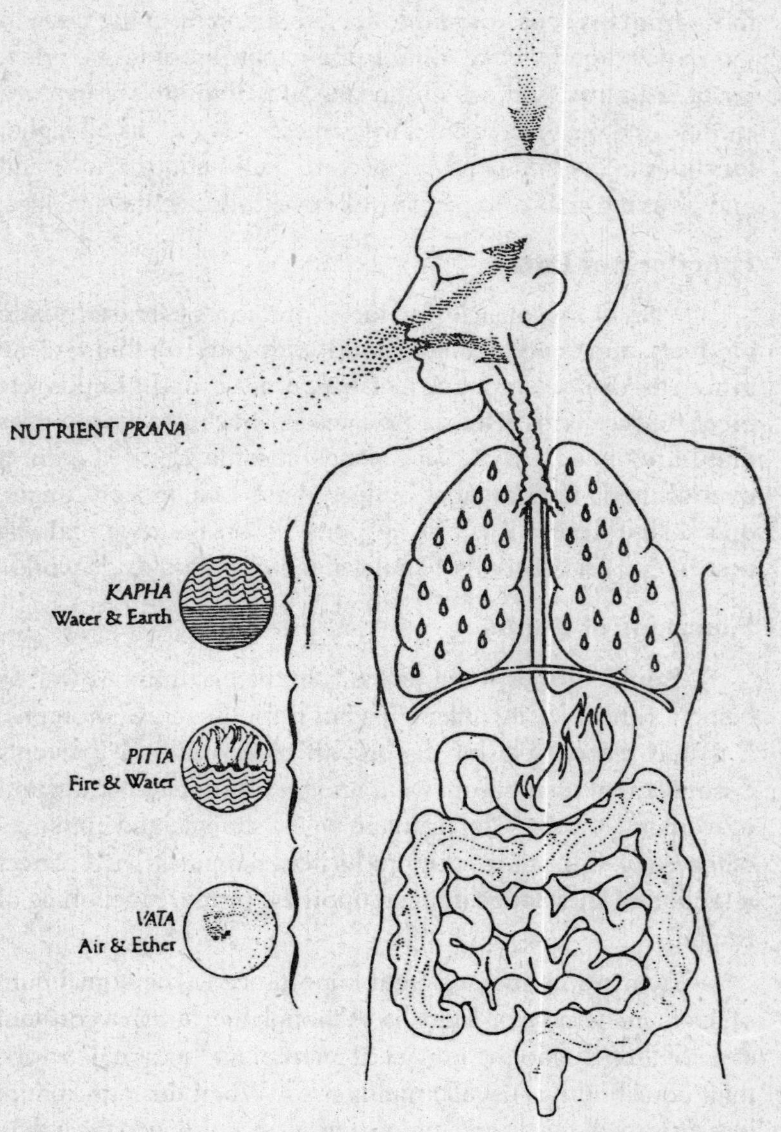

Vata, Pitta, Kapha's seats in the Body

The Human Constitution (Prakruti)

Aspect of Constitution	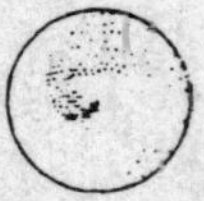 ***Vata***	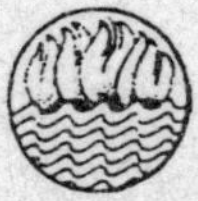 ***Pitta***	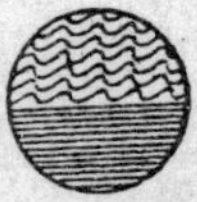 ***Kapha***
Frame	Thin	Moderate	Large
Body Weight	Low	Moderate	Heavy
Skin	Dry, Rough Cool, Brown, Black	Soft, Oily, Warm, Fair Red, Yellowish	Thick, Oily, Cool, Pale, White
Hair	Black, Dry, Kinky	Soft, Oily, Yellow, Early Gray, Red	Thick, Oily, Wavy, Dark or Light
* Teeth	Protruded, Spaces Between Crooked, Gums Emaciated	Moderate in size Soft or Bleeding Gums	Strong, White Full, Well-formed
* Eyes	Small, Dry Active, Brown, Black	Sharp, Penetrating, Green, Gray, Yellow	Big, Attractive. Blue, Thick Eyelashes
* Appetite	Variable, Low	Good, Sharp, Excessive	Slow but Steady
* Disease Tendency	Nervous Disorders, Pain	Heat, Infection, Inflammation	Excess Water, Mucus
* Thirst	Variable	Excessive	Slight
* Elimination	Dry, Hard, Constipated	Soft, Oily, Loose	Thick, Oily, Heavy, Slow

Aspect of Constitution	*Vata*	*Pitta*	*Kapha*
Physical Activity	Very Active	Moderate	Lethargic
Mind	Restless, Active Curious	Aggressive, Intelligent	Calm, Slow, Receptive
Emotional Excesses	Fearful, Insecure, Anxious	Aggressive, Irritable, Jealous	Greedy, Attached, Self-Contented
Faith	Wavering Changeable	Determined	Steady, Loyal
Memory	Recent Memory Good, Remote Memory Poor	Sharp	Slow but Prolonged
Dream	Flying, Jumping, Running, Fearful	Fiery, Angry, Passionate, Colourful	Watery, Ocean, Swimming, Romantic
Sleep	Scanty, Interrupted	Little but Sound	Heavy, Prolonged, Excessive
Speech	Fast, Chaotic, Uninterrupted	Sharp, Clear Cutting	Slow, Monotonous, Melodious
Spending Habits	Spends Quickly, Impulsively	Spends Moderately & Methodically	Spends Slowly Saves
Pulse	Thready, Feeble, Moves Like a Snake	Moderate, Jumping Like a Frog	Broad, Slow, Moves Like a Swan

or vitiated Doshas. Even traumatic diseases which are not initially the result of an imbalance of these Doshas soon become accompanied by one.

TYPES OF THE HUMORS

According to different functions and sites, each humor is divided into Five types.

TYPES OF VATA

The five types of Vata are Prana, Udana, Vyana, Samana, and Apana. All these forms of Vata are responsible for various propulsive movements.

Prana—Udana

These two, having opposite movements, are taken together. Generally speaking the movement of Prana is from the outside to the inside. Prana is responsible for receiving substances like air, water, food, and impressions through the five sense organs from the outside world. Whenever a sound, touch, taste, or smell is attended with full concentration, it has some effect on respiration.

The movement of Udana is from the inside to the outside, mainly through exhalation. Substances received by the stomach in fluid (like alcohol) or solid form (like garlic), if rendered *very* fine during the conversion of food, are eliminated through expiration. Speech is also due to Udana. Remembrance is the bringing out of the knowledge that has been received by Prana. Thus Prana is responsible for intake, Udana for output.

Vyana—Samana

These two types of Vata also have opposite propulsion. Vyana is responsible for propulsion from center to periphery. The movement of the heart in pushing nutritive substances to the periphery is the function of Vyana. It is also responsible for various movements of the limbs and the flow of blood and sweat. Vyana carries afferent impulses from the sense organs to the brain.

Samana, on the other hand, is the propulsive force from the periphery to the center. Efferent impulses in the nerves, bringing ail the fluid pushed out by Vyana back to the center and promoting all fluids into the lumen, are the function of Samana. Thus the action of Samana is the central pull action opposite the outward push of Vyana.

Apana

In contrast to the above two pairs, the function of Apana is to control the movements of constituents like urine, feces, flatus, menstrual discharge, seminal discharge, and the discharge of the fetus. All these are controlled for a particular period of time before being discharged from the body. The overall control of all these substances for a particular period is beneficial to building or maintaining the tissues. Since this control is beneficial to the other types of Vata, it is said that Apana controls all the different forms of Vata.

TYPES OF PITTA

The five types of Pitta are Pachaka, Ranjaka, Alochaka, Sadhaka, and Bhrajaka. All of these are responsible for some type of conversion.

Pachaka Pitta

Pachaka Pitta is responsible for the primary conversion in the body, the digestion of food. Because of its hot and penetrating quality it disintegrates and digests food in the gastro-intestinal tract.

Ranjaka Pitta

Ranjaka Pitta aids in the secondary digestion of food for the formation of tissues. The formation of blood (Rakta) and other tissues in the liver is the chief function of Ranjaka Pitta.

Alochaka Pitta

Alochaka Pitta is responsible for the assimilation and conversion of external impulses that takes place when an object is sensed by the eyes. It is inferred that the sensations of sound, touch, taste, and smell also involve a certain conversion. The factor responsible for this conversion is Alochaka Pitta.

Sadhaka Pitta

Sadhaka Pitta is located in the brain. After sensing any object, its recognition is dependent upon a specific sequence of conversions governed by Sadhaka Pitta. The capacity to appreciate art is another function of it.

Bhrajaka Pitta

Bhrajaka Pitta maintains the temperature and complexion of the skin, and helps in the absorption of massage oils and ointments through the skin.

TYPES OF KAPHA

The Five types of Kapha are Avalambaka, Kledaka, Bodhaka, Tarpaka, and Shleshaka. All these protect various organs from wear and tear due to Vata and the hot and penetrating effects of Pitta. Similarly they help in maintaining the cohesion and interlinking of tissues.

Avalambaka Kapha

Avalambaka Kapha protects the lungs, heart, and proximal portion of the intestines. Due to repeated contraction and relaxation, the lungs and heart are subjected to friction and wear. But the fine, slimy and unctuous secretions inside these organs protect them and preserve their integrity.

Kledaka Kapha

Kledaka Kapha protects the upper and middle abdomen from hot, irritant or cold food as well as from the secretions of Pachaka Pitta.

Bodhaka Kapha

Bodhaka Kapha protects the mouth from pungent, hot, cold or irritating food and drinks. It also helps us to taste the food. Potentially harmful substances are initially rejected by this taste screen.

Shleshaka Kapha

Shleshaka Kapha lubricates all the bony ends of the joints and prevents their friction during movements.

Tarpaka Kapha

Tarpaka Kapha provides various nutrients to the brain cells and gives lubrication and protection to the brain and spinal cord.

DIGESTION OF FOOD

Role of Agni, the Digestive Fire

The agency of conversion in the universe is represented in the physical body by the power of Agni, which literally means "fire." It refers to the principle of transformation in all its potencies and appearances, which we most commonly experience in the outer world of nature in the form of fire. Such a principle of conversion appears throughout the universe in the various changes of substances such as those observed in biochemical, chemical, and nuclear processes. It serves to transform the gross into the subtle, in which process energy is released and new forms are created. In the body, Agni serves to convert food into various body constituents. This conversion takes place by three types of Agni working at three different levels.

Digestive Fire (Jatharagni)

Digestive Fire is the agency responsible for digesting food in the small intestine. It is also called "Kayagni," the bodily fire, as it is the main source of heat in the body. This energy converts food into a uniform suspension or homogeneous mass (Ahara Rasa).

Digestive Power in the Tissues (Dhatvagni)

Dhatvagni is essential for the second stage of conversion. Dhatvagnis are the special digestive agencies for the various bodily tissues (Dhatus). For the formation of each tissue a separate Dhatvagni is required. Thus there are seven Dhatvagnis for the seven tissues. Dhatvagni is dependent on Jatharagni. If the activity of the Dhatvagni is too low or too high it results in the malformation of the particular tissue. If the tissue Agni is too high, the tissue gets burnt up or depleted. If it is too low, an excess of low quality tissue is formed.

Power of Digestion on an Elemental Level (Bhutagni)

Bhutagni is required for the third stage of digestion, the formation of special materials for the sense organs. There are five Bhutagnis for taking the five element portions of the digested food mass (Ahara Rasa) and converting them into nutritive substances for the five sense organs. Some of these specialized materials are the rods and cones responsible for photosensitivity in the eye, special liquids around the taste buds on the tongue, mucous membrane material inside the nose, and the substances forming the architecture of the ear. Such substances specific to each sense organ (Indriya Dravya) are prepared by the Bhutagnis.

PROCESS OF DIGESTION

The process of digestion has two components, namely the primary phase of digestion (Avasthapaka), and post-digestive effect (Vipaka).

The Primary Phase of Digestion (Avasthapaka)

This is also divided into three stages named according to the prevalence of tastes (rasas) operative during them.

The sweet stage of digestion (Madhura Avasthapaka) is the stage of liquefaction. During this stage Kledaka Kapha secretions occur in the stomach and the disintegration of the food takes place. Due to the heavy secretionary action of Kledaka Kapha, there is a reduction of activity in the body after eating.

The sour digestive stage (Amla Avasthapaka) is the stage of acidification. Secretion of Pachaka Pitta, digestive juices and enzymes, which occurs mainly in the small intestine, breaks down the food further. It causes a sensation of thirst and perspiration through its creation of heat.

The pungent digestive stage (Katu Avasthapaka) is the stage of alkalization of food. About four and a half hours after eating, the food passes into the distal part of the gastrointestinal tract, the large intestine, and peristaltic movements are diminished. During this stage there arises a desire to move about in contrast to the first phase of digestion. This stage is due to the transient predominance of Vata.

Post-Digestive Effect (Vipaka)

The post-absorption action of food is also described in three categories, but primary (Avasthapaka) stages occur for every food type. The post-digestive effect can be either sweet (Madhura Vipaka), sour (Amla Vipaka), or pungent (Katu Vipaka), depending upon the quality of the food.

If sweet post-digestive effect (Madhura Vipaka) is formed, the body receives nutrition of all types and excretory products are easily discharged. Sour post-digestive effect (Amla Vipaka) indicates that the body will be poorly nourished but the waste products will be eliminated smoothly. Pungent post-digestive effect (Katu Vipaka) means that the body will neither receive proper nutrition nor it will easily eliminate waste products. Thus the post-digestive effect denotes the ultimate result of the process of digestion in the body.

Movement of the doshas through the cycle of time

	KAPHA	PITTA	VATA
day	7 am – 11 am	11 am – 3 pm	3 pm – 7 pm
NIGHT	7 pm – 11 pm	11 pm – 3 am	3 am – 7 am
SEASON	Feb. 7 – Jun. 7	June 7 – Oct. 7	Oct. 7 – Feb. 7
DIGESTION	1st 1½ hour	2nd 1½ hour	3rd 1½ hour

The Doshas also reflect the rhythms of time. They show how the forces of nature discharge their effects according to the changes of time periods and developments of various processes of transformation.

In the cycle of the day, Kapha is dominant in the morning and evening; Pitta predominates at noon and midnight; Vata is highest at sunrise and sunset, the transitional points of the day. Seasonally, Kapha is highest in late winter and early spring, the seasons of cold and dampness; Pitta is highest in the late spring and summer, the seasons of heat; Vata is highest in the fall and early winter, the seasons of cold and dryness.

In the digestive process, Kapha is highest immediately after eating. Hence nausea right after food intake indicates high Kapha. Pitta is highest two or three hours after eating, at which time it may be experienced as heartburn. Vata is highest at the end of the digestive process, evidenced as symptoms like gas or constipation. It is best to treat the Doshas at their respective times. Hence medicines to decrease Kapha are given in the morning, for Pitta in the afternoon, and for Vata in the evening.

AGGRAVATION OF THE DOSHAS AND THEIR MANAGEMENT

The key to all Ayurvedic treatment is in knowing the imbalance of the humors and how to treat them. For this, one should be able to determine the factors which aggravate them, recognize the symptoms of their aggravated slate; and prescribe those countermeasures which alleviate them.

VATA

Causes of High Vata

Vata becomes vitiated due to cold climate, air-conditioning, drinking cold substances like ice water, refrigerated foods or foods cold in potency like green salads. It is also vitiated by food that is dry, rough or light, like barley and millet of corn etc. Excessive physical exercise, particularly of a strongly aerobic nature, as well as improper movements of the body aggravate Vata, as does mental and emotional stress and strain.

Symptoms of High Vata

These are indicated by a strong desire for warm food and climate, as well as for warm clothing. Physical symptoms are constipation, lack of energy, loss of sleep, fatigue, emaciation, abdominal distention with flatulence, blackish discoloration of feces and urine, defective sensory functioning. Psychological symptoms also arise like fear, anxiety, insecurity, confusion, and irrelevant talking.

Management of Vata

The treatment of Vata is divided into two types based on whether the cause is malnutrition (Dhatukshaya) or obstruction in the channels (Srotorodha).

For malnutrition, the best therapy is tonification (Brimhana). Anti-Vata diet should be given after making certain that the digestive fire is in good condition. Otherwise stimulant or digestion-promoting herbs should be given like dry ginger, cayenne or black pepper. Then light oil massage should be given with warm oils like sesame and fomentation with anti-Vata herbs like Dashamula or Rasna. Sudation or sweating therapy with moist heat is essential. Herbal wines should be taken before food to increase appetite, or after food as a tonic. Draksha or Ashwagandha herbal wine are best. Sitting-type yoga postures with silent meditation are also helpful.

For obstruction in the channels, detoxifying and stimulating herbs should be taken like dry ginger or fennel. Oil massage should use herbs like Nirgundi or Vishagarbha oil. Special alkali medicines may be taken internally to open the channels. Mild laxatives and decoction enemas should be taken. Herbal wines prepared with jaggery and herbs like Rasna and Dashamula should be given. When the system is clean, then anti-Vata diet and tonifying methods can be used.

PITTA

Causes of High Pitta

Pitta is aggravated by food that is hot in temperature, or by hot potency food like chili, black pepper, and mustard, or by too much fried food. Working on night shifts, hot environments or excessive exposure to the sun also increase the Pitta. Psychological factors are anger, irritability and hot temper.

Symptoms of High Pitta

These are desire for cold food, cool environment and cool clothing. Physical symptoms are excessive hunger and thirst, burning sensation in the skin, eyes, or hands. Hypersensitivity may develop in the form of allergic rashes, fevers or giddiness. There is yellowish discoloration of the skin, eyes, urine, and feces. Psychological factors of anger, rage, hatred, and jealousy increase. Besides, many inflammatory diseases also arise.

Management of Pitta

Anti-Pitta diet should be taken with sweet, bitter, and astringent tastes. This includes dairy products like milk, butter and ghee, mung beans, basmati rice, wheat, all sweet fruits, and cool spices like coriander. Bathing or swimming in cool water should be done, followed by light massage with coconut or sandalwood oil. Aromas like rose can be used, like rose water application in the nose. Purgation and blood-letting can be done in more serious conditions. Cool colours like blue, white and purple, and cool gems like sapphire and pearl are good.

KAPHA

Causes of High Kapha

Dietary factors are cold, oily and heavy foods like yogurt, cheese, butter, milk and meat, as well as watery fruits and vegetables like cucumber, melons, oranges, and grapes. Whole grains like wheat and rice in excess also increase Kapha. Cold and damp environments or work situations are additional factors. Psychological factors are greed and attachment.

Symptoms of High Kapha

These are loss of appetite, nausea and possible vomiting, heaviness in the body, pallor of the skin, cold hand and feet, swollen joints, cough with phlegm, excessive sleep, lethargy, and lack of concentration.

Management of Kapha

The person should carry out strong exercise. Deep massage should be done with light and dry oils like mustard. Strong dry sweating or saunas should be taken. Anti-Kapha diet should be taken with dry and hot food, with pungent, bitter, and astringent tastes. For increasing digestion ginger, black pepper and turmeric should be used. Therapeutic vomiting can be given in severe cases.

2

Herbal Energetics, Therapeutics and Theirs' Active Constituents

HERBAL ENERGETICS

Ayurveda approaches herbs through a science of energetics. The properties of herbs are related systematically according to their taste, elements, heating or cooling effects, effect after digestion and other special potencies they may possess. As distance from the complexity of chemical analysis, which often loses us in a maze of details, this simple system of energetics clarifies the basic properties of herbs. It gives us a structure in which they can easily be identified and understood. Therefore they can be used for the individual constitution and condition.

This system of herbal energetics is the main factor in the Ayurvedic understanding of herbs. Chinese herbalism has a similar system of taste and energy. The lack of such a system in western herbalism has placed it at a disadvantage.

TASTE (*RASA*)

The Sanskrit word for taste, *rasa*, has many meanings. All of them help us understand the importance of taste in Ayurveda. *Rasa* means "essence", taste thus indicates the essence of a plant, and so is perhaps the prime factor in understanding its qualities. *Rasa* means "sap", so that the taste of an herbs reflects the properties of the sap which invigorates it.

Rasa means "appreciation," "artistic delight," a "musical note." Thus taste communicates feeling, which again is the essence of the plant. Through it the beauty and power of the plant can be perceived. *Rasa* means "circulation," "to feel lively", "to dance," all of which is reflected the energizing power of taste.

Taste directly affects our nervous system through the *Prana,* the life force in the mouth, which is connected to the *Prana* in the brain. Taste stimulates nerves, awakens mind and senses to make us lively. Thus taste sets our own *rasa* or vital fluid in motion. Through stimulating *Prana,* particularly the gastric nerves, taste affects *agni* and enhances the power of digestion.

It is the good taste of food that is necessary to awaken our *agni* for proper digestion. For this reason, bland food may not be nourishing in spite of its vitamin or mineral content. Without stimulating *agni,* there is no real power of digestion. Ayurvedic medicine has, therefore, always included the science of cooking with the right spices. Together, they are part of the field of Ayurvedic herbal science.

When we are sick, we lose our sense of taste and our appetite. Taste, appetite, and power of digestion are related. Lack of taste indicates fever, disease, low *agni* and high *ama.* To improve *agni* and eliminate disease, it is necessary to improve our sense of taste. This is why spices are such important Ayurvedic herbs. Desire for tasty food indicates hungry *agni* or disease. The problem is that we have perverted our sense of taste with artificial substances.

Taste is the sensory quality that belongs to the element of water. Plants are the life form belonging to the element of water. Taste thus reflects the energies and elements that operate in a particular herb.

Cloud water originally has no taste, but all tastes are latent in it. These are gathered as it falls, as it passes through the five elements in the atmosphere and takes on their qualities.

Ayurveda recognizes six main tastes : sweet, sour, salty,

pungent, bitter and astringent. These are derived from five elements; each taste is composed of two elements. Sweet taste is composed of earth and water; sour of earth and fire; salty of water and fire; pungent of fire and air; bitter of air and ether; and astringent of earth and air.

Sweet taste is basically that of sugars and starches. Sour taste is of fermented or acidic things. Salty is of salt and alkalis. Pungent is the same as spicy or acrid, and is often aromatic. Bitter is of bitter herbs like gentian or golden seal. Astringent taste has a constricting quality, as herbs that contain tannin, like oak bark.

Though the six tastes transmit the properties of the five elements, they are all based on the element of water, which manifests them. It is only when the tongue is wet that we recognize taste.

ENERGY (*VIRYA*)

Virya is the energy, potency or power of herbs, designated in Ayurveda as heating or cooling. Herbs through their taste tend to heat the body or cool it and this produces the most basic energizing effect upon the system.

Pungent taste, as is commonly known in hot peppers, chilis, ginger and other hot spices, has a heating effect. Things sour or acid in taste like citrus or products of fermentation like wine, yogurt or pickles, are heating. Fermentation creates combustion which releases heat. Salt is also heating, which we can experience by the burning sensation it produces on cuts or sores.

Sweet taste is cooling, as sugar counteracts burning sensations in the body. Bitter and cold are often synonymous, as in bitter herbs like gentian and golden seal which reduce fever and inflammation. Astringent taste has a constricting effect, which is the action of something cold like ice, as in such astringent substances like alum, oak bark or witch hazel.

Heating herbs cause dizziness, thirst, fatigue, sweating, burning sensations and they speed the power of digestion. They increase *Pitta*, but generally decrease *Vata* and *Kapha*.

Cooling herbs are refreshing, enlivening, and promote tissue firmness. They are calming and clearing to *Pitta* and to the blood, but generally increase *Vata* and *Kapha*.

"Heating or cooling energy" means that these substances contain, respectively, the energies of fire or water *(agni* or *soma)*.

Through their energy the six tastes fall into two groups: (1) pungent, sour and salty cause heat and increase *Pitta,* and (2) sweet, astringent and bitter cause cold and decrease *Pitta*. Energy, *virya,* tells us the effect of an herb on *Pitta dosha*.

Pungent is the most heating taste, followed by sour and then salty. Bitter is the most cooling, followed by astringent and then *sweet*.

Other Twofold Distinctions

Another important twofold distinction of tastes, though not an independent principle like energy, is whether herbs are drying or moistening.

The main quality of *Vata dosha* is dryness, while that of *Kapha* is wetness. Tastes that are drying (bitter, pungent and astringent) increase *Vata* and decrease *Kapha,* Those that are moistening (sweet, salty and sour) increase *Kapha* and decrease *Vata*.

Pungent is the most drying taste, followed by bitter and then astringent. Sweet is the most moistening taste followed by salty and then sour.

Drying herbs are composed mainly of the element air, while moistening herbs are composed mainly of water. They produce the effects of their element.

Another but less important. twofold distinction is heavy or light— whether herbs tend to increase lightness or heaviness in the body. This distinction is similar to drying or moistening.

Sour taste, owing to its heating potency and its power to increase digestion, tends to be light. Astringent taste, owing to its constricting effect upon the tissues, tends to be heavy.

Sweet is the heaviest taste, followed by salty and then astringent. Bitter is the lightest taste, followed by pungent and then sour tastes that are heavy in quality promote weight and firmness in the body. Those light in quality cause loss of weight, but are stronger in stimulating digestion.

VIPAKA, THE POST-DIGESTIVE EFFECT

The six tastes are reduced to three in their post-digestive effect, *vipaka.* Sweet and salty tastes, have a sweet *vipaka,* sour has a sour *vipaka*, while bitter, astringent and pungent possess a pungent *vipaka.*

These post-digestive effects are related to the processes of absorption and elimination; the final outcome of digestion. The first stage of digestion is in the mouth and stomach; moistening, dominated by the sweet taste. The second stage of digestion is in the stomach and small intestine; heating, dominated by the sour or acid taste. The third stage is in the colon; drying, dominated by the pungent taste. These stages again are *Kapha*, *Pitta* and *Vata,* respectively.

Herbs, particularly in the long-term usage, tend to aggravate the *dosha* whose *vipaka* they possess. Sweet and salty substances promote salivary and other *Kapha* secretions. Sour herbs promote stomach add, bile, and other manifestations of *Pitta.* Bitter, pungent and astringent herbs increase dryness and gas in the colon, thus aggravating *Vata.*

Sweet and sour *vipakas,* owing to their moistening property, allow for easy and comfortable discharge of urine, feces and intestinal gas. Pungent *vipakas,* from their drying property, create difficulty and discomfort in discharge of waste products.

Sweet *vipaka* also promotes the secretion of *Kapha,* including semen and sexual secretions, and allows for comfortable discharge. Sour *vipaka* increases *Pitta* and add formation in the *body,* and reduces semen and sexual secretions but promotes the other tissue-elements of the body.

Pungent *vipaka* tends to cause gas, constipation and painful urination. It reduces semen and sexual secretions and gives difficulty and discomfort in their discharge.

Sweet and also sour *vipakas* aggravate *Kapha,* while they alleviate *Vata.* Pungent *vipaka* aggravates *Vata,* while it alleviates *Kapha. Sour vipaka* aggravates *Pitta* while sweet *vipaka* alleviates it. Pungent *vipaka* tends to aggravate *Pitta* over a period of time.

Post-digestive effect gives us another reference for understanding the effect of herbs, particularly in long term usage.

PRABHAVA, THE SPECIAL POTENCY

Taste, energy and post-digestive effects are only a general schemata for understanding the properties of herbs. Herbs also possess subtler and more specific qualities that transcend thought and that cannot be placed into a system of energetics. *Prabhava* can be called "the special potency" of the herb. It is its uniqueness, apart from any general rules about it.

Some herbs possess a property at variance with its basic energetics. Basic, for instance, which though classified as heating in energy, helps bring down almost any kind of fever, even those cause by heat. Some herbal properties, like strong purgative action, are also not defined by energetics alone. Other herbs, sharing the same energetics, may differ widely in special potencies; one may be a purgative, while another may not be. All this is *prabhava.*

It includes the occult properties of plants, their capacity to affect the mind and psyche on a direct and subtle level. The special and thought transcending power of *mantras* and rituals, and the external use of gemstones to effect inner changes are also *prabhava. Prabhava* includes auric action, astral effect, magnetic effect, and radiation. Even some diseases like cancer originate owing to a kind of *prabhava* or special predisposition whose etiology transcends thought and the reasoning of the materialistic mind.

Ayurveda investigates the occult and spiritual effects of substances, and is not limited to any materialistic or chemical based theory. It understands the value and the limitation of systems, and only uses them as a guide, not as a rigid rule. This spiritual orientation, one could say, is the *prabhava* of Ayurveda, the special power which can be learned from it.

DESCRIPTION OF SIX TASTES

I. Sweet

"The sweet taste (as it is of the same nature as the human body, whose tissues taste sweet), promotes the growth of all bodily tissues and *Ojas*. Aiding in longevity, it is soothing to the five sense organs and the mind, and gives strength and good complexion. Sweet taste alleviates *Pitta, Vata* and the effects of poison. It also relieves thirst and burning sensation and promotes the health and growth of skin and hair. It is too good for the voice and energy.

"Sweet caste is nourishing, vitalizing gives contentment, adds bulk to the *body* creates firmness. It rebuilds weakness, emaciation, and helps those damaged by disease. It is refreshing to the nose, mouth, throat, lips and tongue, and relieves fits and fainting. The favorite of insects, particularly bees and ants, sweet taste is wet cooling and heavy.

Yet when used too much by itself or in excess, sweet taste creates obesity, flaccidity, laziness, excessive sleep, heaviness, loss of appetite, weak digestion, abnormal growth of the muscles of mouth and throat, difficult breathing, cough, difficult urination, intestinal torpor, fever due to cold, abdominal distention, excessive salivation, loss of feeling, loss of voice, goiter, swelling of the lymph glands, legs and neck, accumulations in the bladder and blood vessels, mucoid accretions in the throat and eyes, and other such *Kapha* caused diseases."

In terms of western herbalism, it is nutritive, tonic and rejuvenative. It increase semen, milk and nerve tissue, and promotes tissue regeneration internally or externally. It is demulcent and emollient, moistening, softening and soothing.

Sweet Herbs: Sweet taste is found in herbs that contain sugars, starches or mucilage. It includes bland, starchy and pleasant tastes, and may be mixed with less agreeable secondary tastes. Typical sweet herbs include almonds, comfrey root, dates, fennel, flaxseed, liqorice, maidenhair fern, marshmallow, psyllium, raisins, sesame seeds, slippery elm, and Solomon's seal. Sweet taste in herbs can be increased by processing herbs with various forms of raw sugar, honey, or cooking them in milk.

II. Sour

"Sour taste improves the taste of food, enkindles the digestive fire, adds bulk to the body, invigorates, awakens the mind, given firmness to the senses, increases strength, dispels intestinal gas and flatus, gives contentment to the heart, promotes salivation, aids swallowing, moistening and digestion of food, gives nourishment. It is light, hot and wet.

Yet when used too much by itself or in excess, sour taste makes the teeth sensitive, causes thirst, blinking of the eyes, goosebumps, liquefied *Kapha,* aggravates *Pitta* and causes a buildup of toxins in the blood. It wastes away the muscles and causes looseness of the body, creates edema in those weak, injured or in convalescence. From its heating property, it promotes the maturation and suppuration of sores, wounds, burns, fractures and other injuries and causes a burning sensation in the throat, chest and heart."

Sour taste in terms of western herbalism is stimulant, promotes digestion, increases appetite and is carminative. It is nourishing to all tissue-elements except reproductive tissue (*shukra dhatu*). It promotes metabolism, circulation, along with sensory and brain functioning.

Six Tastes Chart

Rasa	Elements	Energy	Post digestive Effect	Wet/Dry	Heavy/Light
Sweet	Earth and Water	Cooling - 3	Sweet	Wet - 1	Heavy - 1
Salty	Water and Fire	Heating - 3	Sweet	Wet - 2	Heavy - 2
Sour (Acid)	Earth and Fire	Heating - 2	Sour	Wet - 3	Light - 3
Astringent	Earth and Air	Cooling - 2	Pungent	Dry - 3	Heavy - 3
Pungent	Air and Fire	Heating - 1	Pungent	Dry - 1	Light - 2
Bitter	Air and Ether	Cooling - 1	Pungent	Dry - 2	Light - 1

1 - first degree, strong action

2 - second degree, moderate action

3 - third degree, least action

Sour Herbs: Sour taste occurs largely from the presence of various acids in plants, like acid fruit. Sour taste is rarer than sweet. Typical sour herbs include hawthorn berries, lemon, lime, raspberries and rose hips. Sour taste in herbs can be increased by preparing herbs in fermentation as herbal wines or as tinctures in alcohol.

III. Salty

Salty taste is moistening, enkindles digestive fire; it is cutting, biting, sharp, fluid and promotes digestion. It works as a sedative, laxative and deobstruent. Salty taste alleviates *Vata,* relives stiffness, contractions, softens accumulations, and nullifies all other tastes. It promotes salivation, liquefies *Kapha,* cleanses the vessels, softens all the organs of the body, gives taste to food. It is heavy, oily and hot.

Yet when used too much by itself or in excess it aggravates *Pitta,* causes stagnation of blood, creates thirst, fainting and the sensation of burning, erosion and wasting of muscles. It aggravates infectious skin conditions, causes symptoms of poisoning, causes tumors to break open, makes the teeth fall, decreases virility, obstructs the functioning of the senses, causes wrinkling of the skin, graying and falling of the hair. Salty taste promotes bleeding diseases, hyperacidity of digestion, inflammatory skin diseases, gout and other mainly *Pitta* diseases.

In small doses, it promotes digestion and increases appetite; in moderate doses functions as a laxative or purgative; and in large doses is an emetic, promotes vomiting. It is demulcent, softening to bodily tissues and it is calming, mild sedative. It aids in tissue growth throughout the body and promotes water retention.

Salty Herbs: Salty taste is really not a plant but a mineral taste, so it is very rare in plants as a primary taste. Typical salty substances include Epsom salt, Irish moss, kelp, rock salt, sea salt and seaweed. Salty taste in herbs can be increased by adding salt to herbal preparations.

IV. Pungent

The pungent taste is cleansing to the mouth, enkindles digestive fire, purifies food, promotes nasal secretions, causes intestinal torpor, obesity, abdominal swelling and excessive liquid in the body. It helps discharge oily, sweaty and sticky waste products. It gives taste to food, stops itching, helps the resolution of skin growths, kills worms, is germicidal, corrodes the muscle tissue, moves blood dots and blood stagnation, breaks up obstructions, opens the vessels, alleviates *Kapha*. It is light, hot and dry.

Yet when used too much by itself or in excess causes a weakening of virility by its post-digestive effect. By its taste and hot potency, it causes delusion, weariness, languor and emaciation. Pungent taste causes fainting, prostration, loss of consciousness and dizziness. It burns the throat, generates a burning sensations, tremors, and piercing and stabbing pains throughout the body.

It is stimulating, promotes digestions, increases appetite, is diaphoretic and expectorant and is vermicidal. It promotes circulation and generally increases all bodily functions, while reducing all foreign accretions in the body.

Pungent Herbs: Pungent taste arises mainly from various aromatic oils. It is more common than sweet but not abundant. Still, many herbs belong to this category and they are very useful and often become spices and condiments. Pungent taste includes acrid, spicy and aromatic.

Typical pungent herbs include angelica, asafoetida, basil, bayberry, bay leaves, black pepper, camphor, cardamom, cayenne, cinnamon, cloves, coriander, cumin, ephedra, eucalyptus, garlic, ginger, horseradish, mustard, onions, peppermint, prickly ash, rosemary, sage, spearmint, thyme, and valerian.

V. Bitter

Bitter taste, though it does not taste good in itself, restores the sense of taste. It is detoxifying, antibacterial, germicidal, and kills worms. It relieves fainting, burning sensation, itch, inflammatory skin conditions and thirst. Bitter taste creates tightness of the skin and muscles. It is antipyretic, febrifuge; it enkindles digestive fire, promotes digestion of toxins, purifies lactation, helps scrape away fat and remove toxic accumulations in fat, marrow, lymph, sweat, urine, excrement, *Pitta* and *Kapha*. It is dry, cold and light.

Yet when used by itself or in excess, owing to its natural properties of dryness, roughness and clearness, it causes a wasting away of all the tissue elements of the body. Bitter taste produces roughness in the vessels, takes away strength, causes emaciation, weariness, delusion, dizziness, dryness of the mouth and other diseases of *Vata*.

It reduces fevers, is antiinflammatory, antibacterial, detoxifying and germicidal. It is cleansing to the blood and all tissues in general and helps to reduce tumors. It has a reducing and sedating effect upon the body, although in small amounts it is stimulating, particularly to digestion.

Bitter Herbs: Bitter is a very common taste in herbs and plants. It arises from various bitter principles like berberine. Bitters may be simple, like gentian. They may be aromatic (pungent secondarily), like worm wood, or they may be astringent (secondarily) like golden seal.

Typical bitter herbs include aloe, barberry, blessed thistle, blue flag, chaparral, chrysanthemum, dandelion gentian, golden seal, Peruvian bark, rhubarb, rue, white poplar and yellow dock.

VI. Astringent

Astringent taste is a sedative, spots diarrhoea, aids in healing of joints, promotes the closing and healing of sores and wounds. It is drying, firming and contracting. It alleviates *Kapha, Pitta* and stops bleeding. Astringent taste promotes absorption of bodily fluid; it is dry, cooling and light.

Yet when used too much by itself or in excess, it causes

drying of the mouth, produces pain in the heart, causes constipation, weakens the voice, obstructs channels of circulation, makes the skin dark, weakens vitality, causes premature aging. It causes the retention of gas, urine and feces, creates emaciation, weariness, thirst and stiffness. Owning to its natural properties of roughness, dryness and clearness, it causes *Vata-diseases* like paralysis, spasms and convulsions.

Astringent taste is haemostatic, stops sweating, stops diarrhoea, as it promotes absorption of fluids and inhibits their elimination. It is anti-inflationary, vulnerary as it closes wounds and promotes heating by knitting the membranes back together. It constricts the muscles and helps to raise prolapsed organs.

Astringent Herbs: Astringent taste is also very common in herbs, but it is not of such therapeutic importance, as astringent action is used mainly symptomatically. Astringency derives mainly from the presence of various tennins.

Typical astringent herbs include lotus seeds, mullein, plantain, pomegranate, raspberry leaves, white pond lily, white oak bark and witch hazel.

COMBINED TASTES

Tastes of herbs seldom single, though one usually predominates. Sweet and pungent tastes sometimes combine, as with cinnamon, fennel, ginger and onion. Such herbs are particularly good for *Vata*.

Sweet and astringent often combine, as with comfrey, lotus, slippery elm and white pond lily. Such herbs are particularly goods for *Pitta* but may be hard to digest.

Sweet and bitter sometimes combine, as with liquorice. These herbs are also particularly good for *Vata*.

Sweet and sour combine in various fruit like oranges. They are very goods for *Vata*.

Pungent and bitter sometimes combine as with motherwort, mugwort, wormwood and yarrow. Such herbs have a strong effect on *Kapha*.

Pungent and astringent combine occasionally, as with bayberry, cinnamon or sage. They also work on *Kapha.*

Bitter and astringent often combine, as in may diuretics. Such herbs include golden seal and plantain. They work mainly on *Pitta.*

Some herbs posses three or more tastes. For herbs of multiple tastes the energy and post-digestive effect become important for determining their effect. Herbs of multiple tastes often possess powerful or broad spectrum healing action like garlic.

TASTES AND FOODS

Like herbs, foods have therapeutic properties according to the tastes and elements which dominate them. In ayurveda, a special diet is prescribed along with the use of particular herbs. Generally, the patient is told to follow the diet that tends to alleviate his or her particular *Dosha.*

However, particular foods are prescribed therapeutically as herbs, or in combination with herbs. Such substances include milk, honey, *ghee,* raisins, dates and almond. Herbology and nutrition are a single science in ayurveda, and no treatment can be truly efficacious that neglects one or the other. Food deals with the "grosser nutrition" of the body; herbs give subtle nutrition and stimulation to the deeper tissues and organs.

TASTES AND EMOTIONS

Emotions also have a certain taste or flavour and affect the body according to their quantities. These are bitter emotions like grief, or astringent emotions like fear-these aggravate *Pitta.* There are sweet emotions like desire, or salty emotions like greed-these aggravate *Kapha.*

Emotions can have the same effect upon the body as wrong foods, drugs, alcohol, or infections. Psychological factors have the power to overcome physiological factors in treatment. For this reason, ayurveda also has a science of the energetics of the psyche. The unified body-mind science of ayurveda allows us to use herbs to help to counteract mental states and emotional problems.

The science of *rasa*, or taste, and its energetics, comprehends not only the herbs and food but also the mind. Like other aspects of the ayurvedic language of healing, taste has value on all levels of manifestation, both inner and outer.

HERBAL THERAPEUTICS

ALTERATIVE HERBS (*Rakta Shodhana karma*)

Alteratives are herbs those, which cleanse and purify the blood. They produce the following general therapeutic effects:

1. They purify the blood, removing toxins, and tend to have anti-infections and antibacterial action.
2. They help heal and resolve sores, boils, tumours and many kinds of cancer.
3. Typical alteratives work through cooling the blood and so also dispel fevers, reduce *Pitta* and detoxify the liver.
4. They may be used externally on wounds, sores, ulcers, etc. and have anti-inflammatory and vulnerary properties.
5. With their detoxifying action they help to kill worms and parasites, particularly those that invade the blood.
6. They work well in infectious, contagious diseases and epidemics.

Alteratives treat flus, especially those with high fever, sore throat, earache, etc.; in this regard they are a degree stronger than cooling diaphoretics. They treat acne, dermatitis, boils and inflammatory skin conditions. They can be used on herpes and venereal diseases, as well as cancer. They cleanse the lymphatics and strengthen white blood cell count. They attack toxic accumulations, but also have a reducing effect upon the bodily tissues. Some possess diuretic or laxative properties.

Most of the alteratives are cooling, bitter or sometimes

astringent in taste. They decrease *Pitta* and *Kapha*, but increase *Vata*. They are mainly anti *Pitta* herbs.

Typical alternatives are aloe, blue flag, burdock, dandelion, indigo, *manjishta*, neem, plantain, sandalwood and yellow dock.

Many hot, pungent herbs possess a cleansing action in the blood, as well as promoting circulation and resolving blood clots. They are detoxifying, often antibacterial, and help to reduce fevers by destroying the toxin that produces them. They also have an antiparasitical or worm-killing action.

Hot pungent alteratives and cold bitter alteratives can be combined to strengthen the detoxifying power of each. They can be used together in conditions of high *Ama*. This is true even in *Vata* or *Pitta* constitutions until the *Ama* is reduced as in periodic or malarial fevers. Generally speaking, however, cooling alteratives are good for *Pitta,* heating alteratives are good for *Vata,* and both work well on *Kapha.*

Cooling alteratives that have strong antibacterial or antibiotic effect, like golden seal and wild indigo, if used too long or in excess can have the same detrimental effect upon the body as antibiotic drugs, destroying the good as well as the bad bacteria in the body, thus weakening the immune system and causing further infections. They must be used with care, particularly when the patient is weak, deficient or emaciated, as in high *Vata* conditions.

Typical heating alteratives include bayberry, blackpepper, cayenne, cinnamon, garlic, myrrh, prickly ash, safflower and sassafras.

Alterative herbs are often taken in the spring as blood-purifiers. This is a good practice, but should not be done in excess, since they may thing the blood, and are not effective in anaemic or low blood pressure conditions.

ANTIPARASITICAL AND ANTHELMINTIC HERBS (*Krumighna karma*)

Anthelmintics are the herbs that help destroy and dispel worms. In ayurveda, the concept of *krumi*, which often translated as "worm", has broader implications. It includes all parasites, bacterial, fungal and yeast infections, which were accessible to the subtle vision of the yogis. Anthelmintics are useful in these conditions as well. They are valuable in treating the widespread yeast infection of Candida albicans, and related food allergy problems.

Parasitical infections are treated like *Ama,* as undigested food while it stagnates will eventually breed some sort of parasite. They are treated with a detoxifying therapy; tonification would only feed the infestation. For this reason, anthelmintic herbs have an emaciating effect upon the body and can weaken the tissues. In this regard, sperm is also considered a kind of *worm* or *krumi.* Anthelmintic herbs may reduce sperm and deplete vitality. Therefore, these herbs should be used symptomatically and with care, especially when the patient is already weak or emaciated.

Ayurveda identifies parasites with the aggravated *Dosha* through which they are manifested. *Kapha*-type parasites reside primarily in mucus or phlegm, *Pitta*-type parasites in the blood; and *Vata-type* parasites are found in the feces. Care must be taken to treat the aggravated *Dosha* as well as the specific parasites.

Antiparasitical action is possessed mainly by pungent or bitter-tasting herbs, yet it is often more a matter of special potency, *Prabhava,* than of general energetics. So one should be cautious in using hot, pungent anthelmintics on *Pitta-types* or cold, bitter ones on *Vata*-types.

Typical antiparasitical herbs include *ajwan,* asafoetida, cayenne, pepper, cloves, garlic, golden seal, pomegranate, prickly ash, pumpkin seeds, thyme, wormseed and wormwood.

Worms and parasites often cause an acute condition which should be referred to a qualified practitioner.

ASTRINGENT HERBS (*Stambhana karma*)

Herbs astringent in taste exert a firming, condensing and compacting action upon the tissues and organs of the body. They stop excessive discharges and secretions. Although drying, they are also moisture preserving. In addition, they have a healing action upon skin and mucous membranes.

Astringent taste may be differentiated from astringent action; astringent tasting herbs have astringent action while herbs of other tastes may also have astringent effects upon the body.

Astringent tasting herbs are mainly used symptomatically, as in stopping bleeding or stopping diarrhoea. Yet they often do not correct the condition from which the problem arises. Other herbs of different tastes may, in correcting conditions, alleviate these symptoms also. Diarrhoea, for example, may be due to poor absorption in the small intestine. An astringent taste herb like alum or raspberry may suppress the symptom, but will not improve absorption. In this regard, an herb like nutmeg, which is pungent and astringent and which contains heating and digestion promoting action along with astringent action, is more the herb of choice.

It may not always be good to suppress discharges. Diarrhoea caused by *Ama* may be the body's way of naturally cleansing itself. To suppress such diarrhoea with astringent taste herbs would be to hold the toxins in the body and cause further complications. The correct treatment in this case would be to promote the diarrhoea with laxatives until the *Ama* is dispelled. Astringents would only be employed if the diarrhoea continued beyond the point of cleansing.

It is important, therefore, that we do not abuse astringent herbs by using them symptomatically like drugs, without understanding the deeper causes of the disorders they may superficially treat.

Ayurveda distinguishes three different kinds of astringent action: those which stop bleeding, hemostatic herbs (*rakta stambhana*), those which stop excessive discharge of waste materials (*mala stambhana*) and could be called antidiarrhoeal herbs, and the third group vulnerary herbs (*ropana*), which promote healing of tissues, particularly for external usage. Not all of these herbs are astringent in taste.

Haemostatic herbs stop bleeding, usually by cooling the blood. They are related to alterative herbs, blood-purifiers. Since they are mainly anti *Pitta* in action, they can aggravate *Vata*. Their taste is usually astringent or bitter.

Typical hemostatic herbs include agrimony, bistort, cattail, golden seal, hibiscus, *manjishta,* marshmallow, mullein, nettle, plantain, red raspberry, saffron, self-heal, shepherd's purse, turmeric, white oak and yarrow.

Some hot pungent herbs have a hemostatic action, particularly where bleeding is caused by cold, as in some *Vata* or *Kapha* conditions. Such herbs include black pepper, cayenne, cinnamon and the ginger. These stop bleeding in short term usage but in longer usage may promote bleeding by heating the blood.

Bitter tonics and alterative herbs, which generally cool the blood and *Pitta,* may help to stop bleeding by their cooling action even without any more specific haemostatic properties.

Astringent action herbs are those which stop diarrhoea, may also help to eliminate excessive sweating, urination and spontaneous seminal emission. They are usually cooling in energy and astringent to bitter in taste.

Typical antidiarrhoeal herbs include blackberry, comfrey, gentian, lotus seeds, plantain, red raspberry, sumach, white pond lily, white oak bark and yellow dock.

Some warming herbs also stop diarrhoea and other excessive discharges and are usually better for digestion. Such herbs are healthful to *Vata*. They include black pepper, ginger, *haritaki,* nutmeg and poppy seeds.

Vulnerary herbs promote healing of damaged tissue from cuts, wounds, bums, hemorrhaging, etc. They are often used externally in poultices and plasters. Mainly astringent or sweet in taste and cooling in energy, they reduce *Pitta* and *Kapha*. Yet they are not so much for deep seated injuries where there is much tissue damage, because this requires more tonification. Many are demulcent and emollient, softening and soothing to the skin and mucous membranes. Some may contain mucilage.

Typical vulnerary herbs include aloe vera, chickweed, comfrey, honey, marshmallow, plantain, self-heal, shepherd's purse, slippery elm and turmeric.

Some herbs possess all three of these astringent actions and have thereby become famous as heal-all herbs. Such herbs include comfrey, marshmallow, plantain, self-heal and yarrow.

The healing action of astringent herbs is not usually of a nutritive nature. Astringent herbs promote the healing of tissues, but do not actually promote the increase of tissue. This drying action can have not only a healing, but also a wasting effect. Wrong or excessive use of astringent herbs may aggravate *Vata*. This can cause constipation, gas pain, muscle spasms and nervousness.

For this reason, astringent herbs are often used synergistically with nutritive or tonic herbs. The nutritive herbs build up the tissue and the astringents give it firmness and help hold it in the body Herbs that combine astringent and tonic action are thereby powerful rejuvenatives like *amalaki*, *bibhitaki* and *haritaki*, three of ayurveda's most powerful regenerative herbs.

BITTER TONIC AND ANTIPYRETIC HERBS

The Ayurvedic concept of tonic herbs is different than that of most American and European herbal treatments. In western herbalism, the term tonic, implies to an agent that nurtures and strengthens the body, is usually given to cold bitter herbs like gentian or golden seal. These are thought to increase vitality by stimulating digestion. By increasing nutrition, the herbs are thought to strengthen the body and its organs, while at the same lime giving proper tone to muscles and tissues. This herbal action is said to increase the elimination of toxins, waste-products, and to purify the blood. Ionic herbs are thus prescribed for any convalescent or run-down patient.

In Ayurveda, the use of bitter herbs as tonics is not always appropriate or helpful. Bitter taste is the coldest, most drying, most depletive and reductive of tastes. It is not tonic in the sense of being nutritive—promoting tissue growth or building up the body. Its effects are of catabolic or reducing nature detoxifying, promoting the depletion or elimination of tissue, while depressing or sedating most of the organic functions of the body. Its proper use is more to reducing toxins and excesses, not in building up deficiencies. Bitter herbs' are part of a purification, sedation, heat dispelling or reducing therapy, which usage they also share in Chinese medicine.

Ayurveda believes that bitter herbs stimulate digestion, but only in small amounts, and mainly for patients suffering from heat, fever or high *Pitta* conditions. They are not often prescribed for the chronically weak or emaciated. Higher dosages are thought to depress digestion, weaken assimilation and derange peristalsis.

Bitter herbs, by their nature as air and ether, dry up the tissues and vital fluids and may cause rigidity of the muscles or *even* muscle spasms. Rather than promote proper tone of muscles, organs and tissues, under many conditions bitter herbs will reduce it.

Though most western herbalism prescribes these herbs for convalescence and debility, yet ayurveda often regards them as unhelpful in such conditions. Many cases of weakness and convalescence are *Vata* in nature, conditions of chill, fluid deficiency and the wasting away of bodily tissues. They require a warming, moistening and nutritive therapy. Bitter herbs are also *Vata,* airy in nature, and so provide nothing to rebuild the body or increase vital fluids. It is mainly in conditions of lingering fever, remittent or intermittent, or in the debility following a fever or high *Pitta* state that they can be strengthening.

Tonic herbs in ayurveda are generally sweet, nutritive substances that build tissue, strengthen vitality, increase vital fluids, improve sexual energy and aid longevity. They are considered in a separate section on tonic herbs. Bitter herbs can deplete vitality, depress sexual energy and promote the aging-process and they are known as bitter tonic.

One could say, with some justification, that these bitter tonics are tonics for *Pitta,* as they are the strongest herbs to reduce and regulate its function. But their action should not be confused with tonics that are nutritive and rejuvenative.

Bitter tonics are, nonetheless, very important herbal medicines. Ayurveda and western herbalism agree that these arc the strongest herbs to bring down fevers, to cleanse the body and to kill toxins. They reduce fever, *Pitta,* toxins and fat from the body. They are the strongest herbs for clearing the heat.

When the fever is due to an external pathogen and is mainly a surface condition, like the fever due to colds or flus, it should be treated with a diaphoretic therapy by inducing sweating to open the pores, restore circulation and dispel the chill causing it. However, when the fever is high, in the blood or the interior of the body, heating the liver, when there is much thirst, sweating, inflammation or infection, usually a *Pitta* condition, then these bitter tonics are more appropriate.

Bitter tonics do not merely suppress the fever but they destroy the infection which causes it, catabolizing the pathogen. They attack and destroy the *Ama,* the toxins which have entered into the tissues and caused the fever. They are thus indicated in any fever due to *Ama*, which, as in arthritis, may be owing to aggravation of *Vita* or *Kapha*. By their light nature they destroy *Ama*, which is heavy.

In reducing heat, acidity and toxicity, they cool and detoxify the blood; they also possess an alterative or blood-purifying action. One could say that they are like alteratives, but are a degree stronger in action. They regulate liver function, and control and reduce the production of bile and acid in the body. As such, they are indicated in most liver diseases like hepatitis and jaundice, particularly in the initial and acute phases.

They reduce fat and regulate sugar metabolism. In this way they also regulate spleen functioning and may be helpful in such conditions as diabetes. As the strongest herbs to dispel fat and reduce weight, they have a strong anti-*Kapha* action.

This, along with their blood-purifying action, gives them antitumor properties. They may help to reduce both benign and malignant tumors, as in cancer. As they catalyze the catabolic processes of the body, they scrape away heavy accretions and remove congestion in the body.

While being the strongest herbs to decrease *Pitta*, and while having a strong reducing action on *Kapha* as well, they arc also the strongest herbs to aggravate *Vata*. If we use them in *Vata*-caused indigestion i.e., nervous indigestion, which may be thought to be hypoglycemia, they may only induce further nervous derangements and more hypersensitivity.

Typical bitter tonic and antipyretic herbs include aloe, barberry, gentian, golden seal, gold thread, Peruvian bark, white poplar, and, special to India, *chirata*, *kutki* and *neem*.

CARMINATIVE HERBS (*Vata-anuloman*)

Carminatives herbs are the herbs that relieve intestinal gas, pain and distention. They settle digestion and increase absorption and help to dispel water and mucus. *Ama*, stagnating in and clogging the gastrointestinal tract. They promote proper and normal peristalsis.

They are usually aromatic or fragrant herbs that possess a volatile oil that stimulates the gastrointestinal nerves (*samana* and *apana vayus*, the forces of *Vata* that govern the stomach, small intestine and colon) to promote digestion and dispel accumulation of undigested food materials.

Their stimulation of *Vata* also increases *Agni*— just as wind increases fire. In this regard, they resemble with stimulant herbs as well as other herbs possessing actions in both these categories. But while stimulant herbs tend to promote digestion through a direct feeding of *Agni*, these work more indirectly through normalizing *Vata*. As such they are particularly good for digestive weakness owing to nervous upset, anxiety and depression.

They are closely related to nervines as by dissolving blockages in all the channels, *srotas*, they open up the nervous system and relieve spasms and pain. They may also possess diaphoretic and expectorant action, and are often circulatory stimulants. They improve the general spirit and promote the basic energy flow, *prana*, of the body.

All carminative herbs move *Vata*. This stimulating action moves out accumulated *Vata*. Yet their dryness may aggravate *Vata*, if used too long or in excess. Most of these aromatic herbs tend to be heating and are usually pungent in taste. A secondary group, however, is cooling and tends towards bitter taste.

Heating carminatives may aggravate *Pitta* and some promote acidity in which case cooling carminatives would be preferred. Cooling carminatives are more likely to have a long term depleting effect on *Vata*. All aromatic and carminative herbs reduce *Kapha*, owing to their drying property.

Most spices fall in this category of herbs, and used as spices they should be part of the daily diet, particularly for someone with a *Vata* constitution. One to five grams of many of these spices taken with meals can cure many diseases, as most disease arises from indigestion. With food or tonic herbs these spices aid in rejuvenation and correct many congestive diseases and nervous disorders.

Typical heating carminatives include *ajwan*, asafoetida, basil, bay leaves, calamus, cardamom. cinnamon, cloves, garlic, ginger juniper berries, nutmeg, orange peel, thyme, turmeric and valerian.

Typical cooling carminatives are chamomile, chrysanthemum, coriander, cumin, dill, fennel, lime, mustard, peppermint, spearmint and wintergreen.

DIAPHORETIC HERBS (*Svedana karma*)

Diaphoretic herbs induce perspiration and by this action, they restore circulation, dispel fever and dulls, while eliminate toxins from the surface of the body. Strong diaphoretics are called sudorifics. They are surface-relieving agents used in the initial and acute stages of colds and flus, as well as more chronic conditions of asthma and arthritis. The initial or acute stage of colds and febrile diseases paralyzes the defensive energy that moves along the surface of the body. The result is a stoppage of sweating and a blockage of circulation. Diaphoretic herbs, by stimulating, restore the defensive energy of the body.

They produce (a) promote sweating, (b) relieve muscle tension and aching joints, (c) bring down fevers due to external factors associated with colds and flus, (d) promote the eruption and resolution of inflammatory skin conditions, (e) help disperse surface water and facial edema and (f) relieve headaches due to cold and congestion.

Ayurveda recognizes two kinds of diaphoretic herbs according to the *Dosha* on which they work These two kinds are warming and cooling diaphoretics.

Most diaphoretics are of the warming nature. They are generally hot, pungent herbs that decrease *Kapha* and *Vata* but increase *Pitta*. Most colds are of a *Kapha* nature, an invasion of chill and damp *Vata*, or wind, is the factor that carries them into the body. Warming diaphoretics treat the common cold by dispersing wind, chill and dampness. They are generally stimulants, expectorants and may possess antiasthmatic and antirheumatic properties.

Cooling diaphoretics are usually bitter-to-pungent herbs that decrease *Pitta* and *Kapha* but increase *Vata*. They are more for *Pitta*-type colds and are more effective in treating high fever; sore throat and other inflammatory symptoms involving the invasion of toxins in the blood. They are generally alteratives and may possess diuretic properties.

Warming diaphoretics raise body temperature and through sweating, dispel chills. Cooling diaphoretics lower body temperature through sweating, and dispel heat and toxins through the skin. Both dispel water; phlegm and *Kapha*.

Kapha-constitution requires strong diaphoresis owing to its wet attribute. *Pitta* constitution requires moderate diaphoresis of a cooling nature. It can be aggravated by heating diaphoretics, by hot sweat or steam baths, or by hot tubs and saunas, which relieve *Kapha*. *Vata* requires mild diaphoresis of a predominately warming nature to help moisten its surface dryness, but strong diaphoretic methods may dry *Vata* out further.

It should be remembered that colds and flus may not be of the same *Dosha* as the constitution of the person. A *Pitta* person may have a *Kapha* cold-most colds are *Kapha*, at least in the beginning. For such temporary diseases, treatment can be symptomatic.

Diaphoretics cleanse the lymphatics and the plasma, ayurvedic *Rasa Dhatu*. Cooling diaphoretics help open the mind and breath, increase *Prana*, clear the sinuses and the senses and stimulate the nervous system. Cooling diaphoretics have additional cleansing action on the liver and blood.

In ayurveda, diaphoresis is part of the preliminary treatment in *Pancha Kanna*, or purification therapy. After oil massage, which softens the toxins in the body, it is used to melt them and render them mobile for elimination from the body. Diaphoresis usually is followed by emesis, purgation or enema as prime therapy, but it may sometimes be a prime therapy in itself.

It does not require herbs but can be done through fire,

steam, exercise, hot baths and so on. The use of herbal diaphoretics should be included with a hot bath, sleeping under a warm blanket and fasting.

Typical heating diaphoretics include angelica, basil, bayberry, camphor, cardamom, cinnamon, cloves, ephedra, eucalyptus, ginger, juniper berries, sage, thyme and wild ginger.

Typical cooling diaphoretics are burdock, catnip, chamomile, chrysanthemum, coriander, elder flowers, horsetail, peppermint, spearmint and yarrow.

DIURETIC HERBS (*Mutrala karma*)

Diuretic herbs increase urination as they promote the functional activity of the kidneys and urinary bladder. Acting on the water element in all the tissue-elements (*dhatus*) of the body, diuretic herbs reduce and remove toxins. Their action is largely due to detoxification and purgation through the urine. They are purgatives for the water element in the body and as such they reduce the earth element in the body. Hence, like all purgatives, they must be used with caution.

Diuretics decrease water and reduce *kapha,* whose main constituent is water. Generally they are bitter astringent or pungent in taste. Similarly, all diuretics tend to increase the dryness of *Vata.* This action is aggravated by the tastes that relieve *kapha* and dampness. These also reduce *Pitta.* Many or even most of them are stronger in reducing *Pitta* than *Kapha.* This is not just because *Pitta* is also some what oily in nature. It is because urination is also a way of relieving heat from the body, of removing add and toxins from the blood, a way of cooling and purifying the blood.

Heating and drying herbs, pungent taste, bring water up and out of the body through the process of sweating—diaphoretic action. They also work by relieving mucus through the mouth in expectoration. Just as water evaporates upwards by the action of fire, heating and drying herbs purify the system.

Cooling and drying herbs, bitter and astringent tastes—on the other hand—bring water downwards through the urine. Cold herbs cause a descending or contracting action, the way hot herbs create a rising and dispersing action.

Diuretic action is generally cooling and drying—the opposite of the qualities of *Pitta*, heat and moisture. For this reason, diuretics dispel damp heat, as in diarrhea and dysentery, and cool down not only the kidneys and bladder; but also the liver and gall bladder. In increasing urination, they help to dispel kidney and bladder stones, and also stones of the gall bladder. Such stone dispelling herbs are called lithotriptic.

In their more specific *anti-Kapha* action, diuretic herbs dispel edema and water accumulation in the tissues, particularly in the lower half of the body. Facially-accumulated water and water in the head and chest are often better reduced by diaphoretic and expectorant herbs. They help to decrease fat and reduce weight, particularly when fat is mainly composed of water.

They stimulate bladder and kidney function, but are seldom actually tonic or nutritive to the kidneys. Their drying action may cause constipation or dryness of the skin. Scanty urination without water accumulation requires a moistening, not a drying therapy, and in that condition, diuretic herbs are usually contraindicated. *Vata* constitution needs to increase urine by increasing water in the tissues—not a diuretic but a tonic or nutritive therapy. Diuretics are probably the strongest herbs to aggravate *Vata,* and are contraindicated in conditions of convalescent debility and dehydration.

Diuretics can be divided into cooling and heating kinds. Cooling diuretics are often also cooling diaphoretics, alteratives or antipyretic herbs, useful in fevers and infectious diseases, particularly those involving the urinogenital tract (as herpes) or the liver and gall bladder. Warming diuretics, like juniper berries, are often warming diaphoretics, stimulants and expectorants and may have antirheumatic action. They are contraindicated in

Pitta conditions of kidney or gall bladder inflammation unless they are balanced out by a majority of cooling herbs.

A few diuretics are cooling and moistening, apart from their drying action in diuresis, and have a soothing effect upon the mucous membranes of the urinary system. Examples are marshmallow, barley or *goleshura*. Often one such herb is added to a diuretic formula to soothe and protect the kidneys from the drying and scraping action of diuretic herbs that can cause irritation and discomfort.

Typical cooling diuretics include asparagus, barley, burdock, cleavers, coriander, cornsilk, dandelion, fennel, *gokshura*, gravel root, horsetail, lemon grass, marshmallow, plantain, *punarnava* and spearmint.

Typical warming diuretics are *ajwan*, cinnamon, cubebs, garlic, juniper berries, Mormon tea, mustard, parsley and wild carrot.

EMMENAGOGUES (*Raktabhisarana karma*)

Emmenagogues herbs are those herbs that help to promote and regulate menstruation and thereby treat many of the special disorders of the female reproductive system, as uterine tumours or infections. Such herbs are called *raktabhisarana,*, herbs that promote the flow of blood in ayurveda, what could be called "circulatory stimulants."

Emmenagogues are largely pungent to bitter herbs that relieve congestion of the blood, clear blood clots and promote menstruation. They warm the blood and improve its quality, stimulating the heart. They may be heating or cooling in energy, with those cooling in the majority.

The female reproductive system is intimately associated with the blood, it is, therefore, *Pitta* in nature. Imbalances should be examined as increased or decreased *Pitta* conditions. Naturally the same treatment can not work in both cases. Those emmenagogues that are cooling in nature are better for high

Pitta menstrual disorders, those heating in nature for low *Pitta*.

A predominance of cooling emmenagogues is better for menstrual irregularities owing to such conditions as uterine infection or bleeding. Such herbs also help to calm high emotions, anger and irritability. A predominance of heating emmenagogues is better for delayed menstruation due to exposure to cold, overexertion or nervous anxiety. These may also be antispasmodics, relieving uterine cramping and pain. Those which are diuretic treat pre-menstrual water retention. Those which are haemostatic are better for excessive menstruation.

Typical heating emmenagogues are angelica, asafoetida, cinnamon, cotton root, ginger mugwort, myrrh, parsley pennyroyal, safflower; turmeric and valerian.

Typical cooling emmenagogues include blessed thistle, chamomile, chrysanthemum, hibiscus, *manjishta,* motherwort, musta, primrose, red raspberry, rose flowers and yarrow.

Emmenagogues work largely by increasing *apana vayu,* the downward-moving *Vata* governing elimination, urination and sexual functions. As such, they tend to be laxative and to promote the discharge of the fetus. Hence, many are contraindicated during pregnancy.

Ayurveda distinguishes another group of emmenagogues—those which are tonic or rejuvenative to the female reproductive system. These are a subcategory of tonic, rejuvenative and aphrodisiac herbs. They are mainly sweet herbs that build the blood, moisten and nourish the female reproductive organs, and so treat the conditions of organ weakness due to disease, poor nutrition or the effects of aging.

Typical tonic and rejuvenative emmenagogues are aloe are, angelica, cotton root, false unicorn, licorice, lotus seeds, myrrh, peony, *rehmannia, shatavari,* Solomon's wild yam, and such flowers as hibiscus, jasmine, rose and saffron. In this regard, ayurveda also uses various iron preparations.

EXPECTORANT AND DEMULCENT HERBS (*Kasa-Svasahara*)

Expectorant herbs promote the discharge of phlegm and mucus from the body. They not only clear the lungs and nasal passages, but also the stomach. They are useful in respiratory afflictions, chronic or acute colds, flus, asthma, bronchitis, pneumonia. Such problems ayurveda refers to as *kasa* and *svasa,* which mean literally cough and dyspnea. They may also be helpful in digestive problems because mucus has its origin in the stomach and may clog the gastrointestinal tract, giving rise to indigestion and poor assimilation.

Phlegm and mucus can accumulate anywhere in the body, causing various growths or tumours, generally benign. They may accumulate under the skin for example and can clog the channels of the circulatory and other systems, leading to all manner of diseases, including nervous disorders.

Expectorant herbs are of two kinds and work in two different ways. Some expectorants, like ginger remove mucus by a drying action. They are mainly pungent m taste and hot m energy and may also be stimulant, diaphoretic or carminative herbs. A few, *however* like horehound, are bitter in taste and cooling in energy and are particularly good for *Pitta.*

Others, like licorice help to remove mucus by their moistening action. They increase and liquify *Kapha,* promoting its flow out of the body. They are mainly sweet and cold herbs. These are also demulcent and emollient herbs, mucilaginous substances that have a softening and soothing effect upon the skin and mucous membranes.

Warming and drying expectorants dispel chill and dampness, decrease *Kapha* and *Ama,* increase *Pitta* and *Agni,* and are particularly good for *Kapha* or *Kapha- Vaia* type colds and respiratory afflictions.

Cooling and moistening expectorants dispel heat and dryness, liquify *Kapha* and *Ama,* and work more on *Vata* or

Pitta-Vata type colds and respiratory, afflictions of sore throat or dry and hacking cough.

Most expectorants possess cough-relieving action, as coughs are usually caused by mucus blockage or irritation of the respiratory passages. Hence, most cough - relieving herbs are included in this category though some possess more specific action from nervine or antispasmodic properties.

Coughs should similarly be discriminated as wet (productive) or dry (unproductive) and treated with the appropriate kinds of herbs. Cough or cold with clear, abundant phlegm usually indicates *Kapha* disorder, chilldamp. Cough or cold with yellow phlegm or inflammation of the mucous membranes usually indicates fever or *Pitta* derangement, dampheat. Dry cough along with scanty phlegm and chill usually indicates *Vata*, particularly if it is a chronic condition.

Coughs and colds arc basically *Kapha* disorders, as mucus is *Kapha* and *Kapha* has as its site in the stomach and lungs. Chronic colds and mucous congestion are often relieved by therapeutic vomiting, emetic therapy, a kind of radical expectorant action.

Moistening expectorants or demulcents can be used externally to help to heal sores, wounds or ulcers. They are nutritive and promote cell growth, as well as being anti-inflamrnatory.

They are the closest to true tonics in western herbology and in the ayurvedic sense; sweet, nutritive herbs that directly feed and strengthen the organs and tissues. They can be called lung tonics. Some have rejuvenative action. By their softening action, some are laxatives.

The soothing action of demulcent herbs gives them a power to help to calm the heart and nerves. They are effective nervines in *Vata* conditions of dehydration and tissue depletion. Demulcent herbs alleviate dryness, caused friction that irritates physiological function. They feed the mucous membranes and the connective tissue.

Both kinds of expectcrants may be combined to help to balance their action. Hot, dry expectorants, like ginger may be used with a moistening expectorant like licorice, so as not to aggravate *Vata* or *Pitta* by its dryness or heat. Cold, moist expectorants may require the addition of a hot, pungent herb like ginger, as they are heavy and hard to digest and may aggravate *Ama*. The effect of a formula depends upon the predomination of herbs in it and should not be too one-sided in action.

Typical drying expectorants are boneset, calamus, cardamom, cinnamon, cloves, cubebs, elecampane, dry ginger, horehound, hyssop, mustard seeds, orange peel, *pippali,* sage and wild ginger.

Typical moistening expectorants or demulcents include bamboo, chickweed, comfrey root, flaxseed, Irish moss, licorice, maiden hair fern, marshmallow, milk, raw sugar slippery elm and Solomon's seal.

Typical cough-relieving herbs include apricot seeds, bayberry, coltsfoot, ephedra, eucalyptus, grindelia, horehound, mullein, osha, thyme and wild cherry.

LAXATIVE AND PURGATIVE HERBS *(Virechana karma)*

Laxative herbs promote bowel movements, dispel constipation, and help to eliminate food accumulations and toxic build ups from the intestines. They may be weak or strong. Weak laxatives are called simply laxatives or aperients. Strong laxatives are called purgatives or cathartics.

Purgatives promote forceful evacuation, and may cause diarrhoea and griping, with perhaps pain and tenesmus, owing to their irritant effect. As such, they should be used with great care. Purgatives are usually either cold, bitter herbs like rhubarb or hot oils like castor oil.

Mild laxatives are mainly moistening herbs and bulk laxatives, like bran. They work through increasing elimination through greater lubrication of the intestines. Some cold, bitter herbs, like cascara sagrada, also have a mild laxative action, but it is more like a weak purgative, working through stimulating peristalsis.

Laxatives and purgatives are indicated wherever there is constipation, or wherever there is a pronounced coating at the back of the tongue, denoting a buildup of toxins in the colon. Sometimes a person who has regular bowel movements may still have a large accumulation of fecal matter in the colon and so require purgation. Whenever there are toxins in the colon, which may also cause diarrhoea, purgatives can be used. They can also be used in the later stages of a fever to help to clear the toxins out of the body.

Chronic constipation, as well as constipation in the elder age, is usually a *Vata* condition, with its accumulation of gas and dryness in the colon. In this condition, generally mild, moistening or bulk laxatives are prescribed, strong purgatives would cause irritation. However sometimes a strong purge is necessary for high build-up of toxins due to accumulated *Vata.* In such cases, the hot oils, like castor, are specific.

Pitta constitution tends towards diarrhoea due to its damp attribute, but where heat is high it may also cause constipation. Either way, purgatives of a usually cold and bitter nature, which work on the small intestine, are prescribed. Purgation (*virechana*) is the strongest way to eliminate *Pitta,* heat and bile from the body. However, where there is inflammation or ulceraton of the intestinal membranes, which is usually a *Pitta* condition, strong purgatives can cause irritation. For such condition moistening laxatives of a cooling nature, like psyllium seeds, would be indicated.

Kapha constitution may be constipated owing to the accumulation of phlegm, mucus and undigested food particles in the intestines due to deficient digestive power. For this condition, laxatives of a drying nature are indicated; bulk or moistening laxatives would increase congestion.

Laxatives tend to suppress the power of digestion, and may weaken peristalsis in the long run by over stimulation. As such they should be used with stimulant or carminative herbs, like ginger and fennel seeds. Constipation or toxins in the colon can also be treated by increasing the power of digestion, *Agni*. Hot, spicy stimulant-carminative herbs can help to correct constipation in a *Vata* or *Kapha* constitution without actually having to use laxatives. Dryness in the colon may also be related to dryness, in the lungs, and herbs that moisturize the lungs also, like licorice or flaxseed, may be more specific to the condition.

Typical moistening or bulk laxatives are bran, flaxseed, ghee, licorice, prunes, psyllium seed, raisins, shatavari and warm milk.

Strong purgatives include aloe powder, castor oil, croton, epsom salt, mandrake, rhubarb and senna.

Cooling herbs with various degrees of laxative action are aloe, blue flag, cascara sagrada, echinacea, gentian, rhubarb, senna and yellow dock.

NERVINE AND ANTISPASMODIC HERBS

Nervines are herbs that strengthen the functional activity of the nervous system. They may be stimulants or sedatives and can be used to correct excesses or deficiencies of nervous function. They have a strong action on the mind and are useful in promoting mental health and clarity as well as aiding in the treatment of psychological imbalances and mental diseases.

Most nervines are also antispasmodics; herbs that relieve spasms of the voluntary or involuntary muscles and thereby' relieve cramps, stop tremors and convulsions. They may also serve as broncho dilators, stopping spasms in the bronchial tubes, thus proving effective for respiratory afflictions. Others may help to relieve menstrual cramping and headaches.

Many of these herbs are fragrant, aromatic herbs like mint or valerian. This is because aromatic herbs work directly on

Prana, the prime energy of the nervous system, as they are themselves substances that contain much *Prana*, the air element. Such aromatic herbs open the mind and senses, clear the channels, the *srotas,* relieve congestion, stop pain and restore the smooth flow of energy in the body mind system.

Aromatic nervines are often also carminative and stomachic herbs, that dispel intestinal gas and cramping. The basis for this can be seen in light of ayurvedic physiology. *Vata,* the *Dosha* that governs the nervous system, accumulates in the colon, from which it invades the tissue elements of the body. It is also in the colon that the assimilation of nutrients, mainly of oils, occurs for the sustenance of nerve and bone tissue. Hence the treatment of *Vata* in the colon is often a root treatment for *Vata* in the nervous system. *Vata* relieving herbs can treat both.

Generally speaking, in ayurveda nervousness, is supposed as *Vata* or as the mark of a *Vata* constitution, for *Vata* governs nerve responses and, by nature as air or wind, it is impulsive, vaccillatory, hypersensitive. Most diseases of the nervous system are diseases of *Vata.* Hence, in treating nervous disorders, *Vata* is considered firstly. Most nerve pain, lumbago, sciatica, paralysis and degenerative nervous disorders are *Vata* diseases. Yet many emotional or nervous disorders may be caused by the other *Doshas,* as those due to anger which would be a *Pitta* condition. Or *Vata* may be blocked or aggravated by the other *Doshas,* in which case an apparant *Vata* disorder would be due to an underlying excess of *Pitta* or *Kapha.* So, again, primary causes are to be located, rather than evident effects.

Vata emotions, like fear and anxiety, weaken the kidneys and adrenals. They damage the nerves and cause insomnia, mental instability, nerve pain, cramping and numbness, which may lead eventually to the wasting away of nerve tissue. Most nervines, particularly those which are aromatic, move *Vata,* and so help to remove the obstructed *Vata* or life energy behind these disorders.

A few herbs are not only aromatic, but possess *tamasic*, heavy or dulling properties. These are particularly good for both moving and grounding *Vata,* which suffers from "ungroundedness"-from an excess of air and ether. Such herbs include asafoetida, garlic and valerian. Yet where there is a deficiency of nerve tissues, often due to poor nutrition; nutritive herbs are needed—*ashwagandha* or liquorice. Excessive use of aromatic nervines may further weaken the nerves by their drying action; they may also be over-stimulating.

Pitta-type emotions, anger, envy, hatred and so on, heat up the blood, the liver and the heart, creating internal fire. Thereby they can cause hypertension, insomnia, irritability and other mental and nervous imbalances. They can also burn out the nerves, a condition of the high *Pitta,* aggressive, "business executive's" life style. *Pitta*-caused nervous disorders can often be treated with general anti *Pitta* herbs like bitter tonics or purgatives, without having to resort to any specific nervine herbs at all.

Yet many, perhaps most, of the herbs that act upon the mind are cooling in energy. This is because the mind is unbalanced largely by negative emotions, which are like *Pitta* and create heat. A calm and clear mind is usually a cool mind. Hence many herbs for the mind, like gotu kola (Brahmi), are good *anti-Pitta* herbs.

Kapha nervous conditions are more a matter of dullness, lethargy, hypoactivity of the nervous system. Psychologically *Kapha* suffers from greed, desire, attachment and clinging to the past. In terms of the mind and nerves, *Kapha* requires stimulation. Nervines that are aromatic, stimulant and decongestant are best for *Kapha,* and most aromatics, by their drying nature, are good for *Kapha.*

Many herbs that calm the mind to tend to have a positive effect on all three *Doshas,* as it is in the balance of the *Doshas* that the mind is calm. Hence, some nervines may be good for all three *Doshas* (*tridosha herbs*), particularly in small amounts or short term usage. Such cooling aromatics as mint, chamomile or fennel can be widely used as mild nervines. Their drying nature relieves *Kapha*, their cooling energy relieves *Pitta*, and their aromatic property removes obstructed *Vata*.

Like other herbal categories, nervines can be divided into heating and cooling types. Cooling nervines are generally better for *Pitta*, heating for *Vata* and *Kapha*, though both kinds reduce *Kapha* and move obstructed *Vata* to some degree.

Typical heating nervine and antispasmodic herbs are asafoetida, basil, bayberry, calamus, camphor, eucalyptus, garlic, *guggul*, lady's slipper, mugwort, myrrh, nutmeg, pennyroyal, poppy seeds, sage and valerian.

Typical cooling nervine and antispasmodic herbs include betony, *bhringaraj*, catnip, chamomile, gotu kola, jasmine, *jatamamsi*, motherwort, mullein, oatstraw, passion flower, peppermint, sandalwood, skullcap, spearmint, St. John's Wort, vervain and wild yam.

There are other special nervine herbs that are more like drugs and from which many drugs have been derived. They contain certain chemicals or alkaloids on which their action depends. Such special effects of minute chemicals that transcend the energetics of taste are regarded as examples of *Prabhava*. Their action is strong and their side effects cause paralysis. Most are poisons, severely aggravate *Pitta*, and should be used with great care. Examples include dhatura (jimsonweed), digitalis, marijuana and opium.

Metals, minerals and gems have special action on the mind and nervous system. Ayurveda includes within its scope special preparations of these, made non-toxic to the human body. Such compounds relate back to the old alchemical tradition and are called *Siddha Yoga* compounds. These compounds also relate to longevity therapy and are another special feature of ayurveda.

STIMULANT AND DIGESTIVE HERBS (*Dipana-Pachana Karma*)

Stimulants are the herbs that generally stimulate increase or promote all organic functions. They do this primarily by stimulating the power of digestion. Stimulants are mainly hot in energy, pungent in taste, and include most hot spices, peppers and gingers. Their action is to increase internal heat, dispel internal chill, and strengthen the metabolism and circulation.

They are the most powerful herbs to increase *Agni,* the digestive fire, and are thereby the strongest herbs to destroy *Ama,* toxic accumulations. They are synonymous with *Agni Dipana* and *Ama Pachana* herbs in *Ayurveda;* herbs that increase *Agni* and digest *Ama.* They contain large amounts of *Agni,* so that even if the body's *Agni* is low, they can still burn away toxins.

They warm the stomach, increase the appetite, warm the blood, and stimulate the senses. They often have antibacterial or antiparasitical powers and increase the auto-immune system. They do not actually build up the body, but allow for the assimilation of food whereby the body can be built up. They arc often used with tonic and nutritive herbs as well as with foods.

They are the most powerful herbs to increase *Pitta* and decrease *Kapha.* Generally, they decrease *Vata,* but in excess they can aggravate it through their drying property. They are good for *Sama* conditions and can be used in small amounts on *Sama Pitta.* Destroying toxins, also help to relieve fevers, and for this purpose may be combined with bitter tonics and antipyretic herbs.

Many stimulant-digestive herbs have carminative and stomachic properties, but they also stimulate peristalsis (*samana vayu*). Many have diaphoretic properties by heating the surface of the body and promoting sweating. They also increase appetite. Many have expectorant qualities. They help to dispel *Kapha or* mucus from the stomach, lungs and nasal passages, and promote the flow of tears. In promoting circulation, they possess some blood purifying effects.

These digestive stimulants are related to nerve stimulants. They may increase hypertension or cause insomnia. They should be used only to supplement functional weaknesses, not to enable the user to sustain the abuses of excessive activity. Stimulant and digestive herbs are indicated whenever the digestion is to be improved, cold is to be dispelled, toxins and tongue-coating are to be cleared up, and degenerated metabolism and circulation are to be revived.

They are contraindicated in conditions of dehydration, fluid insufficiency, and inflammatory conditions of the mucous membranes. They should not be directly applied to the mucous membranes.

Typical stimulant herbs are *ajwan,* asafoetida, black pepper cayenne, cinnamon, doves, garlic, dry ginger, horseradish, mustard, onions, *pippali* and prickly ash.

TONICS

These are of following types :

A. Nutritive Tonics (Bruhana karma)

The ayurvedic concept of a tonic is a substance that nurtures the tissue elements (*dhatus*) of the body. A nutritive tonic is an herb that nourishes the body and increases weight, density and substance within it. Such herbal foods serve the various *dhatus* or organs that have been depleted or weakened by disease.

Tonics are usually sweet in taste, or in post-digestive effect, which indicates their constructive action. Generally, they have the same nature as *Kapha* and are composed primarily of earth and water. These are usually heavy, oily or mucilaginous. They increase vital fluids, muscle and fat and build the blood and lymph, increasing milk and semen. They are restoratives for conditions of weakness, emaciation, debility and convalescence.

They have a softening, soothing and harmonizing effect, which dispels rigidity and calms the nerves.

Nutritive tonics generally decrease *Vata* and *Pitta* and increase *Kapha*. A few which are heating, like ginseng or sesame seeds, may aggravate *Pitta*. They increase *Ama* and are not the herbs of choice for *Sama* conditions, though they can help to soften the *Ama* where other more primary herbs facilitate its discharge. Nutritive tonics are moistening and cooling in energy—the best herbs to reduce the dryness of *Vata*. Yet they are also heavy and are hard to digest. For the low *Agni*, particularly of *Vata* constitutions, they are usually combined with various stimulant or carminative herbs, for example ginger or cardamom, to aid in their absorption.

For *Pitta* conditions, herbs that combine astringent or bitter with sweet taste, like comfrey root or *shatavari*, are most appropriate. With their cooling energy, they can be used in convalescence from high fever, toxic blood, ulcers or other inflammatory *Pitta* conditions.

Many of these nutritive tonic herbs possess expectorant, demulcent and emollient action. They soothe and nurture the mucous membranes and restore bodily fluids and secretions. As such, they are particularly nurturing for the mucous membranes of the lungs and stomach. They have a healing action on the skin and may help soften and relieve muscle tension and pain.

Typical nutritive tonics are almonds, *amalaki*, angelica, *bala*, coconut, comfrey root, dates, flaxseeds, ginseng, honey, Irish moss, licorice, lotus seeds, marshmallow, milk, raisins, sesame seeds, *shatavari*, slippery elm, Solomon's seal, spikenard, sugar, *vidari kanda* and wild yam.

B. Rejuvenative Tonics *(Rasayana karma)*

Ayurvedic herbology reaches its culmination in the science of rejuvenation. Aimed at renewal of both body and mind, ayurvedic herbology does not seek simply longevity, but moves towards a life of pure awareness, natural creativity, spontaneous delight. The approach is not only towards physical immortality, which on some deeper level of harmony may be possible, but the immortality of the mind, the daily renewal of brain cells. In such a state, the mind and heart are as clear in old *age*, as in childhood.

This science is called *Rasayana. Rasayana* is what enters (ayana), in the essence (rasa). It is what penetrates and revitalizes the essence of our psycho-physiological being. *Rasayana* substances rebuild the body-mind, prevent decay, and postpone the aging. They may even help to reverse the aging process. They do not simply add to the bulk or quantity of the body, but increase its quality. *Rasayana* substances are more subtle, more specific, and more lasting than simple nutritive tonics. Their action sustains the optimal form and function of the various organs, *dhatus* and *doshas* in the body. They are not necessarily sweet and nutritive, though most are sweet at least in *vipaka*, the post-digestive effect. Rejuvenative tonics for *Kapha* may be pungent and hot.

Rasayana substances often have unique potencies. Their action is determined as much by *prabhava* as by the regular rules of taste and energy.

According to ayurveda, plants possess *Soma,* which is the ambrosia or nectar of immortality. It is also the subtle invigorating fluid, *Ojas,* the innermost sap of the body. *Soma* or *Ojas* is the basis for clarity of perception, physical strength, endurance, and longevity of the tissues. It is the subtle essence-energy of the nervous system, the digested essence of all food, impressions and experiences. As such it is our capacity to enjoy life.

The ancient Vedic Science of *Rasayana* was aimed primarily at the mutation of the brain. It attempted to give a physical basis, the right receptacle, for the birth of true awareness in human beings. By transcending the conditioned functioning of the "old brain," with its regressive patterns of fear, desire and ambition based on egoistic function, *Rasayana* performed "miraculous" changes.

Rasayana treatment includes special herbs, but goes far beyond the bounds of any ordinary medical treatment. It includes *mantra* and meditation, which are the real catalysts for this process.

This highest *Rasayana* treatment of inner transmutation is called *Brahma Rasayana. Brahma* means expansion, and refers to the unbounded expansion that is the creative reality of life. Through meditation, we transcend the limitation of the known, the conditioned functioning of the brain.

Typical *Rasayanas* include :

For *Vata: ashwagandha,* calamus, garlic, ginseng, *guggul* and *haritaki.*

For *Pitta:* aloe, *amalaki,* comfrey root, gotu kola (Brahmi), saffron and shatavari.

For *Kapha: bibhitaki,* elecampane, *guggul* and *pippali.*

Other *Rasayanas* include angelica, *bala,* bamboo, *gokshura,* liquorice, *manjishta,* marshmallow, myrrh, oatstraw, onion, rehmannia, sesame seeds, Solomon's seal, spikenard, *vidari kanda* and wild yam.

C. Aphrodisiacs (*Vajikarana*)

A third kind of tonic herb, closely allied with *Rasayanas,* is what is called in Ayurveda *Vijakarana.* These are substances that give the power or vitality of a horse, particularly the horse's great capacity for sexual activity. More commonly, one could call them "aphrodisiacs," though they are much more than superstitious love portions. *Vajikaranas* reinvigorate the body by reinvigorating the sexual organs.

The semen or reproductive tissue (the ayurvedic concept includes both male and female reproductive tissues) is the essence of all the *dhatus,* the cream of all the tissue-elements in the body. It contains the power to create life. This means not only the capacity to bring a new life into existence, to create a child, but also to renew one's own life, to return our cells to the vigour of youth. The same life-creating energy if directed inwards, can aid in the renewal of both body and mind.

Vajikarana substances may be used either to improve sexual vitality and functioning, or to help to direct sexual energy inwards for regeneration. Most of these are not simple aphrodisiacs—substances exciting sexual activity through irritation of the sexual organs but are tonics that actually nurture and give direct sustenance to the reproductive tissues. Others help to promote the creative transformation of sexual energy for the benefit of the body-mind.

By starting in the reproductive system, these herbs invigorate the entire system, just as a tree is invigourated from the roots. They have a strong revitalizing action on the nerves and bone marrow, and increase the energy of the mind. Semen is the *Soma* of the body, which if catalyzed in the right way, by *Rasayana* and *Vajikarana* substances, brings about the renewal of the mind. In a similar way it helps to strengthen the bones, muscles, ligaments and blood.

These can be divided into two types; tonics and stimulants. Stimulants increase the functional activity of the reproductive organs, while tonics increase and improve the tissue-substance that composes them.

Typical aphrodisiacs (Vajikaranas) include angelica, asafoetida, *ashwagandha,* asparagus, cloves, cotton root, damiana, false unicorn, fenugreek, garlic, ginseng, *gokshura,* hibiscus, lotus seeds, raw onions, *pippali,* rose, saffron, saw palmetto, *shatavari,* Solomon's seal, *vidari-kanda* and wild yam. Of these, those which are emmenagogues are more specific for women.

Ayurveda also discriminates those herbs that enhance spermatogenesis, called *Shukrala.* These are the substances that are nutritive tonics to the reproductive secretions, like semen and breast milk. They are mainly those *Vajikaranas* which are nutritive. Such nutritive aphrodisiacs include; angelica, *ashwagandha, bala,* ghee, ginseng, licorice, lotus seeds, marshmallow, raw onions, saw palmetto, sesame seeds, *shatavari,* Solomon's seal, raw sugar, *vidari-kanda* and wild yam.

Those aphrodisiacs whose nature is *sattvic,* and are strong in energy also enhance *Ojas.* Such substances include ashwagandha, *ghee,* lotus seeds and *shatvari.*

ACTIVE CONSTITUENTS

The medicinal effects of certain plants are well known. Senna, for example, has been taken as a laxative for thousands of years, and aloe vera was known to Cleopatra as a soothing skin remedy. It is only recently, however, that the active constituents responsible for the medicinal actions of plants have been isolated and observed. Knowing a little about the chemical contained in plants helps the layman to understand how they work within the body.

Mucilage

It is found in many plants, and is made up of polysaccharides, large sugar molecules that soak up water, producing a sticky jelly-like mass.

Mucilage lines the mucous membranes of the digestive tract, protecting against irritation, acidity and inflammation. This soothing and protective action appears to extend to other areas, including the mucous membranes of the throat, lungs, kidneys and urinary tubules.

Phenols

This group of compounds includes salicylic acid, the natural forerunner of aspirin. Salicylic acid is found in many plants, for example wintergreen (*Gaultheria species*) and white willow (*Salix alba*). Another phenol is thymol a constituent of thyme. Phenols are antiseptic and reduce inflammation when taken internally, yet they have an irritant effect when applied to the skin.

Tannins

Tannins are produced to a greater or lesser degree by all plants. The harsh, astringent taste of tanninladen bark and leaves makes them unpalatable to insects and grazing animals. These contract the tissues of the body hence their use to "ten" leather. They draw the tisues closer together and improve their resistance to infection. Oak bark and black catechu (*Acacia catechu*) are both high Tannins.

Coumarins

Coumarins of different kinds are found in many plant species and have widely divergent actions. The coumarins in melilot (*Melilotus officinalis*) thin the blood, while bergapten, found in celery (*Apium graveolens,*) is used as a sunscreen, and khellin, found in visnaga is a powerful smooth muscle relaxant.

Anthraquinones

Anthraquinones are the main active constituents in herbs such as senna (*Cassia senna*) and Chinese rhubarb, both of which are taken to relieve constipation. Anthraquinones have an irritant laxative effect on the large intestine, causing contractions of the intestinal walls and stimulating a bowel movement approximately 10 hours after being taken. They also make the stool more liquid, easing bowel movements.

Flavonoids

These are found in many plants and have a wide range of actions. They are anti-inflammatory and are especially useful in maintaining healthy circulation. Rutin, a flavonoid found in plants including buckwheat (*Fagopyrum esculentum*) and lemon (*Citrus limon*) strengthens capillary walls.

Anthocyanins

These pigments, which give flowers and fruits a blue, purple or red hue, help to keep the blood vessels healthy. Black berry and grapes (*Vitis vinifera*) contain appreciable quantities of anthocyanins.

Gluconsilinates

These are found exclusively in species of the mustard family. Glucosilinates have an irritant effect on the skin, causing inflammation and blistering. Applied as poultices to painful or caching joints, they increase blood flow to the affected area, helping to remove the build-up of waste products, a contributory factor in joint problems. They also help to reduce thyroid function. Both radish (*Raphanus sativus*) and mustard contain significant quantities of glucosilinates.

Volatile oils

Volatile oils - which are extracted from plants to produce essential oils are some of the most important plant constituents of all. Tea tree for example, is known to contain over 60 different volatile compounds within its volatile oil, many of them being strongly antiseptic. Some volatile oils contain sesquiterpenes, such as azulene, found in German chamomile. These constituents have an antiflammatory effect.

Saponins

There are two types of saponins; triterpenoid and steroidal saponins. The latter get their name from their similarity to the human body's own naturally occurring steroid hormones. Many plants containing steroidal saponins have a marked hormonal activity, liquoirce (*Glycyrrhiza glabra*) being one of the best known. Triterpenoid saponins, for example those in cowslip root are often strong exectorants, and may also aid in the absorption of nutrients.

Cardiac Glycosides

These are found in various medicinal plants, most famously in common foxglove (*Digitalis purpurea*), yellow foxglove (*D.

lutea) and woolly foxglove (*D. lanata*). Cardiac glycosides such as digitoxin, digoxin, and gitoxin have a strong, direct action on the heart, helping to support its strength and rate of contraction when it is failing. Cardiac glycosides are also significantly diuretic. They help to transfer the fluids from the tissues and circulatory system to the urinary tract, thereby lowering blood pressure.

Cyanogenic Glycosides

Though these glycosides are based on cyanide, a very potent poison, they have a helpful sedative and relaxant effect on the heart and muscles in small doses. Wild cherry bark and elder (*Sambucus nigra*) both contain cyanogenic glycosides, which contribute to both plants' ability to suppress and soothe irritant dry coughs.

Vitamins

Some plants also contain significant levels of vitamins. Watercress (*Nasturtium officinale*) for example, contains an appreciable quantity of vitamin E, and the *Amla* has particularly high levels of vitamin C. Most other medicinal plants contain at least some vitamins. While the content may be small, it contributes to overall daily intake.

Bitters

Bitters are varied group of consttituents linked only by their pronounced bitter taste. The bitterness itself stimulates secretions by the salivary glands and digestive organs. Such secretions can dramatically improve the appetite and strengthen the overall function of the digestive system. With the improved digestion and absorption of nuterients that follow, the body is nourished and strengthened. Many herbs have bitter constituents, notably wormwood and chiretta (*Swertia chirata*).

Alkaloids

A very mixed group, alkaloids mostly contain a nitrogen

bearing molecule (NH_2) that makes them particularly pharmacologically active. Some are well known drugs and have a recognized medical use. Vincristine, for example, derived from Madagascar periwinkle (*Catharanthus roseus*) is used to treat some types of cancer. Other alkaloids, such as atropine, found in deadly nightshade (*Atropa belladonna*) have a direct effect on the body, reducing spasms, relieving pain and drying up bodily secretions.

Minerals

Some herbs are particularly rich in minerals. Horsetail (*Equisetum arvense*), for example, has high levels of silica. Dandelion (*Taraxacum officinale*) has large quantities of potassium and unlike other diuretics which flush this mineral out of the body, it helps to maintain high levels of potassium. These plants act as mineral supplements in their own right, while other herbs with a small concentration contribute to overall intake.

3

Growing Drug Plants and Ways to use Them

GROWING DRUG PLANTS

Growing Plants may be more time-consuming than buying them, but it brings with it the unique pleasure of producing own herbal remedies. Many medicinal herbs are easy to grow and will flourish indoors, on a windowsill or in the garden, providing a year round supply of fresh, sweet smelling natural medicines.

HERB GARDEN

Planning a herb garden depends on a range of factors including the space available, aspect, soil, conditions and climate. As a starting point, details of ten of the most common and useful medicinal plants for growing in temperate climates are given in the chart below. Some of them, such as thyme (*Thymus vulgaris*) and sage (*Salvia officinalis*), may be grown indoors. A number of other medicinal herbs, including German chamomile (*Chamomilla recutita*), lady's mantle (*Alchemilla vulgaris*) and lavender (*Lavandula officinalis*) also grow well in a temperate climate and are well worth cultivating. If in doubt about how to care for plants or what will grow well in your garden, consult a nursery.

Outdoor Gardens

Choose a range of hardy herbs to grow in the garden that will establish themselves easily and produce plenty of foliage that can be harvested. Plant exotic or less hardy herbs in sheltered sunny sites or in containers.

Container Gardens

Many medicinal plants such as peppermint (*Mentha piperita*) or bay laurel can be grown in pots, hanging baskets or window boxes. Care must be taken to prevent them from drying out or becoming pot-bound i.e., when the plant becomes too large for the container. Less hardy plants should be moved to sheltered sites or indoors during winter.

Growing Plants Under Cover

Sheltered gardening offers the opportunity to grow more unusual plants. Use the greenhouse to cultivate exotic plants, such as lemon grass (*Cymbopogon citratus*) for medicinal and culinary use, as well as for growing seedlings to be planted out. Tender plants, such as holy basil (*Ocimum sanctum*) thrive indoors, and some indoor plants, such as aloe (*Aloe vera*), have the added advantage of absorbing polluting chemicals from the air.

BUYING HERBS

Reputable herb nurseries are the best place to buy herbs when particular varieties or species are required. But it must be clear about what plants you want before visiting the nursery. When buying for medicinal use, purchase the standard medicinal, rather than an improved or ornamental, variety.

CULTIVATION

The following points are to be kept in mind when planning the garden and choosing herbs.

Site

The majority of medicinal plants prefer a sunny aspect and moderately well-drained soil. It is possible to improve a site, for example by planting hedges as windbreaks. Choose sheltered, sunny corners for delicate and half-hardy herbs, and avoid planting on land formerly used for industrial purposes, which may be contaminated.

Temperature

Some plants tolerate only very specific temperature ranges and many herbs, such as rosemary are only half-hardy herbs, and will not survive exposure to deep or long periods of frost. Protect tender and half-hardy plants from the wind to avoid the wind chill factor. Spring is the best time to plant most herbs. Wintering plants in a greenhouse or cool indoor site is often the only way to keep sub-tropical plants in cool temperate climates, while other herbs will thrive indoors all year round in a warm, sunny position.

Soil

Soils vary greatly depending on the proportions of sand, silt and clay content. Sandy soils drain easily and need feeding, while clay soils can become waterlogged and require drainage.

Pruning

Pruning is used to remove the dead wood and improve the shape, size and quality of growth. It is one of the important garden activities and needs to be done correctly for different woody plants to benefit check the best time of year for each plant. Deadheading plants, especially shrubs, encourages fresh growth. Pruning and tidying the garden regularly also reduces pests and diseases.

Watering

Water well after planting and then, if needed, once a week in the morning or early evening. Do not over water as many herbs produce medicinally active constituents in dry conditions. Water dry pot plants thoroughly before planting.

USEFUL HERBS TO GROW

Plant Name	Time to plant	Cultivation Method	Conditions and Care	Medicinal Uses
Aloe vera (*Aloe vera*)	spring/autumn	offsets	sunny site indoor; pot up as needed; do not overwater	fresh plant gel for minor burn and wounds
Comfrey (*Symphytum officinale*)	spring/autumn	seed/division	warm sunny site; moist soil	ointment or poultice for sprains and bruises (leaf)
Feverfew (*Tanacetum parthenium*)	autumn/spring	seed/cuting/division	well-drained or dry, stony soil in sun	fresh leaf or tincture for headaches and migraines
Lemon balm (*Melissa officinalis*)	spring/autumn	seed/cutting/division	moist soil in sun; cut back after flowering	infusion for anxiety, poor sleep and nervous indigestion; lotion for cold sores
Marigold (*Calendula oficinalis*)	spring/autumn	seed	well-drained soil; full sun; remove dead flowerheads	cream for cuts, grazes, inflamed skin; infusion for fungal infection
Peppermint (*Mentha piperita*)	spring/autumn	cutting/division	sunny but moist site; do not allow to dry out	infusion for indigestion and headaches; lotion for itchy skin
Resemary (*Rosmorinus officinalis*)	spring/autumn	seed/cutting	sunny sheltered site; protect with sacking in winter	infusion as a stimulating nerve tonic and to aid the weak digestion
Sage (*Salvia officinalis*)	autumn/spring	seed/cutting/layering	well-drained or dry, sunny sheltered site	infusion for sore throats, mouth ulcers and diarrhoea
St John's wort (*Hypericum perforatum*)	spring/autumn	seed/division	well-drained to dry soil with sun or partial shade	tincture for depression and menopause; infused oil is antiseptic and heals wounds
Thyme (*Thymus vulgaris*)	spring/summer	seed/cutting/division	well-drained soil, may need a layer or gravel; sunny site	infusion for cough, colds and chest infections; lotion for fungal infections

Weeding and Fertilizing

Weeding is necessary as weeds compete with other plants for nutrients and water. Keep beds and containers as free from weeds as possible. Most medicinal herbs should not be fed or mulched as this reduce their therapeutic strength. However, sandy soils should be fed with a good-quantity fertilizer to maintain the nutrients in the soil.

Pests and Diseases

Use only organic methods to treat pests, diseases and insect infestation. Greenfly can be eradicated using soapy water or water in which garlic skins have been soaked for 2 days. Separate any infected plants to prevent further contamination.

PROPAGATION METHODS

There is a wide variety of propagation methods. Choose the best suited to the plant. When planting, prepare the ground in advance, taking into account the requirements of the individual plant, and the soil, site and time of year, as well as the anticipated size of the mature plant.

Seeds

Seeds can be sown either in containers or in prepared soil in open ground. It is important to time the sowing of seeds to enable seedings to be planted out when weather and soil become sufficiently warm. Annuals and biennials can be grown with ease from seed and will grow vigorously throughout the summer. Check the germination requirements of perennials before buying the seeds, as some varieties germinate easily, while others, can be far more difficult.

Sowing Seeds in Containers

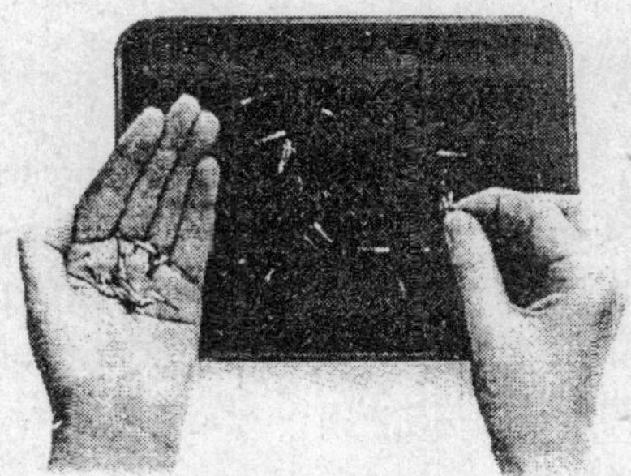

Fill a seed tray with seed compost and water well. Sprinkle on the seeds, covering large seeds with a fine layer of compost. Cover the tray with glass or place in a plastic bag and store in a warm place.

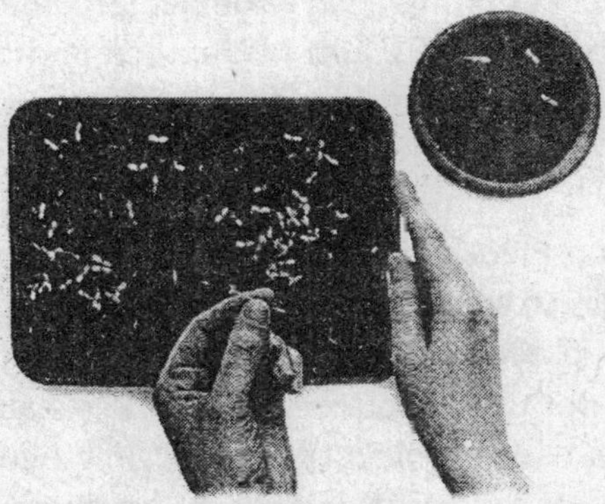

Once the seeds have germinated, fill a number of pots with compost. Gently lift up a seedling, insert it in a small hole in the compost and pack the soil around it. Water thoroughly and do not allow to dry out.

Cuttings

This is one of the most popular methods of propagation which is suitable for woody perennial herbs. Cuttings are usually taken from the stem, although some plants may also be propagated from roots. Choose young healthy plants and take the cutting just below a leaf and stem joint using a clean, sharp knife. Strip off the lowest leaves and dip the stem in hormone rooting preparation before inserting it in suitable compost. Some plants are very difficult to propagate with this way, so check before attempting this method.

Root Division

This is an easy way to propagate plants that form clumps. Divide spring-flowering herbaceous plants in autumn, and autumn flowering herbaceous plants in spring. Carefully lift a mature plant, divide it into smaller sections and replant both the new and the mature plant.

Plants From Produce

Purchase pots of culinary herbs from a grocery or the market, split the seedings into 3 to 4 small clumps and pot them up separately. Fresh roots such as ginger (*Zingiber officinale*) or bulblets, such as garlic (*Allium sativum*) can be planted in pots or in prepared ground outside, if temperature allows.

Layering

Layering involves encouraging a shoot or stem to form roots by making a small slit in its underside and burying it, with the growing tip above ground. When the layer roots emerge, remove and pot up. " Mound layering" is suitable for woody herbs such as usage (*Salvia officinalis*). Pile free draining soil over the base of the plant and when the layered stems form new roots, remove and pot up.

Offsets

Offsets are produced from most herbs that grow from a bulb or corm, such as garlic (*Allium sativum*). These can be detached during dormancy and replanted.

HARVESTING AND PROCESSING

Although, there are some herbs that may be collected throughout the year, but most have a particular growing season and must be harvested and either used immediately or preserved for use in the following year. Herbs need to be processed quickly to prevent deterioration and retain their healing action. Gather only healthy plants, free from disease, insect damage or pollution

HARVESTING FROM THE WILD

Wild plants offer a free and natural source of herbal remedies and give tile satisfaction of collecting herbs in the traditional way. Furthermore, active constituents are often more highly concentrated in wild plants as the herb is generally likely to be growing in its preferred environment.

Identification

Proper identification of wild plants is essential. Use a field or wild flower guide for help, as many plants look similar. If in doubt, do not pick the plant, as poisoning can result from rnisidentification.

Ecological and Legal Factors

While common species such as nettle (*Urtica dioica*) may be readily harvested from tile wild, many rarer species are under great pressure due to the lack of a suitable habitat. Further, it is illegal to uproot any wild plant as certain species may be protected. So, never pick rare or uncommon plants from the wild, even if they are locally plentiful, and do not collect more than you will use. Do not harvest bark from the wild.

Before harvesting, consider where the plant is growing and whether it could be contaminated by pollution. Do not collect from roadsides, close to factories or in areas where crop spraying has occurred.

HARVESTING FROM YOUR GARDEN

Cultivated herbs provide a ready supply of fresh material in a controlled environment. Harvesting garden plants can be combined with pruning the plant, removing unwanted shoots and encouraging bushiness. Cut perennials carefully so that plants can quickly regrow. Some medicinal plants, such as lemon balm provide two or more crops per year.

General Advice

Harvesting Medicinal herbs requires careful planning to ensure the parts are processed in peak condition *and* fast enough to retain their active ingredients.

Equipment

If possible, use a wooden tray or an open basket for collecting the medicinal herbs. This prevents crushing and deterioration of the plant. In the wild, a non-nylon rucksack or canvas sack may be more appropriate. Take a field or wild flower guide to aid the identification. Always make cuts with a sharp knife or scissors to minimize damage to the plant and in general try to handle plants as little as possible. Wear protective gloves if gathering prickly or allergenic plants, such as rue (*Ruta graveolens*) to avoid an allergic reaction.

What To Look For

Collect material from healthy plants that are free from disease, insect damage and, in the case of wild plants, pollution. It is important to discard any damaged plants as they can lead to disease or decay in dried plant material. Do not mix cut plant material to avoid mistakes in identification.

Time To Harvest

Gather herbs in dry weather, preferably on a sunny morning after the dew has evaporated. Picking in the right weather conditions, when the plant is at its peak of maturity, ensures that it will have a high concentration of active constituents. The leaves are best collected as they open during the spring or summer months, flowers as they start to bloom, fruit and berries just as they become ripe, and roots in the autumn once the plant has drawn its vitality back beneath ground. Bark must be gathered with great care if the shrub or tree is to survive-in most cases harvest it in spring or autumn.

Correct Medicinal Part

In many cases, different parts of the same plant, for example the leaves and seeds, can have quite different actions and uses. Make sure that you harvest the correct medicinal part of the plant for your purposes.

Processing Quickly

Only collect plant material that is to be used or processed immediately after harvesting, because the fresh plant material, especially tender flowers and leaves, deteriorates very quickly and the medicinally active constituents are often the first to be affected. In particular, aromatic herbs, which leave their scent in the air or on skin, can lose their volatile oils within hours. Salad leaves and culinary herbs are best eaten straight away to make the most of their nutrients, although they can be stored for a few days in a plastic bag filled with air in a refrigerator.

PROCESSING

Herbs can be preserved in a number of ways, the most common and simple being air or oven drying. A warm, dry place, for example an airing cupboard, is ideal. Use plain paper for drying herbs, never printed newspaper. Dried herbs can be stored for many months in a dark glass jar or a brown paper bag.

Aerial Parts

These include all the parts of the plant growing above ground stems, leaves, flowers, berries and seeds. The stems are normally cut 5-10 cm above ground shortly after the plant has begun to flower, when it is putting most effort into growth. Perennials may be cut higher above ground to encourage further growth. Remove and dry large flowers and leaves separately; smaller ones can be dried on the stem.

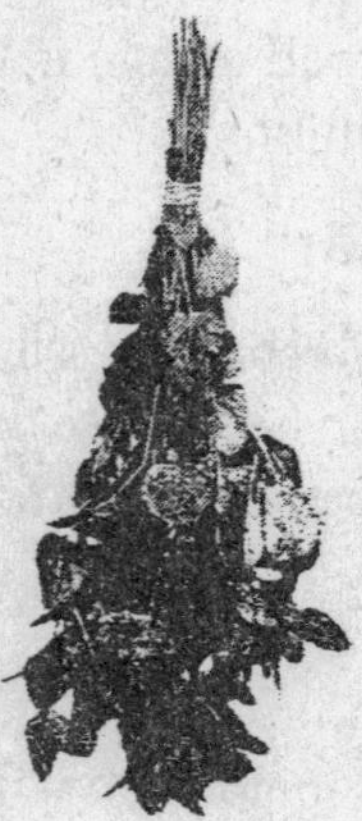

Hang bunches of about 8-10 stems in a warm but not hot, well-ventilated, dark place. Ensure that the stems and leaves are not too tightly packed together. This will enable air to circulate freely around them.

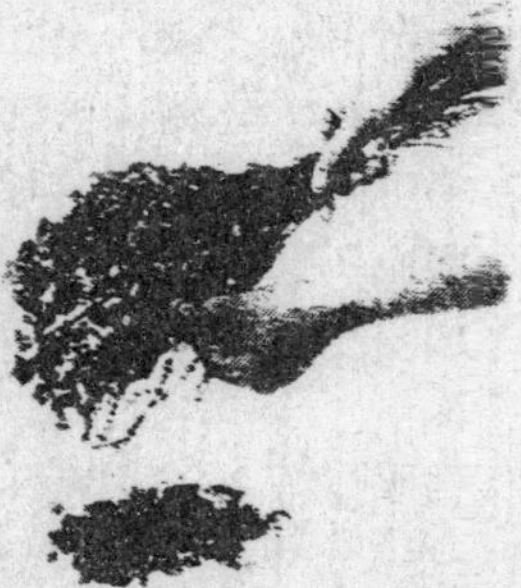

Once brittle but not bone dry, separate small stems, leaves, flowers and seeds from the stems by carefully rubbing the bunches over a large sheet of plain paper.

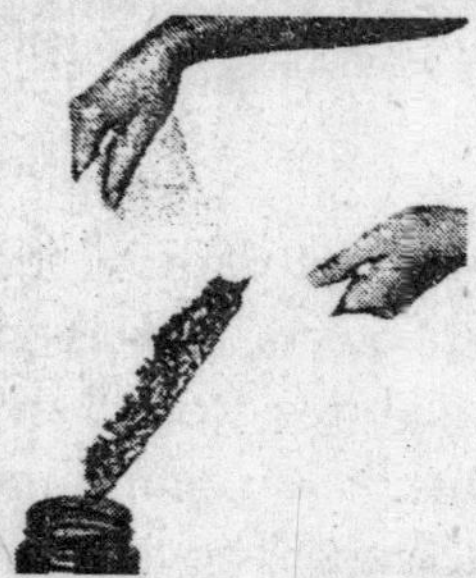

Carefully pour the dried material from the paper into a dark glass jar with a screw top or a brown paper bag.

Large Flowers

In most cases, flowers are picked just after they have opened, usually during the spring or summer. Sometimes only specific parts of the flower are used, such as the petals of marigold (*Calendula oficinalis*), while other flowers are used whole.

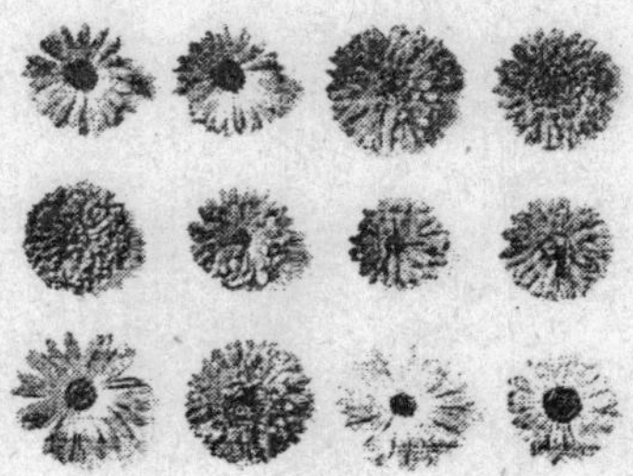

Separate large flowerheads from stems and remove any insects or dirt. Place the flowers on absorbent paper in a dry place, allowing sufficient room between them for air to circulate.

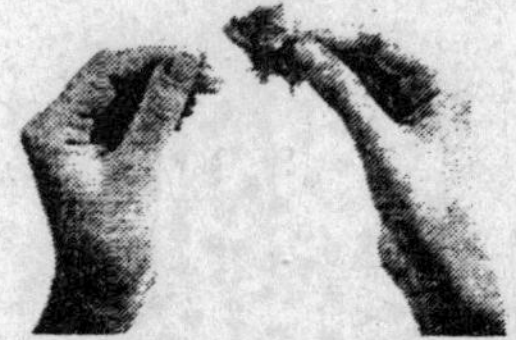

Once dry, store flowerheads in a brown paper bag or dark glass jar. Remove marigold petals from the central part of the flower before storing.

Small Flowers

Small blooms can be picked with the stalk attached and separated later. Hang small flowers, such as lavender (*Lavandula officinalis*) upside down in a paper bag, or suspended over a tray. If the stems are fleshy, dry as for large flowers, above.

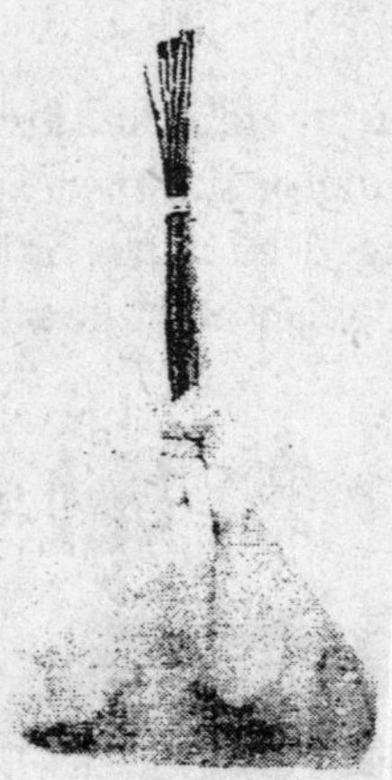

Fruit and Berries

Harvest fruits and berries in early autumn when ripe but still firm. If allowed to become over-ripe, they may not dry properly. They can be picked individually or in bunches.

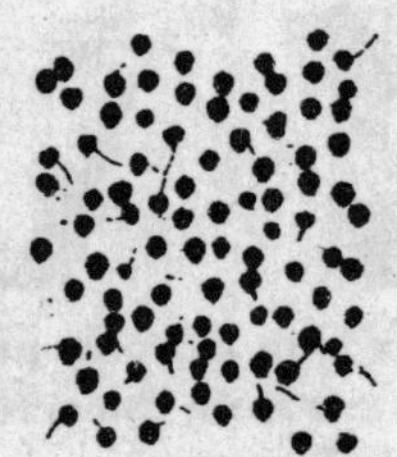

***Place berries* or fruit on absorbent paper on trays. Put in a warmed oven which is turned off with the door ajar for 3-4 hours. Move to a dry, warm, dark site and turn occasionally. Discard any mouldy berries or fruit.**

Roots, Rhizomes, Tubes and Bulbs

The underground parts of the plant are usually gathered in autumn after the aerial parts have withered or become inactive and before the root loses its vitality to aerial growth. Dig deeply around the root, prising it carefully out of the ground. Some tap roots are very difficult to uproot completely. Remove the required amount and replant the remaining underground part.

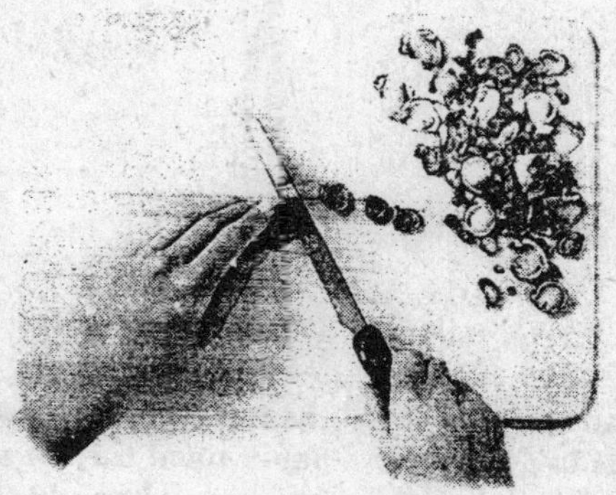

Shake off any soil clinging to the root parts and thoroughly wash and clean them in warm water, removing any small unwanted side roots or damaged soft spots. Chop into small slices with a sharp knife.

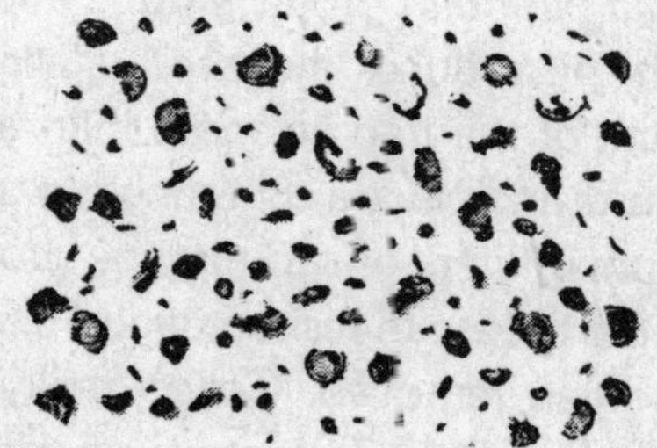

Spread out the root pieces on absorbent paper on a tray and place in a turned off warmed oven with the door ajar for 2-3 hours. Move to a warm place until dry.

Seeds

Collect ripe seed pods, capsules or flowering stems in late summer before the seeds have been scattered.

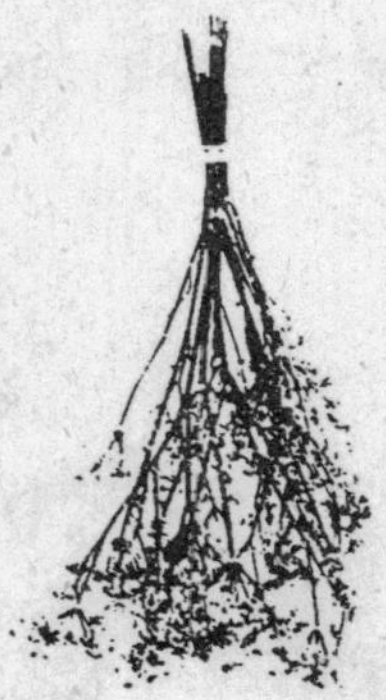

For seeds **that are very small, hang small bunches of seedheads upside down over a paper-lined tray, or place in a paper bag. Allow to dry and gently shake. Remove larger seeds by hand when dry.**

Sap and Gel

Only harvest sap from your own garden. Collect sap in the spring as it rises, or as it falls in the autumn. Trees such as silver birch (*Betula pendula*) produce huge quantities of sap if tapped, although this reduces the tree's vitality. Bore a deep hole into the trunk of the tree no more than a quarter of the diameter of the trunk and place a collecting cup under the mouth of the hole. In spring, liters of sap may be produced and it is essential to stop the hole with resin or wood filler once about a litre of fluid has been removed. Collect milky juices or latex from plants such as dandelion (*Taraxacum officinale*) by squeezing the stems over a bowl. Wear gloves as latex or sap can be corrosive. The gel from aloe (*Aloe vera*) is scraped out after slicing the leaf lengthwise and peeling back the edges.

Bark

Harvest the bark from your own shrubs or trees as it carries the risk of losing the whole plant through over-stripping or "ringing". It is far better to collect bark from outlying branches which can then be prune back. If stripping bark from a plant, gather insects.

lichen and moss from the bark, cut it into small pieces and place on a tray to dry.

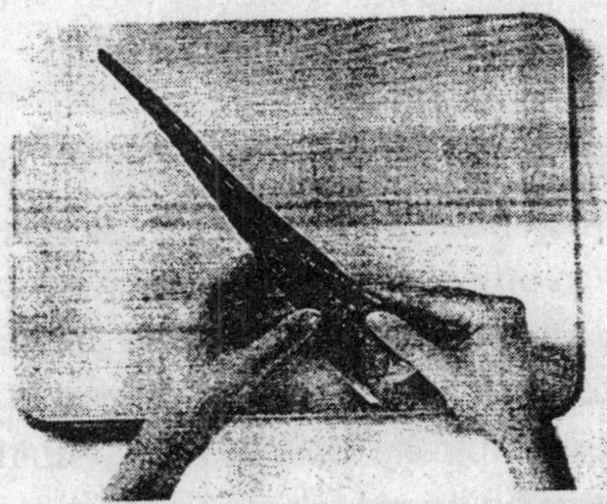

With the fingers and thumb of each hand, carefully slice along the length of an aloe vera leaf and peel back the edges.

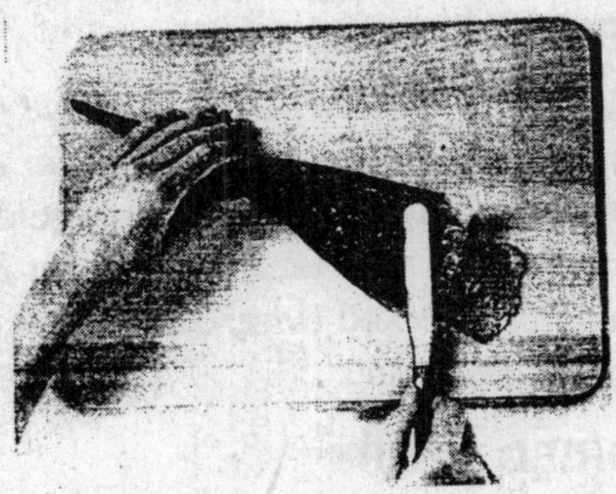

Collect the gel by scraping the blunt edge of a knife along the inside of the leaf. Use aloe vera gel immediately as it cannot be saved.

OTHER WAYS TO PRESERVE THE HERBS

Apart from simply air drying herbs, there are a number of other ways to preserve their medicinal benefits.

Dehumidifying

An effective but expensive way to dry herbs is to use a dehumidifier, which literally sucks water out of the plant. The dehumidifier should be placed in a more or less sealed small room in which the herbs are hung in loose bunches or placed on mesh trays. Herbs will dry quickly with this method and, as no heat is used, there is little deterioration or decay.

Freeze Drying

Freeze-drying retains colour and flavour but is more suited to culinary than to medicinal herbs. Whole springs of herbs such as parsley (*Salvia officinalis*) can be frozen in plastic freezer bags. There is no need to defrost before use as the leaves crumble easily when still frozen. Chickweed (*Stellaria media*) can also be frozen and used topically for itchy and weeping skin conditions. Many plants may be juiced frozen as ice cubes and thawed as required.

Microwaving

It is possible to dry herbs in a microwave oven. The cut parts should be spread out on kitchen paper and dried in the microwave according to the temperature guidelines provided by the manufacturer. This should take about 2-3 minutes, but progress should be checked every 30 seconds, rearranging the parts to ensure even drying.

BUYING DRIED HERBS

Dried herbs are generally available from herbal suppliers some of which offer a mail order service. Buying the herbs from shops is more convenient as they can be examined before purchasing, but mail order companies often have a much higher rate of turnover and may supply better-quality, fresher herbs as a result. To gain the best medicinal effect, good-quality produce is essential. The following points are to be kept before buying the herb:

* Herbs should not be stored in clear glass jars or in direct sunlight, as this causes oxidation, which affects their efficacy.
* Good-quality aromatic herbs should have a distinct scent and taste.
* Check for sings of infestation due to poor drying techniques,

or adulteration. The latter can sometimes be recognized by the inclusion of dried grass or other non-medicinal material in the jar.

* Herbs lose their colour as they age. Look for bright material that has been well dried and stored, and that is not too old. Marigold flowers (*Calendula officinalis*) that are a vivid yellow/orange colour are likely to make good medicine. If they have been kept on a shelf for 18 months, they will probably look drab and pale.

WAYS TO USE HERBS

Storing Herbs

It is vital to store dried herbs properly or they will not last. Leaves, flowers, roots and other parts should be stored in sterilized, dark glass containers with airtight lids. They may also be stored in new brown paper bags which must be kept dry and away from light.

Metal and plastic containers are inadvisable as they may contaminate the herb. Canning jars are excellent for storing herbs or good glass jars with tight fitting lid. In the summer, add a few bay leaves for bug prevention. When working with herbs, it is very important not to use plastic, aluminum, or Teflon containers or utensils. Use enamel, stainless steel, clay or glass. If stored in a cool dark place, herbs can be kept for about 12 months after harvesting. Herbs frozen in plastic freezer bags can be used for up to 6 months. Make sure the container you use is labelled with the herb, source, strength of preparation if appropriate, and date of harvesting. Watch out for insect infestation. If this occurs, put all affected material in a sealed plastic bag and discard. Sterilize the container and check all other herbs for contamination.

Different preparations may be kept for verifying periods of time before they begin to lose their medicinal properties. Infusions should be made fresh each day and decoctions must be consumed within 48 hours. Store both in a refrigerator or in cool place. Tinctures and other liquid preparations, such as syrups and essential oils, need to be stored in dark glass bottles in a cool environment away from sunlight, but can be kept for a number of months or year. Ointments, creams and capsules are best kept in dark glass jars, although plastic containers are also good.

Weights and Measures

For most purposes, ordinary kitchen scales are suitable, although electronic scales are more accurate. Metric measurements of grams and liters are generally much easier to use than imperial measures when making remedies. If it is difficult to weigh a small quantity, such as 10 gm, on your scales, measure double the weight, i.e. 20 gm, then halve the quantity. Liquids can be measured in a kitchen measuring jug, although conical or straight sided glass measures are more accurate. Very small volumes of liquid can be measured in drops.

Measuring Remedies

1 ml	= 20 drops
2 ml	= 1 teaspoon
10 ml	= 1 dessertspoon
20 ml	= 1 tablespoon
70 ml	= 1 sherry glass
150 ml	= 1 cup or wine glass

Never exceed the quantity of herbs used or the recommended dosage. Although these measurements are approximate, they are accurate enough for most purposes and are used as standard. The number of drops to 1 ml depends on the calibre of the pipette or size of the dropper tip being used. This can be checked by counting the number of drops required to fill a 5 ml measuring spoon, 100 drops are equal to 5 ml and then adjusting the drop dosage as necessary.

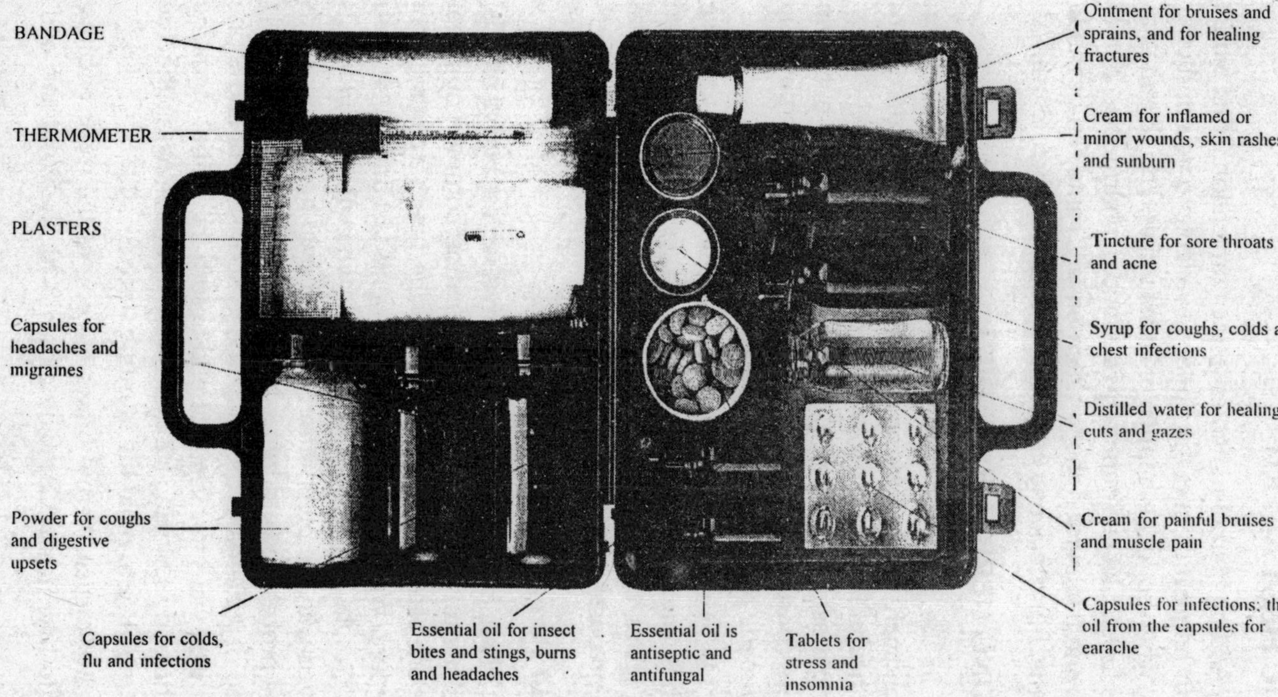

BASIC FIRST AID KIT

BASIC FIRST AID KIT

Adding Herbal remedies to the conventional first aid kit in your home increases the options available to you and your family when accidents happen or illness strikes. The 13 remedies in this first aid kit can generally be found in pharmacies, herbal stores and health food shops. Alternatively, some can be made at home, but check any cautions for each herb before use.

MAKING HERBAL REMEDIES

In the past, medicinal herbs have been made into an extraoridinary variety of formulations not only infusions, decoctions and tincutures, but preparations such as oxymels and elixires. Making most types of herbal medicine is not difficult, but it can be time consuming if there is lack of time or equipment, buy ready-made remedies from a herbal supplier.

Herbs can be smoked like cigarettes or used to make douches, enemas, compresses, bath, gargles, syrup, medicated ghee, jellies, creams, suppositories and oils. Followings are the main preparations made out from the herbal plants :

Liquid Preparations (Teas)

These are called with many names such as herbal blends, herbal brews, herbal mixtures, and the most common one, tea. This is one of favorite ways to take medicine, yet it is a commitment to prepare. We live in a society that wants fast and quick, easy "fix-it" results. Ayurveda teaches that when the individual is involved with the preparation and their own healing, it speeds up the process toward better health. Drinking herbal mixtures instead of water gives the body added nourishment and is one of the best ways to assimilate and absorb the herbal medicine into the body. Drinking tea adds vitamins and minerals that the body may use to build the immune system.

In practice, herbal brews are one of the most effective ways to take herbs. Combine all herbs for the condition and, rather than walking around with a bottle of water, carry a bottle of herbal brew and drink the mixture throughout the day.

Dry Herb Tea

Cut and Sifted

This is one of the best ways to make a tea. Dry herbs for tea are best in the cut and sifted form. The herb has not been ground and still carries all the volatile components. Anytime fresh herbs are available, use them. When making a tea, the roots and bark are best boiled for 10-15 minutes. Leaf and flower teas are made by bringing water to a boil, then adding the herb. Let it steep for 15 minutes. Strain into container; refrigerate for future use. Make up to one gallon at a time. Pitta may drink cool. Vatas should heat before consuming.

Sun Tea

This is done by placing the herb into a jar, adding water, and putting the jar in the sun for 2-3 hours. This method works well with leaves and flowers. For 4.5 litre of water, use 284 ml. Herb, or in smaller amount use 1 teaspoon per cup of water. For variety, or for better flavor, add 1 quart of fruit juice, such as apple, peach, orange, or mango to the gallon of the sun brewed tea. Refrigerate and then use.

Juice Tea

Make any tea of your choice. Strain and then add your favorite fruit juice. This works well for children with a ratio of 30-50% fruit juice and 50-70% herb tea.

Infusions-Tea

This is prepared to keep the volatile components of the herb, as in the boiling process they are lost. The vitamins and minerals are preserved.

For leaves and flowers (they do best in this form):

* Boil water and pour over the dry herbs.

* Steep for 15-20 minutes. Strain.

* Do not use plastic or aluminum.

Beverage teas for the three doshas

The use of herbal teas as beverages, as substitutes or alternatives for coffee or tea, has become very common. Yet without a proper understanding of constitution and condition, the use of such herbal teas may not be entirely health-promoting.

Below is a list of common herbs used as teas or general tonics. Other herbs that may be used as beverages should similarly be related according to constitution and condition so that their real effectiveness can manifest.

This is not to recommend all these herbs for general usage as beverages. Any herb you wish to take as a common beverage should be taken in low dosages and examined for possible long term effects.

KAPHA: Most herbal teas are good for *Kapha,* except those like liquorice, which are sweet and mucus-forming. Important one are :

Alfalfa, basil, blackberry, black pepper, burdock, cardamom, celery seeds, chamomile, cinnamon, cleavers, cloves, dandelion, eucalyptus, ginger, hawthorn, hyssop, juniper berries, lemon, mustard seeds, nettle, orange peel, parsley, peppermint, sage, thyme, wild carrot and wild ginger.

PITTA: Many herbal teas are good for *Pitta, but* those pungent or hot in energy should be avoided. Important ones are:

Alfalfa, blackberry, burdock, chamomile, chrysanthemum, comfrey, coriander, cumin, dandelion, fennel, gotu kola, hibiscus, jasmine, lemon, lemon balm, lemon grass, licorice, lime, marshmallow, nettle, peppermint, raspberry, rose flowers, red clover, red root, saffron, sandalwood and strawberry.

VATA: Many herbal teas are good for *Vata,* but those are bitter, astringent or cold in energy may not be beneficial. Combinations of pungent and sweet herbs are best for *Vata.* Important one are :

Anise, angelica, basil, bay leaves, cardamom, celery seeds, cinnamon, cloves, comfrey root, elecampane, eucalyptus, fennel, fenugreek, fresh ginger, ginseng, brahmi, hawthorn, Irish, liquorice, nutmeg, orange *peel,* safflower, sarsaparilla, Solomon's seal, thyme and wild ginger.

SWEETENERS: *Kapha* constitution should avoid sweeteners in teas, except honey. All sweeteners are good for *Pitta*, except honey. All sweetners are good for *Vata* and help balance out the Vata-increasing properties of some herbs. Refined sugar, however, should be avoided, as it overstimulates the pancreas.

Some teas good in moderation for all constitutions include chamomile, fennel, gotu kola, peppermint, rose flowers, sage, spearmint.

Making an Herbal Brew

1. Mix all herbs together in a bowl. Pray or chant as you sit. to add potency and increase the healing effect.
2. Bring water to a boil and add one teaspoon of herb mix per cup of water. Cover. Remove from heat and allow to steep 1/2 hour or more.
3. Strain into a jar and refrigerate for future use. *Pitta* may drink the blend cool, and *Vata* should warm the blend before consuming.
4. Herbs are best cut and sifted or whole.

Making an Herbal Salve

The basic recipe for making a salve is:

Beeswax	1 part
Medicated vegetable oil	4-6 parts

Medicated vegetable oil is made much like medicated ghee:

Soak herbs in vegetable oil for 30-60 days

Then strain to remove the herbs

OR

Adding essential oils to any vegetable oil will immediately make your vegetable oil medicated.

INFUSIONS

An Infusion is the simplest way to prepare the more delicate aerial parts of plants, especially leaves and flowers, for use as a medicine or as a revitalizing or relaxing drink. It is made in a similar way to tea, using either a single herb or a combination of herbs, and may be drunk hot or cold.

The medicinal value of many herbs lies chiefly in their volatile oils, which will disperse into the air if a lid is not used. Use a teapot, or place a lid or saucer over a cup if making a small quantity. Use water that has just boiled.

Popular herbal teas, are often taken as much four their refreshing taste as for their medicinal value and can be safely consumed in quantities of up to 5 or 6 cups a day. Some herbs, however, such as yarrow, are significantly stronger and must be taken in less frequent doses. Other herbs, such as feverfew are so strong that they are not suitable for use in infusions. Always check the recommended dosage and quantity of herb to use, as infusions have medicinal actions and can produce unwanted effect at the wrong dosage.

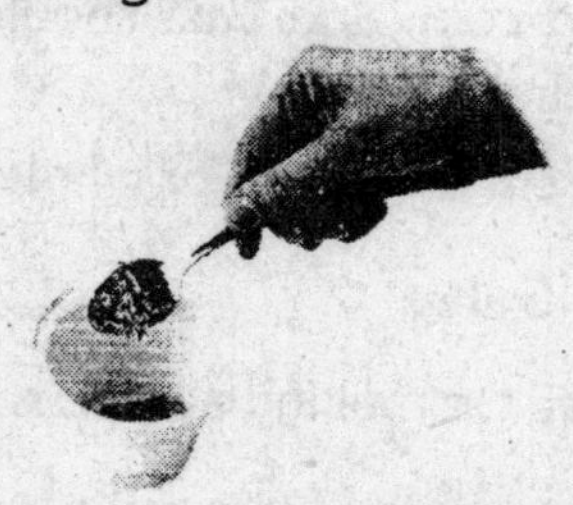

(i) Place the herb in the strainer of the tisane cup and place the strainer in the cup. Fill the cup with freshly boiled water

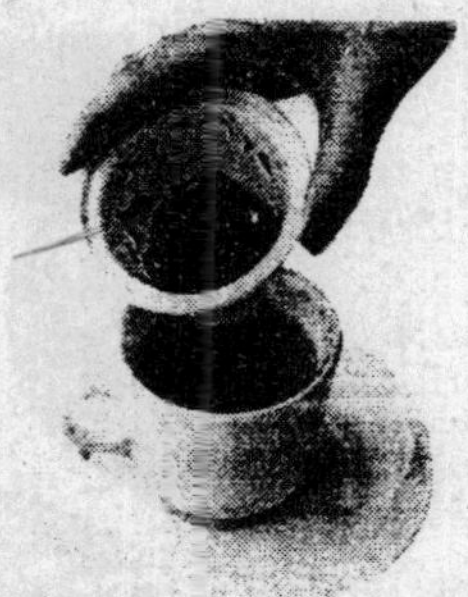

(ii) Cover the cup with the lid and infuse for 5-10 minutes before removing the tisane strainer. Add a teaspoon of honey to sweeten, if desired

INFUSION-PREPARATION

Standard Quantity

Cup 1 teaspoonful (2-3 gm) dried or 2 teaspoonful (4-6 gm) fresh herb (or mixture of herbs) to a cup of water. This makes 1 dose.

Pot 20 gm dried herb or 30 gm fresh herb (or a mixture of different herbs) to 500 ml of water.

Standard Dosage

Take 3-4 doses (500 ml) each day.

Storage

Store in a covered jug in a refrigerator or cool place for up to 24 hours.

Pot Infusion

Warm the pot, then add the herb. Pour in water that has just boiled, replace the lid and infuse for 10 minutes. Strain some of the infusion into a cup. A teaspoon of honey may be added if desired.

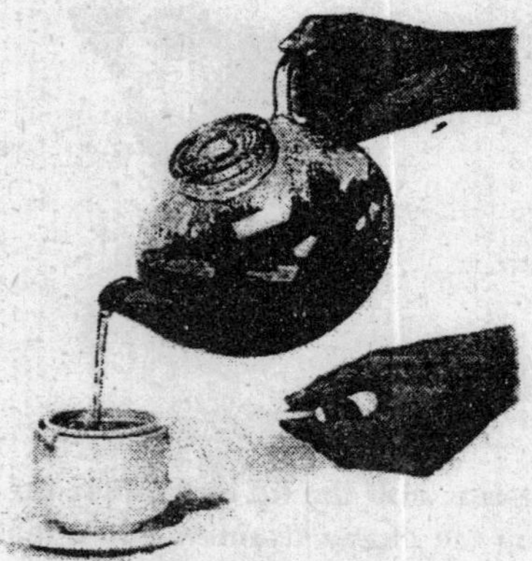

POT-INFUSION

DECOCTIONS

Roots, Bark, Twigs and berries usually require a more forceful treatment than leaves or flowers to extract their medicinal constituents. A decoction involves simmering these tougher parts in boiling water. Fresh of dried plant material may be used and should be cut or broken into small pieces before decocting. Like infusions, decoctions can be taken hot or cold.

Decoctions are generally made by using roots, bark and berries, but sometimes, leaves and flowers may be included. Add these more delicate parts of a plant once the heat is turned off and the decoction has finished simmering and is beginning to cool. Then strain and use as required.

In traditional medicine, decoctions are the main way in which herbal medicines are prepared. Large quantities of herb are often used to produce a highly concentrated liquid, or the decoction is further reduced so that there is only 200 ml of liquid remaining. This increases the preparation's concentration. This process is useful for astringent barks such as babul (*Acacia arabica*) and common oak, which may be used externally to tighten gums or wash weeping skin rashes.

Standard Quantity

20 gm dried or 40 gm fresh herb or mixture of herbs to

750 ml cold water, reduced to about 500 ml after simmering. This makes 3-4 doses.

Standard Dosage

Take 3-4 doses (500 ml) each day.

Storage

Store in a covered jug in a refrigerator or cool place for up to 48 hours.

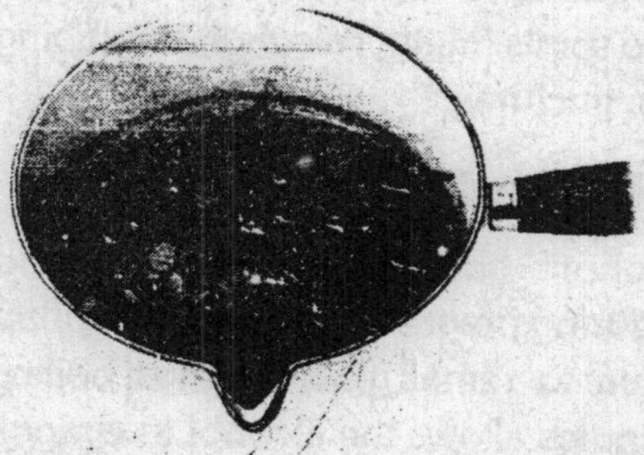

(i) Place the herbs in a saucepan. Cover with cold water cold water and bring to the boil. Simmer for about 20-30 minutes, until the liquid is reduced by about one-third.

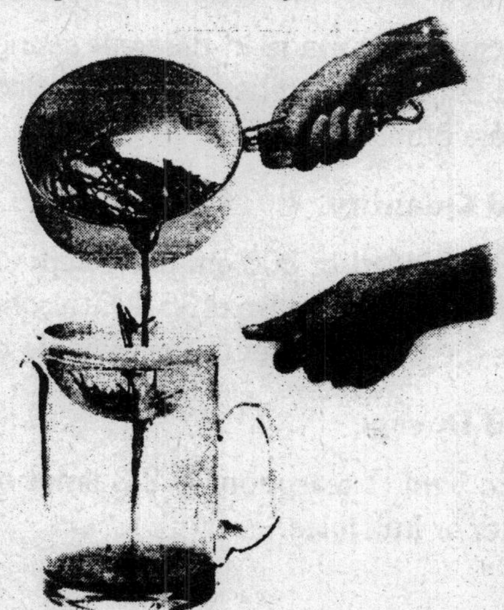

(ii) Strain the liquid through a sieve into a jug. Pour the required amount into a cup, then cover the jug and store in a cool place.

DECOCTION-PREPARATION

TINCTURES

Tinctures are made by soaking a herb in alcohol, which encourages the active plant constituents to dissolve, giving tinctures a relatively stronger action than infusions or decoctions. They are convenient to use and last up to two years. Tinctures can be made using a jug and a jelly bag, instead of a wine press.

Tinctures are strong preparations and it is essential to check the recommended dosage. Never use industrial alcohol, methylated spirits (methyl alcohol) or rubbing alcohol (isopropyl alcohol) in tinctures.

Alcohol-Reduced Tinctures

Alcoholic tinctures should sometimes be avoided, for example during pregnancy or a gastric inflammation. Adding 5 ml of tincture to a small glass of almost boiling water and leaving it for 5 minutes allows the alcohol to evaporate. To make non-alcoholic tinctures, replace the alcohol with vinegar or glycerol.

Tincture Ratios

Tinctures are made in different strengths, expressed as ratios. A 1:5 ratio (1 part herb to 5 parts alcohol) is good to be used, unless otherwise stated.

Standard Quantity

200 gm dried or 300 gm fresh herb chopped into small pieces to 1 litre alcohol vodka of 35-40% alcohol is ideal, although rum hides the taste of bitter or unpalatable herbs.

Standard Dosage

Take 5 ml (1 teaspoonful) 2-3 times a day diluted in 25 ml of water or fruit juice.

Storage

Store in sterilized, dark glass bottles, in a cool dark place for up to 2 years.

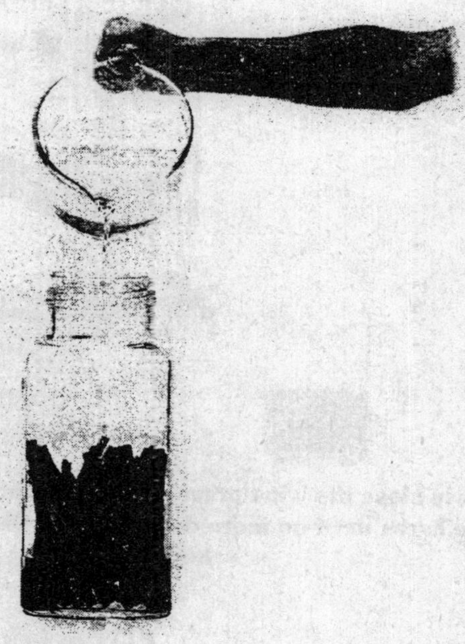

(i) Place the herb in a large, clean glass jar and pour on the alcohol, ensuring that the herb is covered. Close and label the jar. Shake well for 1-2 minutes then store in a cool dark place for 10-14 days, shaking jar every 1-2 days.

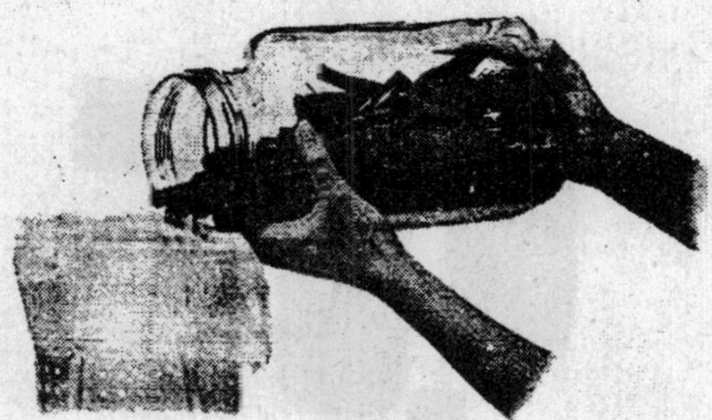

(ii) Set up the wine pres, placing a muslin or nylon mesh bag securely inside. Pour in the mixture and collect the liquid in the jug.

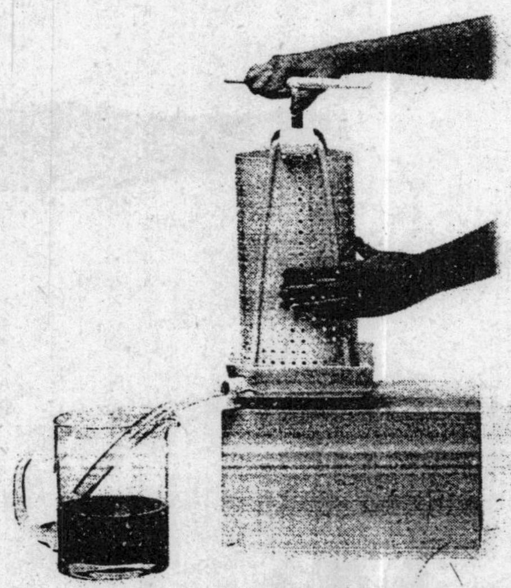

(iii) Slowly close the wine press, extracting the remaining liquid from the herbs until no more drips appear. Discard the leftover herbs.

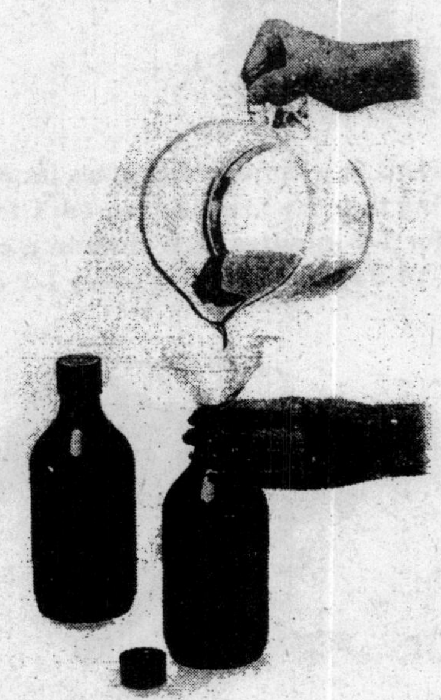

(iv) Pour the tincture into clean, dark glass bottles using a funnel. When full, stopper with a cork or screw top and label the bottles.

TINCTURE-PREPARATION

CAPSULES AND POWDERS

Powdered herbs are most easily taken as capsules but can be sprinkled on food or taken with water. Externally, they can be applied as a dusting powder to the skin or mixed with tinctures as a poultice.

Reputable herbal suppliers are the best place to buy powder the better the grade and quality. Gelatin or begetarian capsule cases are also available from specialist outlets. Powdered slippery elm makes a useful base for poultices and astringents may be applied to weeping skin or mixed into ointments for haemorrhoids and varicose veins.

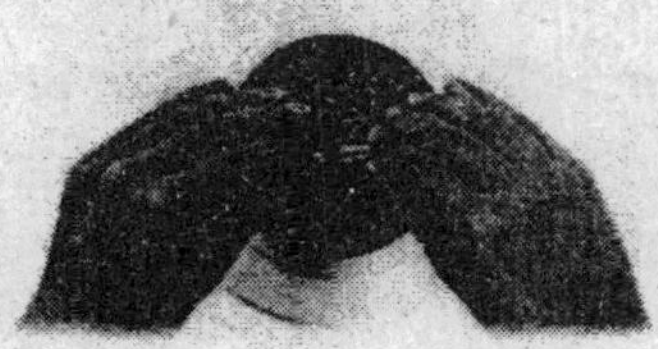

(i) Pour the powder into a saucer and slide the capsule halves towards one another, scooping up the powder or use a capsule-making tray.

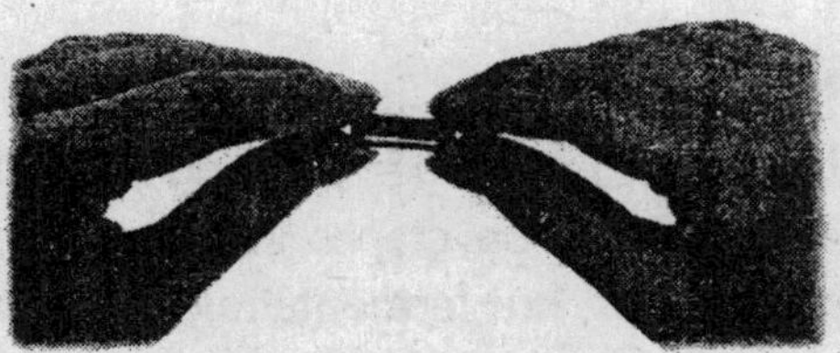

(ii) When the halves of the capsule are full of powder, slide them together without spilling the powder and store.

MAKING CAPSULES

Standard Quantity

Fill size capsules which contain approximately 250 mg of powdered herb.

Standard Dosage

Take 2-3 capsules twice a day.

Storage

Store in airtight, dark glass containers in a cool place for up to 3-4 months.

TONIC WINES

Tonics Wines are an agreeable way to take strengthening and tonic herbs to increase vitality and improve the digestion. Neither strictly medicinal, nor simply appealing to the palate, they are easy to prepare at home. Tonic wines are made by steeping the tonic herbs, such as angelica or bitter herbs, such as southernwood in red or white wine for several weeks.

A simple and effective way to make a tonic wine is in a jar or a ceramic vat with a tap at the base to enable the wine to be drawn off without distrubing the herbs. Wine can be added periodically to keep the herbs covered, although, in time, this will reduce the wine's tonic effectiveness. If exposed to the air, the herbs may go mouldy, making the remedy not only ineffective but unsafe to take.

Herbal Wines

Herbal wines are made by fermenting the herb in the same way that wine is produced from grapes. With the correct equipment this is a simple process, but fermentation alters the activity of the herbs and tends to reduce their medicinal value.

Standard Quantity

100 gm dried or 200 gm fresh tonic herbs or 25 gm dried bitter herbs and 1 litre of red or white wine.

Standard Dosage

Use a ceramic vat with a tap at its base, or a sterilized

glass jar. Store for 3-4 months, ensuring wine covers the herbs. If the herbs go mouldy discard the remedy.

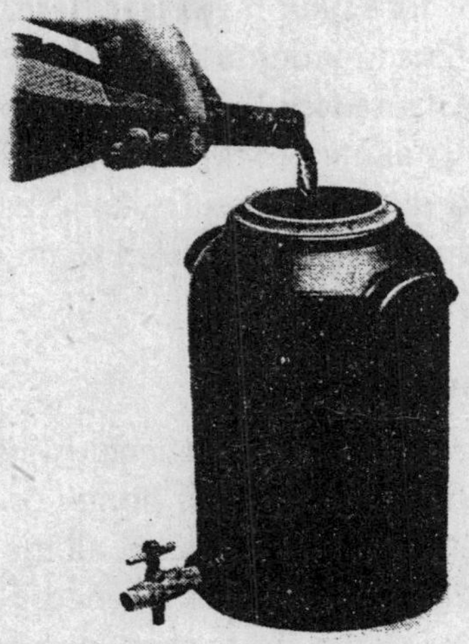

(i) Place the herb in a large clean jar or vat. Pour in enough wine to cover the herb completely. Close the jar securely, shake carefully and leave to stand.

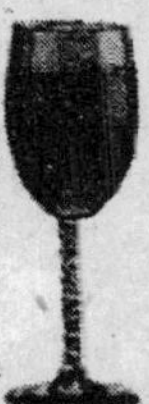

(ii) Allow the wine to mature over 2 or preferably 6 weeks, then 'take a dose from the tap or jar. Regularly top up the mixture with wine.

TONIC-WINES PREPARATIONS

SYRUPS

Honey and unrefined are effective preservatives and can be comibined with infusions or decoctions to make syrups and cordials. They have the additional benefit of having a soothing action and therefore make a perfect vehicle for cough mixtures as well as relieving sore throats. With their sweet taste, syrups can disguise the taste of unpalatable herbs and are therefore greatly appreciated by the children.

A syrup is made with equal proportions of a herbal infusion or decoction and honey or unrefined sugar. When making an infusion or decoction for a syrup, it needs to be infused or simmered for the maximum time in order to optimize its medicinal action. Infusions should be infused for 15 minutes and decoctions should be simmered for 30 minutes. Press the soaked herb through the strainer or sieve to remove as much liquid as possible. Small amounts of neat tincture can be added to the cooled syrup to increase its effectiveness.

Syrups made with Tinctures

Syrups may also be made with tinctures instead of infusions or decoctions. Combine 500 gm of honey or unrefined sugar with 250 ml of water. Gently heat until all the sugar or honey has dissolved and the mixture has thickened. Remove from the heat. Once cool, stir 1 part of the tincture, or mixture of tinctures, into 3 parts of the syrup and bottle as directed opposite.

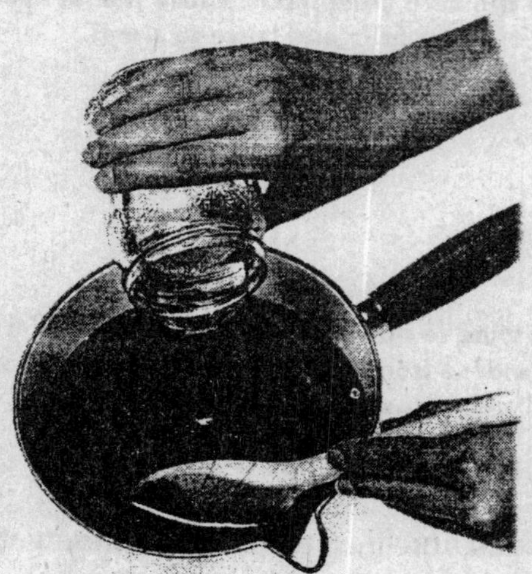

(i) Pour the infusion or decoction into a pan and add the honey or sugar. Gently heat, stirring constantly until all the honey or sugar has dissolved and the mixture has a a syrupy consistency. Remove from the heat and cool.

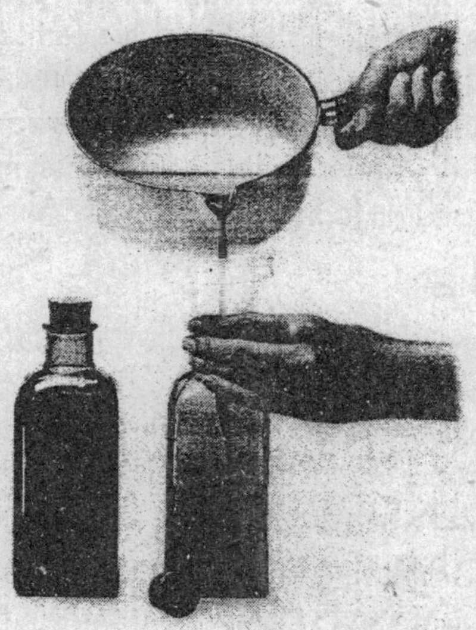

(ii) Pour the cooled syrup into sterilized glass jars using a funnel and store in a cool dark place. Seal the jars with cork stoppers, as syrups are prone to ferment and may explode if kept in screw-topped bottles.

SYRUP-PREPARATION

Standard Quantity

500 ml infusion or decoction infused or heated for the maximum time. 500 gm honey or unrefined sugar.

Standard dosage

Take 5-10 ml (1-2 teaspoonfuls) 3 times a day .

Storage

Store in dark glass bottles with cork tops in a cool place for up to 6 months.

INFUSED OILS

Infusing a herb in oil allows its active, fat-soluble ingredients to be extracted; hot infused oils are simmered, while cold infused oils are heated naturally by the sun. Both types of oil can be used externally as massage oils or added to creams and ointments. Infused oil should not be confused with essential oil, which is an active constituent naturally present in a plant and has specific medicinal properties and a distinct aroma. Essential oil may be added to an infused oil to increase its medicinal efficacy.

Hot Infused Oils

Although hot infused oils can last up to a year, they are most potent when used fresh. If only using infused oils very occasionally, make a smaller quantity than the standard amount with the same proportion of herb to oil. The wine press may be replaced with a jug when cool enough to touch, squeeze the oil through the jelly bag.

Many herbs make effective hot infused oils especially spicy herbs such as ginger (*Zingiber officinale*), cayenne (*Capsicum frutescens*), and pepper (*Piper nigrum*). These oils can be rubbed into the skin to relieve rheumatic and arthritic pain, improve local blood flow and relax muscles. Other hot infused oils from leafy herbs, such as comfrey (*Symphytum officinale*), speed wound healing. Oil infused with mullein (*Verbascum thapsus*), is used for earache and ear infections, and chickweed (*Stellaria media*), ointment may be produced from a hot infused oil.

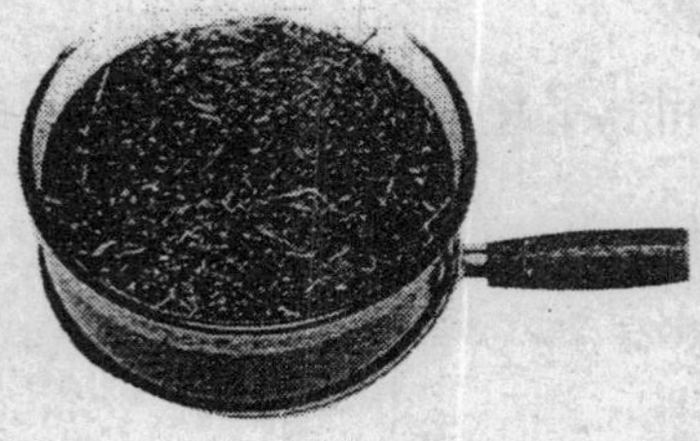

(i) Stir the chopped herb and oil together in a glass bowl over a saucepan of boiling water. Cover and simmer gently for 2-3 hours.

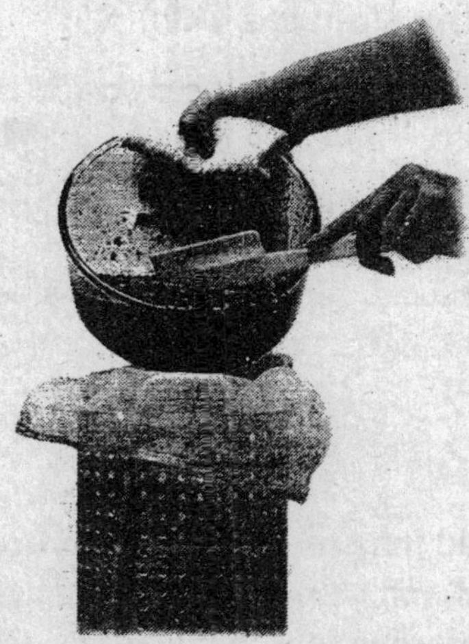

(ii) Remove from the heat and allow the mixture to cool, then pour into the wine pres or jug if not available with a jelly bag in place. Collect the strained oil in a jug, pressing all the liquid out of the herbs.

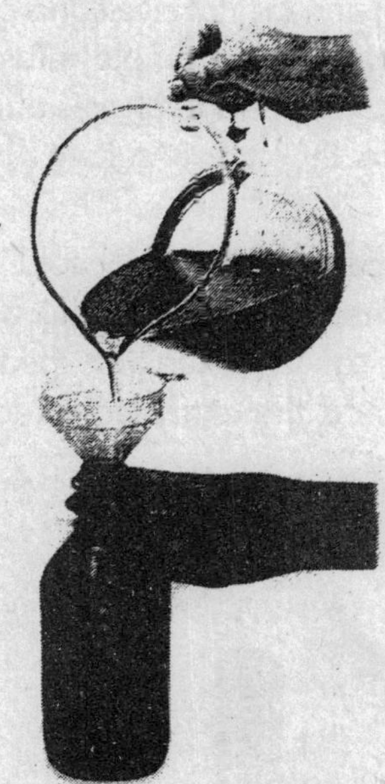

(iii) Pour the infused oil into clean, dark glass bottles, using a funnel. Seal and label each bottle.

INFUSED-OIL-PREPARATION

Standard Quantity (Infused Oils)

250 gm dried or 500 gm fresh herb to 750 ml olive, sunflower or other good-quality vegetable oil.

Storage

Store in sterilized, airtight, dark glass bottles for up to 1 years; dark glass bottles for up to 1 year; for the best results, use within 6 months.

Cold Infused Oils

Making a cold infused oil is a slow process and involves leaving a jar packed with herbs and oil to stand for several weeks. Sunlight encourages the plant to release its active constituents into the oil. It is the most suitable method of oil infusion for fresh plant material, especially the more delicate parts such as flowers. St Jhon's wort (*Hypericum perforatum*), marigold (*Calendula officinalis*), and melilot (*Melilotus officinalis*) are three of the most commonly produced cold infused oils. St Jhon's wort oil is anti-flammatory and analgesic and may be applied topically or taken internally, after consulting a herbalist, for peptic ulceration.

Olive oil is particularly suitable for cold infusion as it rarely turns rancid. The intensity of sunlight and length of time a herb is infused for affects the concentration of its medicinal constituents. For greater strength, add the extracted oil to a fresh suply of herbs and infuse again.

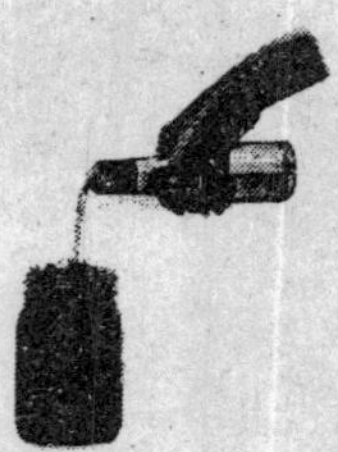

(i) Place the herb in a clear glass jar. Pour in oil until it completely covers the herb, close the jar and shake well. Place the jar in a suny spot, such as on a windowsill, and leave for 2-6 weeks.

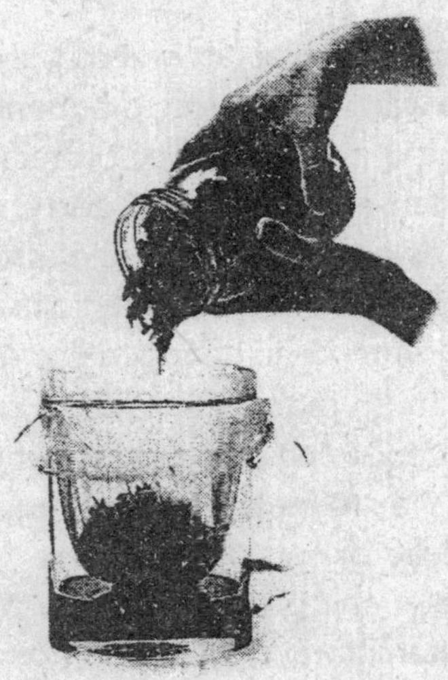

(ii) Pour the oil and herb mixture into a jelly bag, securred to the rim of a jug or bowl with string or use a wine press. Allow the oil to filter through the bag.

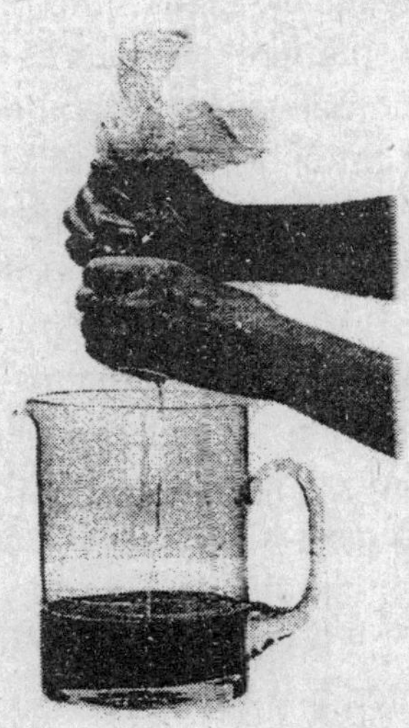

(iii) Squeeze out the remaining oil from the bag. Pour the infused oil into dark glass bottles, label and store. Alternatively, repeat the whole process with the infused oil and fresh herbs.

COLD INFUSED OIL-PREPARATION

OINTMENTS

Ointments contain oils or fats heated with herbs and, unlike creams, contain no water. As a result, ointments form a separate layer on the surface of the skin. They protect against injury or inflammation of damaged skin and carry active medicinal constituents, such as essential oils, to the affected area. These are useful in conditions such as haemorrhoids or where protection is needed from moisture, as in chapped lips and nappy rash.

Ointments can be made with dozens of bases and they vary in consistency, depending on the constituents and proportions used. The simplest way to make a soft, all-purpose ointment is to use petroleum jelly or soft paraffin wax. Petroleum jelly is impermeable to water and provides a protective barrier for the skin. Single herbs or mixtures of herbs may be used as required, provided they are finely cut, and essential oil can be stirred into the ointment just before straining.

Different Consistencies

A solid and relatively grease-free ointment will spread easily and is useful for preparations such as lip balms. This can be made by using alternatives to mineral oils. Melt 140 gm of cocunut oil with 120 gm of beeswax and 100 gm of powdered herb. Simmer gently for 90 minutes in a glass bowl set in a pan of boiling water, or a double boiler, then strain and pour into jars.

A less solid ointment, for conditions such as skin rashes, can be made by combining olive oil and beeswax. Melt 60 gm of beeswax with 500 ml of olive oil and 120 gm of dried or 300 gm of fresh herb in a glass bowl. Cover and place in a warm over for 3 hours, then remove, strain and pour into jars. This ointment can also be made by combining 500 ml of hot infused oil with 60 gm of melted beeswax.

Standard Quantity

60 gm dried or 150 gm fresh herb or mixture of herbs to 500 gm of petroleum jelly or soft paraffin wax.

Standard Application

Apply as little 3 times a day.

Storage

Store in sterilized, dark glass jars with lids for up to 3 months.

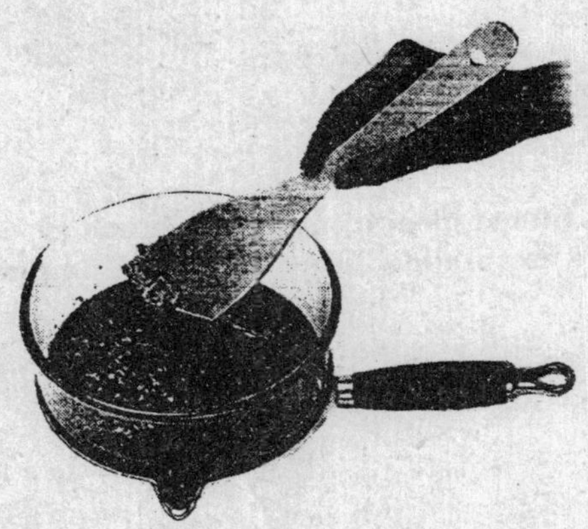

(i) Melt the petroleum jelly or wax into a glass bowl set in a pan of boiling water, or use a double boiler. Add the finely cut herb and simmer for 15 minutes, stiring continuously.

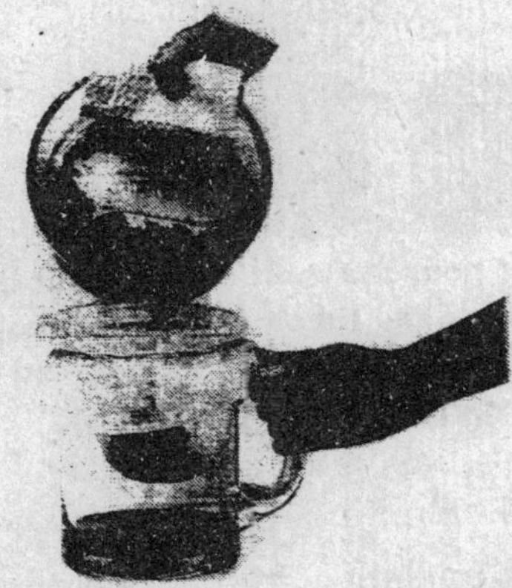

(ii) Pour the herb mixture into a jelly bag secured to the rim of a jug with string, and allow the liquid to filter through.

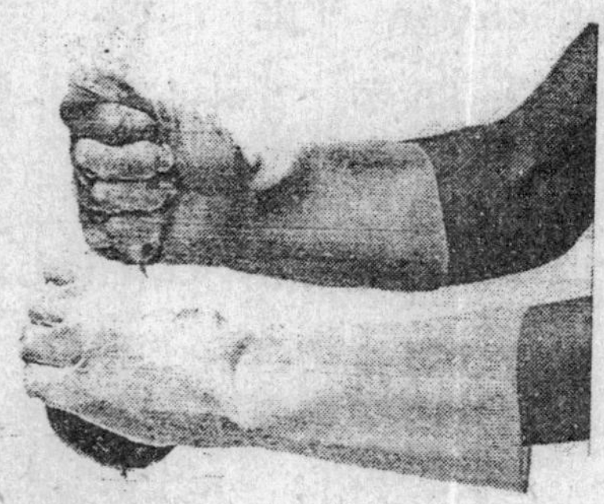

(iii) Wearing rubber gloves, squeeze as much of the hot herb mixture as possible through the bag into the jug.

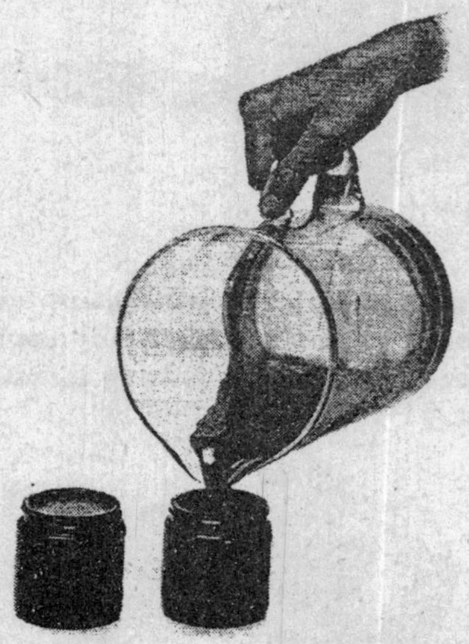

(iv) Quickly pour the pour the molt en ointment into jars before it sets in the jug. Place the lid on each jar without securing it firmly. When cool, tighten the lids and label.

OINTMENT-PREPARATION

POULTICES

A Poultice is a mixture of fresh, dried or powdered herbs that is applied to an affected area. Poultices are used to ease nerve or muscle pains, sprains or broken bones, and to draw pus from infected wounds, ulcers or boils.

A Poultice of self-heal relieves sprains and fractures, while St Jhon's wort can help ease muscle or nerve pains.

Drawing Boils & Infected Wounds

Slippery elm powder mixed with marigold (*Calendula officinalis*) tincture or myrrh (*Commiphora mukul*) tincture makes a useful poultice for drawing boils and wounds.

Standard Quantity

Sufficient herb to cover the affected area.

Standard Application

Apply a new poultice every 2-3 hours. Repeat as often as required.

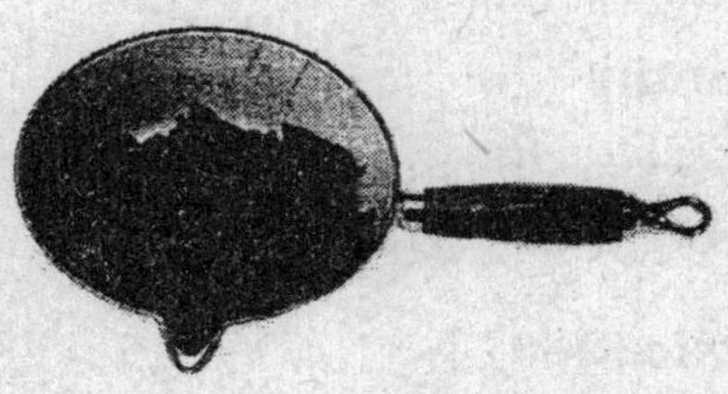

(i) Simmer the herb for 2 minutes. Squeeze out any excess liquid, rub some oil on to the affected area to prevent sticking and apply the herb while a hot.

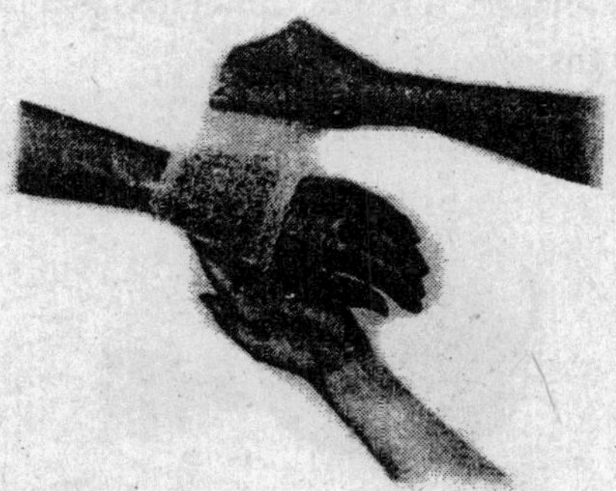

(ii) Bandage the herb securely in place using gauze or cotton strips. Leave on for up to 3 hours, as required.

POULTICE PREPARATION

CREAMS

Making a Cream involves combining oil or fat and water in an emulsion. If the process is rushed, the oil and water may separate. Unlike ointments, creams blend with the skin and have the advantage of being cooling and soothing while at the same time allowing the skin to breathe and sweat naturally. They can, however, deteriorate quite quickly and are best stored in dark, airtight jars in a refrigerator.

Small quantities of additional ingredients such as tinctures, powders and essential oils can be added to a cream before or after it is put in jars. Adding an essential oil, such as 1 ml of tea tree to 100 ml cream, counters mould growth and lengthens shelf life, as does 5 ml of borax. Other receipes for making cream use infusions, tinctures or infused oils.

Standard Quantity

30 gm dried or 75 gm fresh herb, 150 gm emulsifying wax, 70 gm glycerine and 80 ml water.

Standard Application

Rub a little into the affected area 2-3 times a day.

Storage

Store in sterilized, airtight, dark glass jars in a refrigerator for up to 3 months.

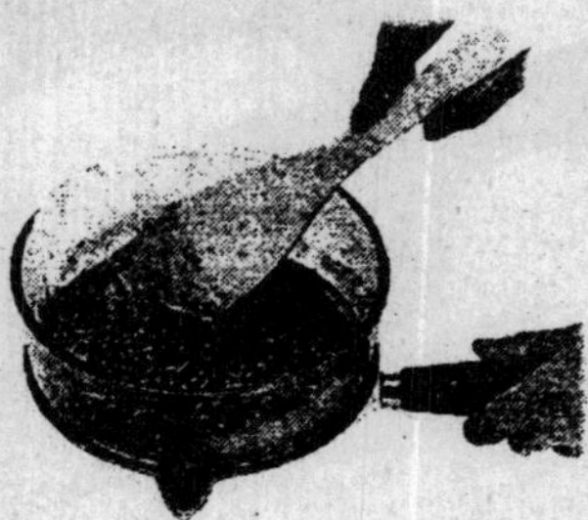

(i) Melt the emulsifying wax in a glass bowl set in a pan of boiling water or a double boiler. Add the glycerine, water and herb while stirring, and simmer for 3 hours.

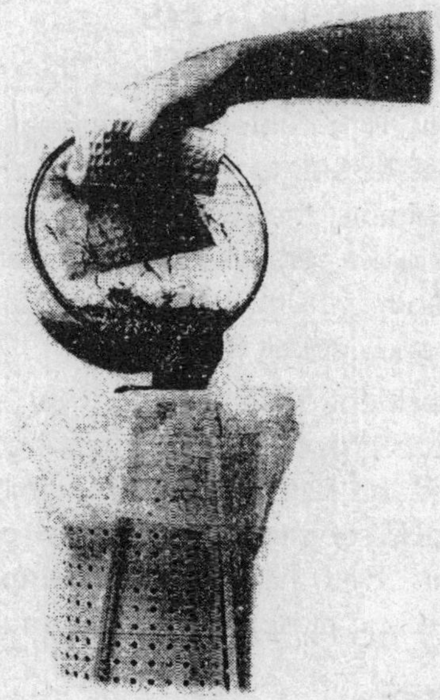

(ii) Strain the mixture through a wine press or a jelly bag. Stir slowly but continuously until it cools and sets.

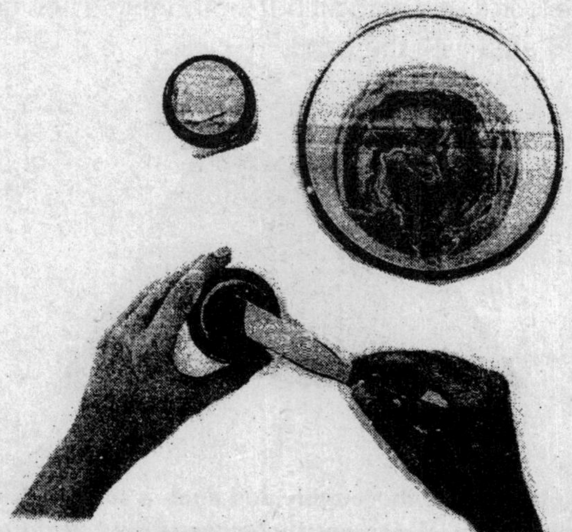

(iii) With a small knife or spatula, place the set cream into dark glass jars. Tighten the lids and label. Store in a refrigerator as soon as possible.

CREAM-PREPARATION

COMPRESSES AND LOTIONS

Lotions are water-based herbal preparations such as infusions, decoctions or diluted tinctures that are used to bath inflamed or irritated skin. Compresses are cloths soaked in a lotion and held against the skin. Lotions and compresses are both simple ways to use herbs externally and can be very effective in relieving sewlling, bruising and pain, soothing inflammation and headaches, and cooling fevers.

After an accident or sports injury, bruising and swelling can often be reduced or prevented if a hot compress is swiftly applied, provided the skin is unbroken. Cold compresses are particularly useful in soothing inflammation, cooling fevers and easing headaches. Both hot and cold compresses should be frequently soaked and re-applied for maximum benefit.

Applying A Lotion

As specified, make an infusion or decoction and strain it well. Alternatively, dilute a tincture with water. Soak a clean cloth in the lotion and wring it out thoroughly. Then gently bath the affected area with the cloth.

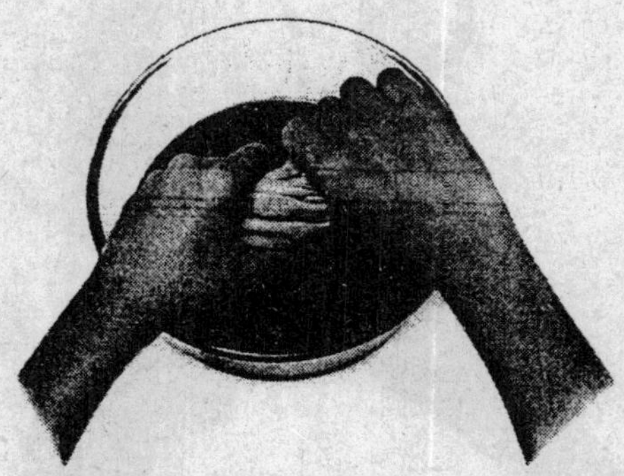

(i) Wash your hands thoroughly and soak a soft cloth or clean flannel in the lotion. Wring out the excess liquid. Before applying, rub some oil on the affected area to prevent sticking.

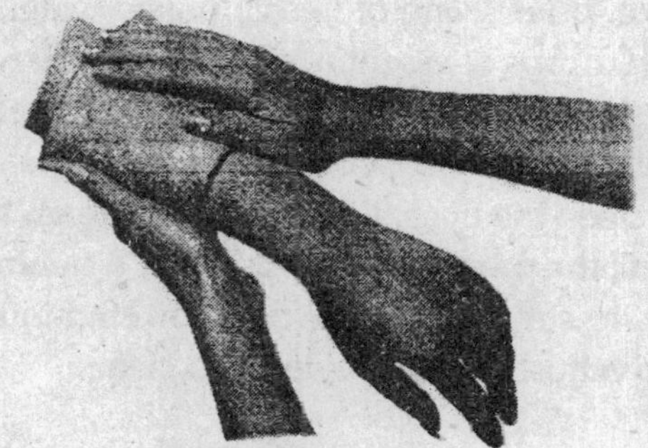

(ii) Place the compress against the affected area. For pain and swellings, secure the compress with plastic film and safety pins and leave for up to 1-2 hours, Re-apply as required.

APPLYING COMPRESSES

Standard Quantity of Lotion

500 ml infusion or decoction, or 25 ml tincture in 500 ml water.

Standard Application of Compress or Lotion

Use as required. Prepare a fresh compress or lotions in sterilized bottles, with lids, in a refrigerat or for up to 2 days.

OTHER PREPARATIONS

Diffierent herbal preparations suit different ailments. Most of the following preparations provide localized relief. Steam inhalations, for example, help clear various respiratory complaints; gargles and mouthwashes soothe sore throats and mouth ulcers; massage oils can ease aching muscles; and skin washes relieve inflamed skin conditions.

Steam Inhalations

Steam inhalations are an effective way to clear catarrh, and relieve sinusitis, fever and bronchial asthma. The combination of steam and antiseptic ingredients clears the airways throughout the respiratory system.

To make. pour 1 litre of freshly boiled water into a large bowl. add 5-10 drops of essential oil and stir well. Alternatively, make an infusion of 25 gm of herb to 1 litre of water, brew for 15 minutes, and pour into a bowl. Cover the head and bowl with a towel, close the eyes, and inhale the steam for about 10 minutes or until the preparation cools. After a steam inhalation, it is advisable to stay in a warm room for 15 minutes to allow the airways to adjust and any catarrh to clear.

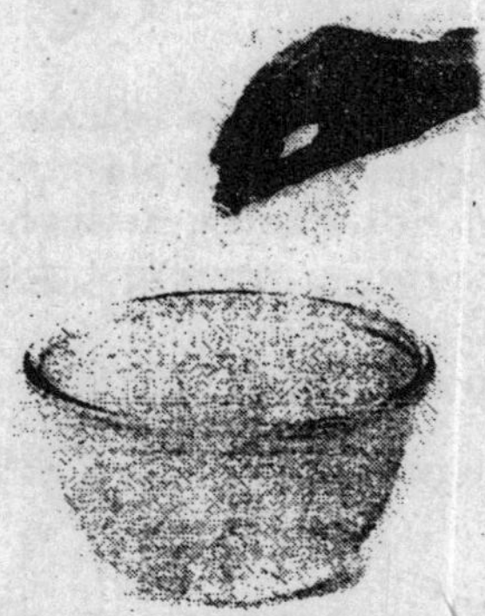

***Inhalations using* essentials oil relieve many respiratory complaints.**

GARGLES & MOUTHWASHES

Gargles and mouthwashes usually contain astringent herbs which tighten the mucous membranes of the mouth and throat. Astringent herbs such as myrrh can be made more palatable and more effective for sore throats by adding a little liquorice or a pinch of cayenne preparation. As gargles and mouthwashes are made from infusions, decoctions, or diluted otinctures, they can generally be swallowed for internal treatment. But do not exceed the daily internal dose of a herb.

To make, prepare an infusion but allow it to stand for 15-20 minutes in order to increase its astringency. Strain, then gargle, or rinse the mouth with a cupful. Alternatively, use a decoction or dilute about 5 ml of tincture in 100 ml of hot water and use in the same way. Repeat as often as required unless specified.

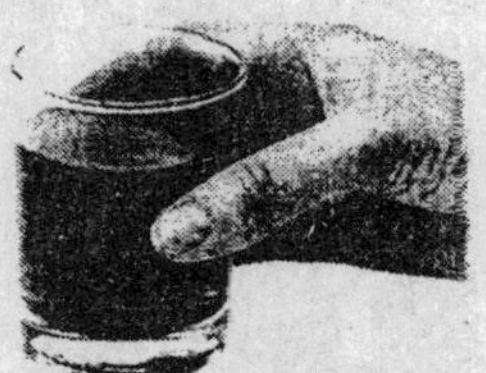

***Infusions* made with antiseptic herbs make useful gargeles and moulthwashes for sore throats and mouth ulcers.**

Pessaires And Suppositories

Pessaries and suppositories are waxy pellets containing essential oil or fine powder. They are used when oral medicine is likely to be broken down during digestion before reaching its intended site. Pessaries are inserted into the vagina and suppositories into the anus where they melt at body temperature. The herb is quickly absorbed into the bloodstream providing fast relief. It is best to buy ready made suppositories.

To make pessaries, use a pessary mould or make 24 moulds from cooking foil shaped around a thimble. Mix 10 gm of soft soap, 50 ml of glycerine and 40 ml of methylated spirits and pour into the moulds. Leave for a few minutes to coat the moulds then pour out the excess and leave to harden. Melt 20 gm of cocoa butter, remove from the heat and add 30 drops of essential oil or 5 gm of powder. Pour into the shells and leave to set for 3 hours, before removing the pessaries. Store ill a cool place in a pot lined with greaseproof paper for up to 3 months.

Essential Oils

Essential oils can be used in massage to soothe minor aches and pains. Before use, they should lie diluted with a carrier oil as they can irritate the skill. Essential oils deteriorate rapidly after dilution, so it is best to mix small quantities as you need them.

For massage, mix 5—10 drops of essential oil with 1 tablespoonful of carrier oil, such as wheatgerm or almond oil, and massage gently into the skill.

Oil burner, use 5-10 drops of neat essential oil mixed with water. Burn for 30 minutes.

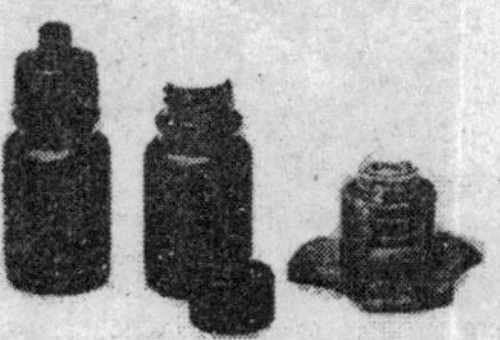

***Essential oil area* used in baths, oil burners and in massages to relieve tension and stress.**

BATHS & SKIN WASHES

Herbal baths and skin washes can relieve many conditions, including aching limbs and stuffy sinuses. They are made from diluted essential oils or infusions. Eyebaths soothe sore, inflamed or irritated eyes.

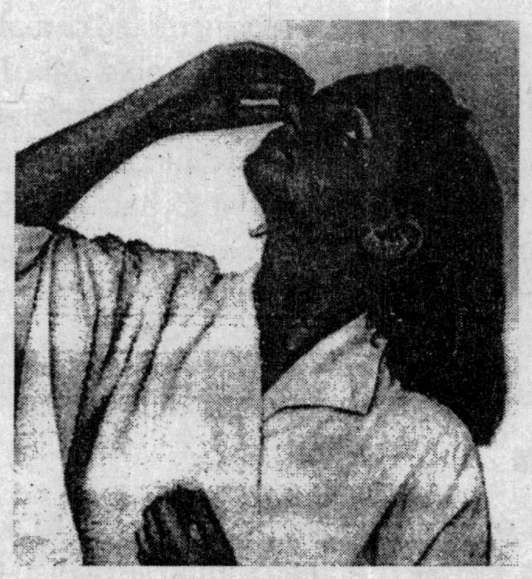

***Eyebath is applied* to the affected eye find the head is tilted well back.**

To make a herbal bath, add 500 ml of strained infusion or 5-10 drops to essential oil to a running bath.

To make a skin wash, make an infusion, strain it and bathe the affected area.

To make an eyebath, make a small quantity of an infusion or use a herbal teabag. Strain the liquid carefully into a sterilized eyebath. Alternatively, add 2-3 drops of a tincture to an eyebath filled with water that has just boiled. Allow to cool and place the eyebath firmly over the eye. Tip the head back and bath the eye by continuously blinking. Repeat up to 3 times a day.

General Cautions

Eyebaths should be very weak, so as not to sting the eyes. Always use boiled, cooled water in a sterilizer container. Do not bath eyes over a period of more than 2-3 weeks at a time. If bathing eyes frequently, add a tiny pinch of salt to each eyebath to counter leaching of salts and minerals from the eye.

Cold macerations

Heat destroys the active constituents of some herbs and a cold maceration is more appropriate than decoction.

To make, pour 500 ml of cold water on to 25 gm of herb and leave to stand overnight. Strain and use as the decoction.

Juices

The juices extracted from many herbs can be taken internally or applied externally.

To make, pulp the plant preferably using a mechanical juicer. Otherwise use a food processor. Squeeze the pulp through a jelly bag to collect the juice. Some herbs need to be cooked in order to extract their juice.

Part II
Description and Discussion of Common Drug Plants

4

Description and Discussion of the Common Drug Plants

ACONITE

***Aconitum napellus* Linn.**

(Famliy: Ranunculaceae)

Description : It is a perennial herb. The stems are often decumbent in small stage, glabrous or slightly pubescent. Leaves are variable in size, palmatipartite; segments linear. The flowers are dull greenish - blue and are borne in simple or sparingly compound racemes. The follicles are 3-5 with numerous seeds.

Flowering is during September-October and fruiting later.

There are four varieties of this species viz. *napellus* proper, *rigidum, multifidum* and *rotundifolium.*

Distribution : It is known to found in alpine and sub-alpine belts of the Himalayas in India.

Parts Used : Leaves and roots are used.

Medicinal uses : The roots are generally used after processing in combination with other medicines in small doses as tonic and a remedy for fever, nervous debility, rheumatism and cardiac diseases. But in larger doses, it becomes toxic; milk is prescribed as antidote for its poisoning. Aconitine, one of main alkaloids of its roots, is used externally in various forms of neuralgia, tetanus, acute and chronic rheumatism, gout, and erysipelas and in affections of the heart characterized by increased action. This is also given internally in very small doses in fever to lower the temperature, for relieving pains, cystis, diarrhoea and cough irritation but its repeated internal dose of 1.0 - 2.0 mg may cause toxic symptoms.

Its other species *Aconitum balfourii* Stapf. *Aconitum bisma* (Ham) Rapaics, *Aconitum chasmanthum* Stapf. ex Holmes, *Aconitum deinorrhizum* Stapf., *Aconitum falconeri* Stapf. and *Aconitum ferox* Wall. ex. Ser. are also used under the same name.

AGNIMANTHA

Clerodendrum multiflorum (Burm.f.) O. kuntze

(Syn. _C. phlomidis_ Linn.f.)

(Family : Verbenaceae)

Description : It is a large bushy shrub with pubescent leaves. Leaves are ovate-sinuate or serrate, 5.0 x 3.7 cm and mature puberulous or pubescent beneath. The flowers are white and aromatic on slender pedicels and are borne in terminal leafly rounded panicle, composed of axillary 3-9 flowered cymes. The fruits are black obovoid with 4-kernels and about 5.0-10.0 cm across.

Flowering is during April-May and fruiting during May-June.

Distribution : The plant is found throughout India; chiefly in Uttar Pradesh, Bihar, West Bengal and Deccan Peninsula.

Parts used : Leaves, bark and roots are used.

Medicinal uses : Its leaves are alterative and bitter tonic and their juice is given in syphilis. The root-decoction is slightly astringent, demulcent and stomachic and is used as bitter tonic for children during convalescence from measles and is also given in gonorrhoea. The bark and roots of the plant are known for their bitter and tonic properties and are used in nervous disorders and debility. Besides, various plant parts are used in fever, post-natal complaints, cholera, and anthrax.

AJAKARNA

***Vateria indica* Linn.**

(Family: Dipterocarpaceae)

Description: This is a large and very handsome tree with white bark and clothed young branches and inflorescences. Leaves are 12.5-20.0 x 5.0-10.0 cm, elliptic – oblong, shortly pointed or obtuse, cordate or rounded at the base and glabrous; lateral nerves in 12-15 pairs and very prominent. Flowers are about 0.6 cm in diameter in large 15.0-20.0 cm long terminal panicles with caducous and acute bracts. Capsules, the fruits are 6.5 x 3.8 cm, oblong, fleshy and 3-valved with 1 seed in each valve.

Flowering and fruiting is during hot season.

Distribution: It is found in western parts of the country from Kanara to Travncore between 1200-1400 m, chiefly in evergreen forests but occasionally along rivers in deciduous forests.

Parts used: The bark and the resin are used.

Medicinal uses: The bark of the plant is known as acrid, alexipharmic and bitter and is used to cure the cough, anaemia, ear diseases, urinary discharge, skin eruptions, ulcers and wounds. The resin obtained from the plant is of three kinds: reddish, dark and slightly white and possesses alexipharmic, bitter, carminative, expectorant and detergent properties. This is used in chronic amenorrhoea, bronchitis, hemicrania, piles, rheumatism and tuberculosis glands; its smoke is good in painful piles and beneficial to the foetus in pregnanat women. The resin mixed with wax and oil forms a good resinous ointment which is used as a substitute for officinal resin, and its fine shavings are administered internally to check the diarrhea.

AJWAIN

***Apium graveolens* Linn.**

(Family: Apiaceae)

Description: This is an annual – biennial, erect and glabrous herb with fistular and angular stem. Leaves are pinnate; leaflets 1.0-1.6 cm long, oval – obovate and usually 3-lobed, incised and glabrous; petioles upto 1.0 cm long or lacking in upper leaves. The umbels are leaf opposed and 12-15 rayed. Involucre and involucel are absent. Umbellules are 20-25 flowered. The flowers are white and fruits ovoid to suborbicular with prominent ridges.

Flowering and fruiting is during March – June.

Distribution: A native of Europe, now got naturalized and is found distributed in the foot of North Western Himalays and outlying hills in the Punjab and Uttaranchal.

Parts used: The roots and seeds are used.

Medicinal uses: Its roots are described as alterative and diuretic and are given in anasarca and colic. Besides, the seeds possess antiseptic, carminative, cordial, emmenagogal and stimulant properties and are used as tonic, in asthma and bronchitis and also for liver and spleen diseases.

ALOE

Aloe barbadensis Mill.

(Syn. *A. vera Tourn.ex Linn.; A. indica Royle; A. littoralis Koening*)

(Family: Liliaceae)

Description : It is a perennial and succulent herb, about 30-60 cm high. Stem is short, thick and somewhat divided. Leaves are sessile, crowded and lanceolate. Scape is longer than the leaves and branched. Inflorescence is of long and dense racemes. Bracts are short-lanceolate and membranous. Flowers are pendulous, imbricate and yellow.

Flowering and fruiting is in late winter.

Distribution : Many of the forms of the plant are naturalized in India and are found in a semi-wild state in all parts from the dry west-ward valleys of the Himalayas. Also planted in gardens.

Parts used : Pulp, expressed and dried juice of leaves and the roots are used.

Medicinal uses : The plant is known to be used in menstrual diseases and stomach pain, after pregnancy as a tonic, in fever and in uterine disorders. Pulp is used in menstrual suppressions and it keeps the nervous system under control when applied on head. The mucilage is used in painful inflammation. The dried juice is given in consipatiion and fresh juice as cooling in fevers. Aloe meat is eaten to alleviate colds and with salt to keep blood in good condition and to relieve constipation. Aloe steeped with *Stemodia maritima* (Gomabush) is drunk to ease swellings and dropsy. Leaves are used as a poultice in swellings. Aloe extract and vitamin therapeutically are used for glaucoma patients. Besides, the roots of aloe are used in colic pain.

According to Wahid and Siddiqui (1961), the plant in Unani medicine, is used as antiseptic, germicidal and blood purifier and in chronic ulcers to stimulate healing But it should be used with caution during pregnancy since in doses of 0.6 gm a day is very unsafe for pregnant women and is likely to produce abortion.

AMALAKI

***Emblica officinalis* Gaertn.**

(Syn. *Phyllanthus emblica* Linn.; *Cicca emblica* Kurz.)

(Family: Euphorbiaceae)

Description : The plant is a moderate-sized deciduous tree with greenish-grey or red bark which is peeling off in scales and long stripes. Leaves are pinnate, distichously closeset, linear-oblong and obtuse. Flowers are greenish-yellow and are borne in axillary clusters along the branchlets; males are on slender pedicels and females are sub-sessile and few. Fruits are of three 2-valved cocci, globose, fleshy and obscurely 6-lobed when ripe. The seeds are trigonous.

Flowering is during February-May and fruiting in October-March.

Distribution : It is found wild or cultivated throughout tropical parts of India.

Parts used : Fruits, seeds, flowers, leaves, bark and roots are used.

Medicinal uses : The fruits are antidiarrhoeal, astringent, antidysenteric, antiscorbutic, carminative, cooling, stomachic and tonic and unripe fruits are aperient. These are useful in urinary problems and are prescribed in anaemia, jaundice and dyspepsia in combination with iron. Fermented liquor prepared from its fruits is used in jaundice, dyspepsia and coughs. Its seeds are used as a collyrium in eye complaints and their infusion is given in asthma, bronchitis and fever. The infusion of its seeds is also useful in diabetes. Seeds fried in ghee and ground in 'conjee' are applied as lep to the forehead to stop nose-bleeding.

Its flowers are used as cooling, refrigerant and aperient and the juice of its leaves is applied externally to ulcers and their infusion mixed with fenugreek seeds is given in chronic dysentery. Besides, the bark and roots are used as astringent. The juice of the bark combined with honey and turmeric is used as a remedy for gonorrhoea. Its root-bark rubbed with honey is used in aphthous stomatitis.

APAMARGA

Achyranthes aspera **Linn.**

(Family: Amaranthaceae)

Description : It is a stiff erect herb about 30-90 cm high with erect and simple or slightly branched stem. Leaves are 3.8-12.5 x 5.0-7.5 cm, opposite, elliptic, obovate or suborbicular, usually rounded at apex and tomentose or velvety on both surfaces. Flowers are bisexual, greenish-white and are borne in long spikes which elongate in fruits and reach upto 50 cm in length. Fruit is an oblong utricle which is enclosed in hardened perianth and disarticulating easily and carry spinous bracteoles with it. The seeds are subcylindrical with a truncate brown apex.

Flowering is in winter and fruiting in summer season.

Distribution : This is a common weed found throughout India upto 1000 m usually in dry area and along the road sides.

Parts Used : Whole plant is used.

Medicinal uses : The entire plant is considered pungent, purgative, diuretic and astringent and is used in dropsy and haemorrhoids. The decoction of the plant is useful in pneumonia, cough and kidney stones and ash of the plant is given in haemorroids. The dried plant is useful in colic and gonorrhoea and also acts as laxative. The ashes of the plant with water and jaggery are effective in ascites and anasarca; sesamum oil medicated with ashes of the plant is used as eardrops. Achyrol, its leaf-extract is used in leprosy and the juice of the leaves is in eczema and leprosy. Leaves made into a paste with water are applied to bites of poisonous insects, wasps and bees etc. The roots are given in stomach pain and their paste is applied to remove opacity of cornea and to wounds as haemostatic besides, their decoction in diarrhoea. The root-paste is given to stop bleeding after abortion. Powdered roots mixed with honey are given internally in haemorrhoides. A pinch of its root powder in combination with pepper powder and honey forms a good remedy for cough.

The seed-paste is applied against insect-bite. Its seeds are rubbed with rice-water and are prescribed to patients of bleeding piles and the powder of its seeds is soaked in butter milk is given in biliousness. Its flowers are ground and mixed with curd and sugar, are given in menorrhagia and the flower tops are used in treatment of rabies. A decoction of the whole plant is diuretic and efficaceous in renal dropsies and in combination with that of Kakajanga (*Leea aequata*) useful in insomnia. It is also stated that the fresh juice of its leaves thickened into an extract by exposure to the sun and then mixed with a little opium, may be beneficially applied to primary syphilitic sores. Besides, the powder of roots with bangbhasm is used as aphrodisiac to increase sexual desires.

APRAJITA

Clitoria ternatea Linn.

(Family: Fabaceae)

Description : It is a perennial climbing herb with slender, terete and downy stems. Leaves are pinnately 3-7 foliolate; leaflets ovate or oblong, obtuse and subcoriaceous. The flowers showy, blue or white and solitary or axillary; bracteoles large and obtuse. Pods, the fruits are linear and compressed. Seeds are 6-10, black and smooth.

Flowering is during May-June and fruiting in winter.

Distribution : It is a common garden plant and also occurs among hedges all over the tropical regions from Himalayas to Chennai.

Parts used : The roots, root-bark, leaves and seeds are used.

Medicinal uses: Its roots are known as bitter, refrigerant, opthalmic, laxative, intellect promoting, alexeteric, diuretic, anthelmintic, depurative, aphrodisiac and tonic and are used in ophthalmopathy, tubercular glands, amentia, hemicrania, burning sensation, strangury, helminthiasis, elephantiasis, leprosy, leucoderma, inflammation, vitiated conditions of 'pitta', bronchitis, asthma, pulmonary tuberculosis, ascitis, visceromegaly, ulcers and fevers. The root-bark is used as diuretic and laxative. Besides, the leaves are used in otalgia, hepatopathy and eruptions and the seeds as aperient and powerful purgatives.

ARAGWADHA

***Cassia fistula* Linn.**

(Family: Fabaceae)

Description : It is a moderate sized and wholly glabrous tree with greenish-grey bark and about 3.7-4.8 m in height. Leaves are paripinnate and 5.0-12.0 cm long; leaflets 8-16, acuminate and ovate-lanceolete. The flowers are yellow in lax pendulous racemes and fragrant. Pods, the fruits are about 30-40 cm long and 2.0-2.5 cm across, cylindrical, smooth, hard, indehiscent and yellowish-grey. The seeds are about 0.6 cm in diameter, compressed and albuminous and are parallel with septa.

Flowering is in April-July and fruiting during August-September. The fruits may be seen hanging on the plants throughout the year.

Distribution : It is cultivated as an ornamental plant for attractive yellow blossoms in pendant racemes and grows wild in many parts of India.

Parts used : The pods, flowers, leaves and root bark are used.

Medicinal uses : An ethanol extract of its pods and of stem- bark is considered hypoglycaemic, antiviral and anticancer. It is used in cancer, epilepsy, convulsions and delirium febris, pimples, burns, syphilis, dysuria, haematuria, gravel and diarrhoea. The pulp of fruits is used as a tonic and in chest infection and with sugar is taken in constipation; also useful in heart and chest diseases. A paste of its leaves is applied to the ringworm lesions and the leaves are mixed with bark and rubbed with oil, are used efficaciously in Chilblains ringworm, pyoderma, insect bites, eczema, scabies and psoriasis. The seeds are emetic and are used in jaundice and the bark paste is given internally in blindness. Besides, the fruits are said to be applied in snake-bite.

The gum of the seeds is used as a substitute for Gaur gum obtained from *Cyamopsis tetragonoloba* (Farooqi, 1995).

ARJUNA

***Terminalia arjuna* (Roxb.) W. & A.**

(Family: Combretaceae)

Description : It is a large tree often with buttressed trunk, smooth grey bark and drooping branchlets, about 20-25 m high. Leaves are usually sub-opposite, oblong or elliptic-long, pale dull green above and pale-brown beneath, 10.0-20.0 cm long and hard. The flowers are yellowish-white and are borne in shortly panicled-spikes. The fruits are 2.5-5.0 cm long drupes, ovoid or obovoid-oblong, fibrous woody, glabrous and with 5-7 equal, hard, coriaceous and thick narrow wings.

Flowering is in April-May and fruiting during September-November.

Distribution : It is common on the banks of rivers, streams and dry water-courses in Sub-Himalayan-tract and Central and South India and in West Bengal.

Parts used : Fruits, leaves and bark are used.

Medicinal uses : The fruits are used as tonic and deobstruent. Externally, its leaves are used as a cover on sores and ulcers and their juice is used in earache. The bark is antidysenteric, antipyretic, astringent, cardiotonic, lithotriptic, styptic and tonic. The powder of its bark acts as a diuretic in cirrhosis of liver and gives relief in symptomatic hypertension. A decoction of its thick bark made with milk is given every morning on an empty stomach or its powder with milk and gur as a cardiotonic. About 500 mg bark powder can be used three times daily, but it may cause mild gastric intolerance and constipation in some persons. The powder of the bark is also given with honey in fractures and contusions with ecchymosis. The extract of its bark is used for cleaning sores, ulcers and cancers etc. as astringent. An ointment made from the bark mixed with honey is used to cure acne. The ashes of its bark are prescribed in scorpion-stings. Besides, a linctus made from the bark, soaked and dried seven times successively in the leaf juice of *Bansa* (*Justicia adhatoda*) and well mixed with honey, sugar-candy and cow's ghee is prescribed in cases of phthisis; it stops the blood in the sputum and clears up and cures the sores.

ARK

***Calotropis procera* (Ait.) Ait. f. ssp. *hamiltonii* (W.) Ali (Syn. *C. hamiltonii* W.; *C. procera* auct. non (Ait.) f.)**

Description : This is a middle-sized shrub. Its young parts are covered with adpressed white tomentum and young leaves are hoary and glabrous when full grown. Leaves are 10-18 cm long, ovate-obovate or obvate-oblong and acute. Inflorescence are covered with woolly tomentum. The flowers are purplish-red and silvery outside with odour; buds are hemispherical. The fruits are about 6.5-9.5 x 2.5-5.0 cm and recurved. Seeds are numerous, ovoid and 0.6 cm long with a bright silky white coma.

Flowering and furiting is during February - September.

Distribution : This is known to occur more or less throughout India in warm dry places from the Punjab to Western, Central and Southern India. Abundant in the Sub-Himalayan tracts and the adjacent plains in the North-East.

Parts used : The flowers, leaves, latex and root-bark are used for the medicinal purpose.

Medicinal uses : Its flowers are known as digestive, stomachic and tonic and are useful in asthma, cold, cough and anorexia. A powder of its flowers with black pepper is given with ashes of barley seeds in cholera. The leaves are roasted and are applied to painful joints or swellings. The powder of leaves boiled in sweet oil is used in skin eruptions, eczema, toothache, ulcers and wounds. The tinctures of its leaves is given in intermittent fever. The latex obtained from the plant is considered irritant and purgative. It produces abortion when a stick smeared with it is applied locally to induce uterine contractions. It is given orally with 'gur' in bite of rabid dog and is also used in piles along with powdered 'javakhar' and 'batasha'. Besides, its root bark is considered antidysenteric, antispasmodic, diaphoretic, emetic, expectorant and purgative and is used in piles and syphilis and its paste is applied in hydrocele and elephantiasis.

ASHOKA

***Saraca asoca* (Roxb.) De Wilde**

(Syn. *S. indica* auct. non Linn.)

(Family: Fabaceae)

Description : It is a small evergreen tree about 5-8 m in height. The bark is with warty surface and dark brown to grey or almost black. Leaves are equally pinnate and 15-20 cm long; leaflets 6-12, oblong-lanceolate, glabrous and 7.5-20.5 x 1.3 cm. The flowers are orange or orange-yellow and very fragrant and are borne in axillary corymbs. Pods are flat, oblong, woody and 7.5-25.0 × 3.8-5.0 cm. Seeds are ellipsoid-oblong and compressed.

Flowering is in March-April and fruiting during August-September.

Distribution : It grows wild along streams or in shady evergreen forest upto an altitude of 750 m in Central and Eastern Himalayas as well as in the Khasi, Garo and Lushai hills.

Parts used : The stem-bark, flowers and seeds are used.

Medicinal uses : Its stem-bark is used to cure colic, dysentery, dyspepsia, piles, ulcers and uterine problems, particularly in menorrhagia due to uterine fibroids, leucorrhoea and menstrual pain. The flowers are pounded and used in blood dysentery, diabetes, as excellent uterine tonic and in syphilis. Besides, its seeds are considered diuretic and their powder is given in gravels and strangury.

Its bark is adulterated with that of *Polyalthia longifolia* and the fruits are chewed as substitute of areca fruits.

ASHWAGANDHA

Withania somnifera Dunal

(Family: Solanaceae)

Description : It is an erect and much-branched perennial undershrub about 0.5-2.0 m high with glutinous cell sap. Leaves are entire, ovate, subacute and 4.0-15.0 x 2.5 - 6.0 cm. Flowers are in 3-5-flowered axillary fascicles. Berries, the fruits are red and globose and are enclosed in the much enlarged, inflated, membranous, 5-angled and pubescent calyx and about 0.6 cm across. The seeds are numerous, discoid, 0.25 cm across and yellow.

Flowering is in July - August and fruiting during January-February.

Distribution : It occurs throughout the drier and subtropical parts of India.

Parts used : The fruits, seeds, leaves and roots are used.

Medicinal uses : The fruits of the plant are used as diuretic and in chest complaints. Its seeds are hypnotic and diuretic and are used in chest complaints and cogulating milk. Leaves are antipyretic, anthelmintic and bitter and after bruising these are applied in carbuncles, scabies, ulcers and painful swellings and their fomentation is used for sore eyes and swollen hands and feet. The roots are said to be adaptogenic, aphrodisiac, deobstruent, alterative, diuretic and tonic and are used in cough, dropsy, leucorrhoea, hiccough, menstrual problems, to restore loss of memory, in nervous exhaustion, spermatorrhoea and seminal debility. The powder of its root is given daily with sugar, honey and long pepper in the doses of 1.7 gm in spermatorrhoea and debility. A decoction of the roots are used with long pepper, ghee and honey in scrofula and consumption. The root is also used for toning up the uterus of women who is habitual of miscarriage.

According to Wahid and Siddiqui (1961), the plant is also used is unani system of medicine.

ASHWATHA

***Ficus religiosa* Linn.**

(Family: Moraceae)

Description : It is a large or medium-sized deciduous tree with speading branches and about 10-12 m high. Bark is grey with brownish specks, smooth and 1.3 cm thick. Trunks are irregularly shaped. Leaves are alternate, 10.0-17.5 x 7.5-12.5 cm, broadly ovate or rotund, caudate and somewhat pendulous; upper surface glaucous, 5-7 veined and long petioled. Male flowers are very few and sessile: sepals 3, stamen 1 and filament short. Female and gall flowers: sepals 5, style short and lateral. Fruits are sessile in axillary pairs, depressed-globose, 1.3 cm across and dark purple when ripe.

Flowering is during summer and fruiting in rainy season.

Distribution : It is found wild or cultivated throughout India; also as an avenue tree, or along road-sides. It is an important host-plant for the summer brood of lac insects and epiphytic when young.

Parts used : The fruits, seeds, leaves and bark are often used.

Medicinal uses : Its bark is astringent and is used in gonorrhoea. Pulverised bark is applied externally on unhealthy ulcer and wounds to promote granulation and found very effecaceous when rubbed with honey to apthous sores of children. The dried bark in powdered form is used in anal fistula and in the form of a paste, as an absorbent in inflammatory swellings. Tender and fresh leaves are beneficial when used alongwith butter fat to cover the inflammatory ulcers. The oil medicated with its leaves is used as eardrops in earache. Leaves and its twigs are also used as laxative. The fruits are also used as mild laxative and digestive. The seeds are laxative and in powder form these are given for three days during menses as to sterilize women if given for long time. Besides, various parts of the plant are used in otitis media, suppurativa, mouth sores, atrophy, emaciation or cachexy, rheumatism, small pox, carbuncle, mucus in urine, spermatorrhoea, gravel, cholera and rinderpest.

According to Bhandari (1993), its bark along with the barks of *F. virens, F. racemosa, F. bengalensis* and *Azadirachta indica*, pass by the name *panchaval kala*, is used in combination for gargle in salivation, as a wash for ulcers and as a injection in leucorrhoea. Water in which the freshly burnt bark has been steeped is said to cure the case of obstinate hiccup. The powder of the dried bark is also used in anal fistula. For the purpose, *hakim* introduced a metallic tube something like a blow-pipe into the fistula and putting a small quantity of the powder into it, blew the same into the fisula.

ATIVISHA

Aconitum heterophyllum Wall. ex. Royle

(Family: Ranunculaceae)

Description : It is a perennial, erect and showy herb with about 30 - 90 cm height. The stems are simple or branched from base, glabrous and puberulous above, broad, ovate or orbicular or somewhat 5-lobed and toothed, above 3-fid or entire. The flowers are 2.5 cm long, blue or greenish blue with purple veins and helmet shaped.

Flowering is in July-August and fruiting during October-December.

Distribution : It is common in subalpine and alpine Himalayas of Sikkim and adjoining Tibet between 3300 - 4600 m.

Parts used: Dried tuberous roots are used.

Medicinal uses : The roots of the plant are considred aphrodisiac, digestive, febrifuge and bitter tonic and are used in throat infections, abdominal pain and gastralgia in the doses of 0.7-2.0 gm. A plain powder of its roots mixed with honey is given to children suffering from cough, coryza, in fever and vomiting.

BAKUCHI

***Psoralea corylifolia* Linn.**

(Family : Fabaceae)

Description : It is an erect, annual herb about 0.5-1.2 m high with grooved stem and branches. Leaves are simple, 3.5-7.5 x 2.5-5.0 cm, broadly elliptic and inciso-dentate. Flowers are bluish purple or yellow in axillary long - peduncled heads. Pods are indehiscent, ovate, mucronate, somewhat compressed and about 0.5 cm long. Seed is one, smooth and adhering to the pericarp.

Flowering and fruiting is during April-June.

Distribution : It is found wild on road sides and waste places almost throughout the India.

Parts used : Seeds of the plant are used.

Medicinal uses : Its seeds are considered deobstruent, anthelmintic, stomachic, diuretic and diaphoretic and are used in febrile conditions, leprosy, leucoderma and other cutaneous diseases. The powder of its seeds is recommended much by the *Vaidyas* in leprosy and leucoderma internally and in the form of a paste, these are applied externally. Besides, an ointment prepared by mixing one part of an alcoholic extract of its seeds with two parts of Chaulmogra oil and two parts of lanoline, is rubbed once or twice daily in leucoderma, white leprosy, psoriasis and other skin diseases and febrile conditions.

BAKUL

***Mimusops elengi* Linn.**

(Family: Cucurbitaceae)

Description : It is a large evergreen tree with about 16 m height and dark grey bark. Leaves are coriaceous, shining, elliptic and glabrous with undulate margins. The flowers are white and fragrant in axillary fascicles of 2-6 flowers and drooping. The fruits are ovoid, 1.7-2.0 cm long and 1-seeded berries and are reddish-yellow when ripe.

Flowering is in March-April and fruiting during April - June.

Distribution: It is found cultivated throughout the tropical India, particularly in Deccan Penninsula and Andamanns; also planted along road-sides.

Parts used : Seeds, flowers, fruits, bark and leaves are used.

Medicinal uses : Its seeds are knwon as purgative and after brushing they are applied locally within the anus of children in cases of constipation. Its powder of the seeds is used as snuff to relieve headache. Its flowers are used as astringent. The flowers and fruits together with other astringents are used in a lotion for wounds and ulcers. Its fruit-pulp is considered astringent and is used in curing chronic dysentery and the bark is astringent, febrifuge and tonic and is useful in fevers and is also given internally to increase fertility in women. Besides, the decoction of the bark is used as a gargle in the diseases of gums.

BALA

***Sida cordifolia* Linn.**

(Family: Malvaceae)

Description : It is a small erect, branched and stellate-tomentose herb or shrub. Leaves are ovate-oblong to cordate and very downy on both surfaces. Petioles are as long as the blade. The flowers are yellow and small and are borne solitary or in fascicles. Capsules, the fruits are 0.7 - 0.8 cm in diameter.

Flowering and fruiting is during August - December.

Distribution : It grows wild throughout the tropical and subtropical India, ascending upto 1050 m.

Parts used : The entire plant is used.

Medicinal uses : The juice of entire plant mixed with water is given in rheumatism, gonorrhoea and spermatorrhoea. Its seeds are considered aphrodisiac and are useful in colic, tenesmus and gonorrhoea. An infusion of its leaves is prescribed as febrifuge and also as vegetable to patients suffering from piles. Its roots ae considrered astringent, diuretic and tonic and their infusion is given successfully in nervous and urinary diseases, cystitis, strangury, bleeding piles, haematuria, leucorrhoea, chronic dysentery and in asthma as cardiac tonic. The juice of its roots is used in healing of wounds. A strong decoction of its roots is used as diaphoretic, antipyretic, stomachic and tonic. The roots mixed with asafoetida and rock salt are given in hemiplagia, facial paralysis, stiff necks and noises in the ear with headache. Besides, a paste of its roots made with juice of Palmyra palm is used in elephantiasis.

Its root-bark with sesamum oil and milk is in used facial paralysis and sciatica and in powder form, is given with milk and sugar for the relief in micturition and leucorrhoea.

BANAFSHA

***Viola odorata* Linn.**

(Family: Violaceae)

Description : This is a small glabrate or pubescent perennial herb with short tufted root stock. The root is as thick as a crow's quill, crooked, with a number of radicals having a spongy bark. Leaves are all radical, ovate, 1.2-2.5 cm in diameter and toothed. The flowers are violet coloured and aromatic and become brown or brownish-yellow when old.

Flowering and fruiting is during March-June.

General distribution : It is found distributed in Kashmir Himalayas at an altitude between 1524-1828 m.

Parts used : Panchang (i.e., all five parts viz., roots, stem, leaves, flowers and fruits) and flowers, commonly known as '*Gule banfshah*' are used.

Medicinal uses : The *panchang*, commonly known as '*banafshah*' is aperient, antipyretic, cooling, demulcent, diaphoretic, emollient, expectorant, febrifuge and purgative in action. This is used in piles, asthma, consipation, cough, fever, headache and in skin diseases. Besides, its flowers are considered emollient and demulcent and are used in billiouness, lung problems, prolapse of the rectum and uterus and in restraining suppuranation besides, cough, kidney problems and liver affections.

BARBERRY

***Berberis aristata* DC.**

(Family : Berberidaceae)

Description : It is an erect and glabrous, spinescent shrub attaining a height of 3-6 m. Leaves are acute to obtuse, entire or toothed and elliptic - obovate. Flowers are yellow and are borne in corymbose racemes. Berries, the fruits are bright red and obovid or oblong-obovoid.

Flowering is in April-June and fruiting during August - October.

Distribution : It is almost found in open places along shrubberries in Himalayas between 2000 -3300 m. .

Parts used : Root-bark, stem and fruits are used.

Medicinal uses : The root-bark is known for its alterative and deobstruent properties and is used in skin diseases, menorrhagia, diarrhoea, jaundice and affections of the eyes. A paste of its root-bark is applied externally on ulcers for healing and an extract prepared from root bark is used as a local application in affected parts of the eyelids and opthalmia. The decoction of its root-bark is also given in malarial fever and in enlargement of liver and spleen. The roots of the plant in combination of opium, rocksalt and alum are considered useful antiinflammatory agent. Besides, a decoction of the stems of the plant mixed with that of haldi (*Curcuma longa*) is recommended in gonorrhoea. Its fruits are also given to children as a mild laxative.

Commercially, it is sold in the market under three name viz., *Daruhaldi*, *Rasaut* and *Zirisk*. *Daruhaldi*, is the pieces of 2.5-5.0 cm diameter covered with a soft corky light brown bark beneath this there is a hard layer of stony cells, forming complete coating to the stem and it is marked by longitudinal furrows corresponding to the medullary rays which are prominent and close grained and contain many stony cells. All parts of the wood are impregnated with yellow colouring matter, which is freely soluble in water. Wood extract known, as 'rasaut' is a dark brown extract of the consistency of opium, having a bitter and astringent taste and is readily soluble in water. Zirisk is a moist mass of small black and almost abortive fruits but some of them may contain one or two seeds with a thin roughish testa beneath which is a membraneous covering exist.

BAYBERRY

***Mryica esculènta* Buch.-Ham.ex D. Don.**

(Syn. *M. nagi* Hook. f.)

(Family: Myricaceae)

Description : It is a small or medium sized, evergreen tree with rough and brownish-grey bark reaching a height of 3-15 m. Leaves are oblong-obovate, lanceolate, serrate, crowded at the end of branches and 7.5-15.0 x 2.5-5.0 cm. Flowers are unisexual in axillary spikes. Male spikes are 0.7 cm long and arranged recemosely on a common axillary stalk and female spikes are erect, axillary and 1.3-2.5 cm long. The drupes are ellipsoid or ovoid, reddish or cheese coloured when ripe and composed of spindle shaped fleshy fibres radiating from rugose nut.

Flowering is during October - November and fruiting later.

Distribution : This is found abundantly in subtropical Himalayas between 2100-3500 m, Khasia Hills and Sylhet.

Parts used: Thé bark, seeds and fruits of the plant are used medicinally.

Medicinal uses : In ayurveda, its bark is described as acrid, bitter and pungent and is used to cure '*kapha*' and '*vata*' diseases, asthma, fever, piles bronchitis, anaemia, dysentery and ulcers and in Unani system of medicine, the bark is known to possess astringent, bitter, carminative and tonic properties and is used for liver complaints, headache, inflammations, piles, gleet and in chronic bronchitis and also as uterine stimulant. It is chewed to get relief in toothache and a lotion prepared from it, is used to wash sores. An oil prepared from its bark, is dropped into ear in earache and the pessaries made of its bark are used to promote menses. A paste of its seeds with stimulant balsams is mixed with ginger and is used externally as a rubefacient application to fore arms, calves and extremities during collapse stages of cholera and with asafoetida and camphor is applied over piles successfully. Besides, its fruits yield a wax, which is externally used for healing ulcers.

BHALLATAKA

***Semecarpus anacardium* Linn.**

(Family: Anacardiaceae)

Description : It is a medium-sized, dioecious and deciduous tree with rough dark-coloured bark. Its young branches, inflorescences and undersides of leaves are clothed with fine pale pubescent. Leaves are crowded towards the extremities of the branches and are large, oblong-obovate, rounded at apex, cartilagious at margin and coriaceous. Flowers are greenish-yellow, fasciculate and are arranged in erect, compound and terminal panicles. The drupes are about 2.5 cm long, obliquely oval or oblong, smooth, shining and purplish-black and are seated in an orange cup.

Flowering is during May-June and fruiting in Novermber-February.

Distribution : It is known to occur in Sub – Himalayn tracts form the Beas eastwards, ascending in the outer hills upto 1200 m, Assam, Khasia hills, Chittagong, Central India, Gujarat, Konkan, South Maharashtra and Kanara and deciduous forest of the Chennai.

Parts used : Fruits and bark are the parts, used medicinally.

Medicinal uses : Its fruits are used in asthma, ascites, epilepsy, neuralgia, psoriasis and rheumatism and also as abortifacient and vermifuge. A decoction of its fruits mixed with milk and butterfat is used efficaciously in asthma, gout, hemiplegia, sciatica and syphilis. Its fruits are bruised and are applied to *os uteri* to procure abortion and also given as vermifuge. Oil obtained from its nuts is used as vesicant and externally in rheumatism and leprous nodules. A paste containing equal parts of the juice of its nuts, *Plumbago zeylanica, Baliospermum montamum, Euphorbia ligularia, Calotropis gigantea,* sulphate of iron and molasses, is applied over scrofulous glands of the neck. Besides, ripe fruits are boiled with cow's dung, washed and mixed with butter to purify and then used internally in dyspepsia, nervous debility and skin diseases; also given to relieve asthmatic attacks. A brownish gum exudate obtained from bark is found useful in nervous debility and in leprous, scrofulous and venereal diseases.

BHANG

***Cannabis sativa* Linn.**

(Family : Cannabinaceae)

Description : It is a tall annual herb, about 1.2-4.9 m high with angular stem. Leaves are palmate, alternate or lower one opposite and 5.0-20.0 cm long; the lobes of of the upper leaves are 1-5 and in lower 5-11, linear laneeolate, sharpely toothed, long-pointed and narrowed at base. The flowers are small, greenish and unisexual. The males are borne in long dropping panicles and female in short axillary spikes. The fruits are 0.3 cm across, ovate and flat and are enclosed in persistent perianth.

Flowering and fruiting is during March-May.

Distribution : It is a native of Central and Western Asia, now naturalized in the Sub-Hamalayan tract and abundant in wastelands from Punjab Eastwards to Bengal and Bihar extending Southwards. Commonly occurs in waste places, along roadsides and becomes gregarious along irrigation chanels. Cultivated also in Almora, Garhwal and Nainital etc. in Uttaranchal for the narcotic drug.

Parts used : The seeds, leaves, dried flowering or fruiting tops of the female plant and resionous exudate, are used for medicinal purposes.

Medicinal uses: The plant is considered as tonic, analgesic and antiseptic and is useful in gonorrhoea, menorrhagia, diarrhoea, cholera, hydrophobia, tetanus and rheumatism. Its leaves are used in ear troubles and their juice is applied on cuts after mixing with sugar. The juice of leaves is also used to destroy the worms and vermin. The crushed leaves are applied on skin in skin diseases. The chronic use of cannabis is also said to be useful in patients of diabetic hypertension. The leaves are also used as snuff and are given internally about 2.5 gm per day to relieve pain and swelling orchitis.

Narcotic drugs *Bhang, Ganja* (Marijuana) and the *Hashish* (Charas) are prepared from this plant. *Bhang*, deep green in colour, consists of its dried leaves. Female flowering tops of the plant are stimulant, sedative and antispasmodic and the *Ganja* is prepared from those dried flowering or fruiting tops of female plants from which no resin has been removed. *Charas* is the resinous exudate from leaves, which has a powerful smell and dark green or brown in colour. *Bhang* and *Ganja* are used as appetizer and nervous stimulant and in bowel complaints. Bhang is made into a paste with water then is mixed with milk and sugar and is taken as intoxicating liquor producing euphoria. *Charas* is used for soothing activity in cases of mania and hysteria and also in asthma and tetanus. Like opium, it does not produce loss of appetite or constipation.

BHARANGI

Clerodendrum serratum **(Linn.) Moon**

(Family : Verbenaceae)

Description : It is an erect shrub with thick woody rootstocks. Leaves are sessile, usually in whorls of 3, 10.0-20.0 × 4.0 - 6.0cm, oblong-elliptic or obovate with a subcordate or rounded base and glabrous. The flowers are bluish or purplish-white and are borne in axillary cymes forming a terminal leafy panicle. The fruit is a succulent drupe which is globose and black when ripe.

Flowering is during May -August and fruiting in September-November.

Distribution : It grows more or less throughout India.

Parts used : Whole plant is used.

Medicinal uses : The roots of the plant are bitter, acrid, thermogenic, anti-inflammatory, digestive, carminative, stomachic, anthelmintic, depurative, expectorant, sudorific, antispasmodic, stimulant and febrifuge and their decoction is given for asthma, bronchitis and other catarrhal affections of the lungs. Its leaves are used in fevers and boiled with oil and butter are made into an ointment which is applied externally in cephalagia and ophthalmia. Besides, the plant is also used in dropsy, anasarca, rheumatism, hemiplegia, sores, prolapus ani, fistula ani, cholera and rinderpest.

BHRINGRAJ

Eclipta prostrata **(Linn.) Linn.**

(Syn. *E. alba* (Linn.) Hassk.; *Verbesina prostrata* Linn.)

(Family: Brassicaceae)

Description : It is a prostrate, decumbent - ascending or erect, annual or perennial herb. Stems are creeping and rooting at the base. Leaves are sessile, ovate - lanccolate, elliptic - oblong or oblong, acute or obtuse, narrowed to the base and entire or serrate. The floral heads are axillary and terminal and 0.6 - 1.0 cm across on 5.0- 7.0 cm long peduncles. Involucral bracts are 2-seriate, ovate-lanceolate, acute, and appressed-pubescent and 0.3-0.6 cm long. Marginal flowers are white and with 2-dentate and 0.25 cm long ligules. The fruits are achenes, oblong - turbinate and tuberculate with thickened margins and about 0.2 cm long.

Flowering and fruting is during the greater parts of the year.

Distribution : The plant is found distributed throughout India upto 1980 m in the Himalayas.

Parts used : The whole plant is useful.

Medicinal uses : The entire plant is used as tonic and deobstruent in hepatic and spleen enlargement and as emetic. A juice of entire plant in combination with aromatics is administrated for catarrhal jaundice. Its roots are emetic and purgative and are applied externally as antiseptic to ulcers and wounds of cattles.The juice of its leaves along with honey is used as a remedy to catarrh in infants. Crude extract of gum resin from herb possesses anticancerous activity against Ehrlich ascites carcinoma. The pulp of the bruised herb roasted in ghee is applied to wounds and burns. The powder of the herb cure patients suffering from infective hepatitis. Besides, the aqueous extract of the herb is myocardial depressant and hypotensive and their juice is used to cure shoulder pain caused by carrying heavy loads.

The fresh plant mixed with sesamum oil is externally applied in elephantiasis and the juice of the plant in anus to remove anal worms.

BHUMYAMALAKI

Phyllanthus fraternus Webster

(Syn *P. niruri* sensu Hook. f.)

(Family: Euphorbiaceae)

Description : It is an erect and glabrous annual herb about 10-30 cm high. Leaves are subsessile, elliptic-oblong or linear-oblong, dark green above, glaucous on the lower surface, 0.5-2.0 × 0.2-0.5 cm. The flowers are axillary and yellowish or whitish. The male flowers are 1-3, stamens 3, disk-lobes 6, glandular. The female flowers are soliary, and style free, appressed to the ovary. The fruits are depressed, globose, smooth capsules, which are 0.2-0.3 cm across. Seeds are trigonous, brown with 6-7 straight longitudinal ribs.

Flowering and fruiting is during May-September.

Distribution : It is common throughout India in hotter parts from the Punjab to Assam and south wards to Travancore, ascending the hills upto 914 m.

Parts used : The whole plant is used.

Medicinal uses : The whole plant as antipyretic, antiseptic, astringent, cooling, deobstruent and diuretic and it is useful in dropsy, gastro-intestinal problems as colic, diarrhoea, dysentery, dyspepsia, gonorrhoea, menorrhagia, and other gential diseases and in jaundice. The decoction of entire plant is given in jaundice and gonorrhoea and the juice as an efficaceous dressing is applied for offensive sores and mixed with some bland oil is used in opthalmia. Its leaves are stomachic and diuretic and after mixing with salt are applied locally to skin affections, swellings and ulcers in the form of a poulitice. A decoction of the leaves is used as refrigerant for the scalp. Its leaves boiled with milk are given in dropsical disorders and urinary complaints and the infusion of its young shoots is given in dysentry. Besides, its fresh roots are given in jaundice, with rice water in menorrhagia and with milk as a galactagogue.

BIBHITAKA

***Terminalia bellirica* (Gaertn.) Roxb.**

(Syn. *T. bellirica* var. *laurinoides* Cl.; *Myrobalanus bellirica* Gaertn.)

(Family: Combretaceae)

Description : It is a large deciduous tree with bluish or ashey-grey bark and about 20-25 m high. Leaves are clustered at the ends of the branchlets and are coriaceous, pale beneath, broad elliptic or obovate-elliptic, 8.0-20.0 cm long and often with unequal base. The petiole is 2.5-7.5 cm long and usually glandular. Spikes are slender, interrupted and 8.0-15.0 cm long. The flowers are about 1.25 cm across and dirty-grey or greenish-yellow with offensive smell. The fruits are 2.5 cm long, ovoid, ellipsoidal or globose and grey velvety with 5, more or less indistinct furrows. The nuts are thick walled and hard.

Flowering is during April-June and fruiting in December-January.

Distribution : It is found distributed throughout the forest of India upto 914 m elevations and along the foot hills of the Himalayas.

Parts used : Fruits, bark and gum are used.

Medicinal uses : Its fruits are considered bitter, astringent, tonic, laxative, antipyretic and antidiarrhoeal and are used in piles, dyspepsia, leprosy, billousness, headache, hoarseness and eye diseases. The ripe ones are used as an astringent in combination with chebulic myrobalan and half ripen fruits are used as a purgative. The oil obtained from its fruits is applied to hairs and rheumatic swellings. The fruits pulp mixed with honey is used in opthalmia. However, the excessive eating of the seed pulp may cause intoxication.

Besides, the kernels of its fruits are used as narcotics; the bark as diuretic and gum yielded by the tree as demulcent and purgative.

BILWA

Aegle marmelos Correa ex Roxb.

(Family : Rutaceae)

Description : This is a small or medium-sized deciduous and aromatic tree about 10 m high with straight sharp, axillary and 2.5 cm long spines. Leaves are trifoliolate, with 2.5-6.0 cm long and terete petiole; leaflets are ovate-lanceolate, lateral sessile, terminal long and acuminate, 5.0-10.0 × 2.5-6.0 cm, cuneate to obtuse at the base. The flowers are greenish-white, sweet scented and about 2.5 cm in diameter and are borne in axillary panicles. Fruits are 5.0-10.0 cm across, globose, grey or greyish-yellow, hard with orange coloured sweet pulp. Seeds are numerous, oblong and compressed and are embedded in aromatic pulp; testa woolly and mucilaginous.

Flowering is during April-May and fruiting in March-April in next year.

Distribution : The plant is common throughout India in dry hilly areas, gardens and along road-sides; also cultivated in various places in India, especially near temples.

Parts used : Fruits, seeds, flowers, leaves, bark and roots are usable.

Medicinal uses : The ripe fruits of the plant are alterative, cooling, laxative and nutritive and are useful in habitual constipation, chronic dysentery and dyspepsia. Its unripe fruits are used as antidiarrhoeal, astringent, demulcent, digestive and stomachic. Its seeds are used as laxative. The flowers are used as antidiarrhoeal and antitematic and the leaves as expectorant, febrifuge and the fresh ones in dropsy and effectively in bronchial asthma. Its fresh leaf-extract is reported to reduce the period of convalescence in patients suffering from cholera or cholearic diarrhoea. The leaf-juice is applied externally in abscess and their ash is to kill worms and injuries caused by animals. Besides, the bark of the root and that of stem is beneficially used in intermittent fever, melancholia, palpitation of heart and in stomach pain.

The pulp of its fresh fruits mixed with milk when administered with Cubeb powder acts as diuretic and astringent on the mucuous membranes of the generative organs, therefore, useful in gonorrhoea.

BLACK PEPPER

***Piper nigrum* Linn.**

(Family: Piperaceae)

Description: This is a climbing and perennial shrub with stout and trailing branches, which roots at the base. Leaves are entire, 12.5-17.5 x 5.0-12.5 cm, cordate or rounded and equal or unequal with acute base and sometimes glaucous beneath. The flowers are minute, borne in spikes and are usually dioecious but female often bears anthers and male a pistillode. Fruits are globose or ovoid and bright red when ripe. The seeds are usually globose with hard albumin and thin testa.

Flowering is in the rainy season and fruiting during autumn.

Distribution: It is found wild from North Kanara to Kanyakumari; also cultivated in Assam, Karnataka, Kerala and Maharashtra.

Parts used : Its fruits are used medicinally.

Medicinal uses: The fruits of the plant are known to have aromatic, astringent and stomachic properties and are used in the treatment of dyspepsia, flatulence, malarial fever, paralysis and arthritis. Externally, these also find a useful application in sore throat, piles and skin diseases.

BRAHMI

***Centella asiatica* (Linn.) Urban**
(Syn. *Hydrocotyle asiatica* Linn.)
(Family: Apiaceae)

Description : It is a prostrate perennial herb. Stem is creeping with long stolons and nearly glabrous or hairy on young parts. Leaves are long-petioled, reniform or orbicular, crenate and lobed and glabrous. The flowers are 3-6 and are borne in umbel in the axils of small bracts and purple whites. The fruits are sub-cylindric, curved, slightly compressed, reticulate and 0.2 x 0.3 cm and each is with 9 curvilinear subsimilar ridges within the commissure.

Flowering is in July - August and fruiting later on during October - December.

Distribution : It is found throughout in India in marshy places upto 1828 m.

Parts used : The whole plant is used.

Medicinal uses : The juice of its leaves is given in fever and is also useful in cataract and other eye problems; also taken as tonic for improving memory and both externally as well as internally are useful in syphilitic skin diseases. The leaves are known to contain an alkaloid which produces toxic symptoms similar to those of strychnine; the leaves also have diuretic action.

Besides, the plant is also useful in treatment of swollen painfull joints as external application and internelly is used as alterative and tonic in diseases of skin, nerves and blood.

BRIHATI

***Solanum ferox* Linn.**

(Syn. *S. indicum* Linn.)

(Family: Solanaceae)

Description : It is an erect, stellate-tomentose and armed herb or undershrub. Stems are acuteate with hooked prickles.

Leaves are ovate-oblong, sinuate-pinnatifid with subcordate or rounded or truncate base, subacute or obtuse, stellate-pubescent and 6.0-12.0 x 5.0-8.0 cm. The flowers are in lateral cymose corymbs. The fruits are orange-yellow, fulvous, 0.8 cm across and spreading. Seeds are 0.2 cm across and smooth.

Flowering and fruiting can be seen throughout the year.

Distribution : It occurs throughout India ascending upto 1524 m on the Himalayas.

Parts used : Fruits, roots and seeds are used medicinally.

Medicinal uses : The fruits are used in asthma, chest pain, cough, dropsy, rheumatism and sore-throat. Its roots are considered carminative and expectorant and are used in difficult parturition, toothache, fevers, worm complaints, colic, dysuria and inchuria. Besides, the seeds are used as appetizer.

CALAMUS

***Acorus calamus* Linn.**

(Famliy: Araceae)

Description : It is a semi-aquatic plant with underground stem and rootstocks. Leaves are bright green, acute, thickened in the middle with wavy margins and 0.9-1.8 cm long. Spathe is 15-75 cm long and spadix is 5.0-10.0 x 1.3-2.0 cm, obtuse and slightly curved. Sepals are as long as the ovary and scarious; anthers yellow. The fruits are turbinate and prismatic with pyramidal tips.

Flowering is during June-July and fruiting later.

Distribution: This is found almost throughout India in marshy places, ascending in the Himalayas up to 1828 m in the Sikkim.

Parts used: Its rhizomatous rootstocks are used medicinally.

Medicinal uses: In ayurveda, its rootstocks are known to possess anthelmintic, bitter, carminative, diuretic, emetic, laxative and pungent properties and are used to improve appetite and in abdominal pains, inflammations, fevers, epilepsy, bronchitis, delirium, hysteria and dysentery; whereas in Unani system of medicine, its rootstocks are described as alexiteric, carminative, expectorant and laxative and are used for general weakness, stomatitis, leucoderma and kidney problems. An infusion of rootstocks of this plant is given in dyspepsia, flatulence and in loss of appetite; also in hysteria and neuralgia and as antispasmodic in tertiary fevers. This is administered with liquorices in cough, fever, capillary bronchitis and colic. In cases of irritation of throat and cough, its rootstocks are simply chewed to copious salivation. Besides, these with *bhang* and *ajowain* in equal parts are used as a fumigation to get relieve in painful piles.

CAMPHOR

***Cinnamomum camphora* (Linn.) Nees & Eberm.**

(Family: Lauraceae)

Description : It is a tall evergreen tree with about 30 m height and 1.5-2.5 m girth in wild state. The bark is aromatic, rough from outside and smooth inside. Wood is yellowish-brown and strongly aromatic. Leaves are coriaceous, glaucous, aromatic; usually 3-veined and 5.0-10.0 cm long. The flowers are small and unisexual; female flowers are usually larger than the males. The fruits are seated on more or less enlarged perianth and are globose, ovoid, 0.6 cm across and aromatic. All parts of the plant possess special odour.

Flowering is in March-April and fruiting in July-August.

Distribution : A native of Japan, China, and Taiwan, now got naturalized and is planted some gardens in India upto 1200 m in the North Western Himalayas.

Parts used: The wood and leaves are used.

Medicinal uses : The camphor is considered as sedative, anodyne, antiseptic, diaphoretic, anthelmintic, stimulant and carminative and is used in insecticidal preparations. The vapours of camphor are inhaled in cold and affections of chest. A liniment prepared by dissolving one part of camphor in four parts of olive oil, is used externally in muscular strains, rheumatism and inflammations. The camphor is also used against carbuncles. The camphor now a days is prepared synthetically also.

According to Singh (1983), the camphor is obtainted naturally from *Cinnamomum camphora*, besides, it is also obtained from *Dryobalanops aromaticus* and *Ocimum killimau-oscharicum*.

About 0.2 gm camphor is mixed with 0.02 gm of opium and made into pills. One pill daily is used at night for spermatorrhoea and polyuria. The camphor mixed with 'gulabjal' is dropped in nostrils in nose bleeding. In asthma, camphor in 0.2 gm doses with equal quantity of asafoetida is made into pills, which are taken after every second or third hour during a paroxysm, and affords in some instances great relief. These pills also sometimes relieve violent palpitation of the heart. In cough of children, camphor liminent previously warmed, is rubbed over chest at nights gives relief. In painful affection of the uterus, camphor in 0.3-0.4 gm gives much relief. In advanced stages of fever,, smallpox and measles when the patient is low, weak and exhausted and when at the same time there is delirium, muttering and sleeplessness, 0.1 gm of camphor with an equal parts of asafoetida may be given after every third hour and turpentine stupes or mustard poultice being applied to the feet or over heart portion at the same time give much relief. But it should be used with great caution and discontinued if cause headache or increased heat of the scalp. Besides, its young sprouts and young leaves are eaten boiled and old leaves are dried and powdered and are used as a spice.

CARDAMOM

Elettaria cardamomum Mat.

(Family: Zingiberaceae)

Description: It is a somewhat woody or fleshy and branching plant with 1.8-2.7 m high stem, which is clothed below with spongy sheaths. Leaves are subsessile, 30.0-60.0 x 7.5 cm and oblong-lanceolate. Panicles are numerous to one leafy stem, 30.0-60.0 cm long; bracts linear-oblong, persistent, 3.8-5.0 cm long. Capsules, the fruits are subglobose or oblong, about 1.3 cm long and marked with many fine vertical ribs.

Flowering is during April-June and fruiting in October-December.

Distribution: It is found wild or cultivated in the Malabar area and the Western Ghats between 900-1500 m.

Parts used: Its seeds, roots and the fruits are used.

Medicinal uses: In ayurveda, its seeds are known for their bitter, cooling, fragrant and pungent proepeties and are used as abortifacient, to clear the head, brain and the mouth and also in asthma, bronchits, piles, pruuitus, stanguary, scabies and the diseases of the kidney, rectum and in throat problems. The seeds are also used in compound preparations. Besides, the roots and fruits are also used in medicines because of their laxative and tonic properties. Its fruits are internally administered in the diseases of the liver and the uterus and externally are applied to tumours of the uterus.

CASTOR

Ricinus communis Linn.

(Family: Euphorbiaceae)

Description : It is a tall glabrous and glaucous annual shrub reaching a height upto 4.0 m. Leaves are palmately 7-many lobed; lobes are oblong to linear, acute or acuminate and gland-serratted. The flowers are large and monoecious in terminal subpanicled racemes. Fruits are capsules of 3-2-valved cocci, globosely oblong and smooth or echinate. The seeds are oblong, smooth and mottled.

Flowering and fruiting is during the greater part of the year, chiefly in winter.

Distribution : It is a native of Africa, now cultivated

almost thronghout the India in gardens and field; also runs wild in waste lands.

Parts used : The seeds, leaves and root-bark are used.

Medicinal uses : Its seeds are purgative and couter-irritant and are said to be used in scorpion-sting and as fish poison. An oil, derived from the seeds known as castor oil, in a doses of 5-20 ml is used as a purgative; and the seed-paste as a poultice is applied on sores and gout or rheumatic swellings. Its leaves are known for their anodyne and galactogogue propereties and externally are applied to boils and sores in the form of a poultice. Besides, its root -bark is considered emetic and purgative and is used in lumbago and in skin diseases; also effective in reducing fat of the body.

CATECHU

***Acacia catechu* (Linn.) Willd.**

(Family: Fabaceae)

Description : It is a moderate-sized tree with thorny branches. Bark is rough, dark, grey or greyish-brown and about 1.2 cm thick, exploiting in long narrow strips. Leaves are 10.0-17.5 cm long, pinnate with a pair of recurved prickles at base of rachis and pinnae 40-80; leaflets are 60-100 small and ligulate. Flowers are pale-yellow in axillary cylindrical spikes. Pods, the fruits are thin, glabrous, lustrous, straight, star-shaped, dark brown and 5-6 seeded. The seeds are flat, dark-brown and orbicular.

Flowering is in rainy season and fruiting during November-January.

Distribution : It occurs in drier regions of Sub-Himalayan tract upto an altitude of 1200 m from Punjab to North-Eastern states, Madhya Pradesh, Gujarat, Andhra Pradesh and Tamil Nadu.

Parts used : The bark and the heartwood, are the parts used generally.

Medicinal uses : Its bark is known as astringent and is

useful in passive diarrhoea usually in combination with cinnamon or opium. The decoction of bark is given internally in leprosy. The *katha*, obtained from heartwood of 20-30 years old trees is astringent, cooling and digestive and is used in relaxed condition of throat, mouth, gums, cough and in diarrhoea. This is also applied externally to ulcers, boils, and eruptious of the skins. In cracked nipples and sores of various etiology, a decoction of bark is used as compresses. For leprosy, the decoction of the entire plant (root, leaf, flower, bark and fruit) can be given as drink with meals along with washing of the affected part with it and application of ointment of catechu to ulcers.

Kheersal, a product met within some older trees in the form of white crystalline deposit of catechism is used for treatment of cough and sore throat. Its decoction with that of *chirayata* is used in spleen enlargement during chronic fever. Besides, a mixture of catechu and myrrh called, *kathbol* is generally given to women after confinement as a tonic and to promote the secretion of milk.

CAYENNE

***Capsicum annum* Linn.**

(Syn. *C. frutescens* sensu Cl.)

(Family: Solanaceae)

Description : It is an erect herb or undershrub. Leaves are entire or repand and ovate. The flowers are white and 2-3 in axillary fascicles. The fruits are red and pungent berries and are variable in form and size. Seeds are many, discoid and smooth or subscabrous.

Flowering and fruiting is almost throughout the year.

Distribution : It ils extensively cultivated throughout India.

Parts used : The fruits are used.

Medicinal uses : Its fruits are considered stimlulant, stomachic, antidiarrhoeal and carminative and are used in atonic dyspepsia, putrid sore throat, scarlatina, hoarseness, yellow diarrhoea and piles. A decoction of its fruits with opium and fried asafoetida is given in cholera. Externally, a paste of the fruits is used as a rubifacient and as a local stimulant for the tonsils in tonsillitis.

CHAKUNDA

***Cassia tora* Linn**

(Family: Fabaceae)

Description : It is an annual bushy foetid herb or undershrub about 30-150 cm high with flexous stem. Leaves are paripinnate and 2.5-3.8 cm long; leaflets ovate - oblong, obtuse rounded and glabrous above. The flowers are small, yellow and 5-6 gogether. Pods, the fruits are slender, sub-4-angled and 12.5-15.0 x 0.8 cm. The seeds are many, dark brown and broadly ovoid.

Flowering and fruiting is throughout the year, chiefly during July - December.

Distribution : It is found distributed throughout the tropical parts of India.

Parts used : Leaves, seeds and root are used.

Medicinal uses : The decoction of leaves is used as laxative. The leaves are pounded and when applied on cuts, act like tincture of iodine; also applied on eczema and other skin diseases. Tender leaves are taken internally to prevent skin diseases. Its leaves are prescribed in decoction form in 60 gm doses for children suffering from feverish attacks while teething and boiled in caster oil they are applied to foul ulcers; also on inflammation caused by any irritant.

Its seeds after boiling with tea are taken for cold and their powder is given in abnormal delivery and with turmeric and mustard oil are used against eczema. Its seeds are steeped in the juice of *Euphorbia nerrifolia* to make a paste with cow's urine, which is applied as an application to cheloid tumours. The seeds are also useful in leprosy and psoriasis, when ground with sour butter milk or lime juice and applied to ease the irritation of itch or skin eruptions. Besides, the roots are rubbed into a paste with lime juice and are used for ring worm; also applied for buboes in plaque. An oil called *Chakramarda* oil containing *Cassia tora* and *Eclipta prostrata* is very useful application in obstinate skin diseases such as ring worm etc.

According to Farooqi (1995), its seed gum, known as Chakunda gum is used as a substitute for Gaur gum.

CHAVYA

Piper chaba Linn.

(Family: Piperaceae)

Description: It is a climbing and glabrous rather flesh shrub. Leaves are oblong, ovate or lancolate, acuminate and cordate with unequal rounded base; nerves at base are 3, with 2 pairs from midrib, 12.5-18.0 x 6.3-7.0 cm. Peduncles are 1.3-2.5 cm long. Fruting spikes are cylindro – conic, widest at the base and bright red, about 2.5-7.5 cm long. The drupes are very small and globose sunk.

Flowering is in rainy season and fruiting during winter.

Distribution: This is cultivated in various parts of the India.

Parts used: Its fruits and the roots are used.

Medicinal uses: The fruits of the plant have stimulant and carminative properties and are used in haemorrhoidal affections. Besides, the roots are known as alexeteric and are used in asthma, bronchitis and consumption; also as carminative, anthelmintic, expectorant and to improve appetite and taste.

The plant is used as a substitute for *Piper longum*.

CHIRETTA

Swertia chirayita (Roxb. ex Flemming) Karsten

(Family: Gentianaceae)

Description: This is an annual herb with subterete stem

reaching a height of 5.0-12.0 cm. Cauline leaves are subsessile, elliptic, acute and 5-nerved; the lower are often much larger and sometimes petioled. Flowers are green-yellow in many-flowered, leafly and large panicles; often fascicled. Capsules, the fruits are sessile and ovate with polyhedral and smooth seeds.

Flowering is during July-August and fruiting in September-October.

Distribution : It is known to found in temperate Himalayas between 1200-3000 m from Kashmir to Bhutan and Khasia Hills.

Parts used : Whole plant is used medicinally.

Medicinal uses : In ayurveda, the plant is known for its antihelmintic, antipyretic, antiperiodic, bitter, cooling, galactagogue and laxative properties and is used to cure asthma, bronchitis, biliousness, burning sensation, inflammations, leucoderma, pain of the body, piles, urinary discharges and ulcers; while in Unani system of medicines, it is considered as astringent, bitter, stomachic and tonic and is used to improve eye sight, as a sedative to pregnant women, pain of joints, leucoderma and skin diseases. An infusion of the plant is generally used as antidiarrhoeal, febrifuge, stomachic and tonic. Besides, the infusion is also taken daily in the morning on an empty stomach to keep fit and healthy.

It is used as a substitute of Quinine (Garg, 1992).

CHITARK

***Plumbago zeylanica* Linn.**

(Family: Plumbaginaceae)

Description : It is an erect or straggling perennial undershrub. The stems are glabrous with diffuse branches. Leaves are alternate, ovate, narrowed into the petiote, acute and 2.5-10.0 x 1.5-6.0 cm. Flowers are white and are borne in terminal and axillary racemes combined into a leafy panicle. Fruits are oblong, acute and longitudinally furrowed capsules, which are a enclosed by persistent viscid calyx.

Flowering is during August - September and fruiting during winter.

Distribution : It is found throughout India including West Bengal, Bihar and Peninsular India; also grown in gardens.

Parts used : Roots and leaves are used.

Medicinal uses : Its roots are used in skin diseases, diarrhoea, dyspepsia, piles and anasarca; also to excite digestion. A paste of its roots with vinegar, milk or salt and water is used externally in leprosy and other skin diseases and also as abortifacient and in rheumatism. In combination with other ingredients, it is prescribed for epilepsy and hysteria, nervous affections, obesity, prurigo and indolent ulcers. An infusion of the roots is used in black-water fever and influenza. Besides, its leaves are also eaten for abortion.

CINNAMOMUM

***Cinnamomum zeylanicum* Blume**

(Family: Lauraceae)

Description: It is a moderate and evergreen tree with rather thick, smooth and pale bark and compressed twigs and glabrous young parts except the buds, which are finely silky. Leaves are opposite or subopposite, rarely alternate, hard and coriaceous, ovate or ovate – lanceolate, subactue or shortly acuminate, glabrous and shining above and 7.5-20.0 x 3.8-7.5 cm with acute or rounded base. Flowers are numerous, in silky–pubescent lax panicles usually longer than the leaves; peduncles long, oftern clustered and glabrous or pubescent. The fruits are 1.3-1.7 cm long, oblong or ovoid – oblong, minutely apiculate, dry or slightly freshy and dark purple surrounded by the enlarged camapnulate perianth.

Flowering is in January-February and fruiting during May-August.

Distribution: It is found wild in the southern coastal regions of western India upto 2000 m; also cultivated in southern parts of the country.

Parts used : The bark is used.

Medicinal uses: In ayruveda, the bark of the plant is described as anthelmitic, aphrodisiac, bitter, pungent and tonic. It is used to cure *vata* diseases, biliousness, thrist, parched mouth, bronchitis, diarrhea, itching and the diseases of the heart and rectum and that of urinary tracts. An oil obtained from its bark is used as styptic, carminateive and in the loss of appetite, flatulence, eructations, vomting and toothache.

CINNAMOMUM LEAF

***Cinnamomum tamala* (Buch.-Ham.) Nees & Ebern.**

(Family : Lauraceae)

Description: It is an evergreen tree with rough stem and grey brown wrinkled bark upto 12 m high. Leaves are acute or acuminate, entire, scarcely shining above, glaucous beneath and 3-nerved; petioles 0.8-1.8 cm long. Flowers are pale-yellowish and often unisexual, in terminal and axillary 15-30 cm long and lax panicles. The drupes are ovoid, succulent and purplish blace upto 1.0 cm long and supported at the base by perianth.

Flowering is during February – April and fruiting in June–July.

Distribution: It is found in tropical and subtropical Himalayas, between 1000 – 2600 m and in Sylhet and Khasia hills between 1000 – 1400 m.

Parts used: The bark and the leaves are used.

Medicinal uses: Its bark is is used in gonorrhoea and the leaves as carminative and stimulant in rheumatism, colic and diarrhea; also in scorpion stings. As its bark and leveas possess aromatic property hence much used as flavouring tea and in various food preparations. Besides, its bark is also chewed medicinally in dyspepsia and throat irritations.

CITRON

***Citrus aurantifolia* (Christm.) Swingle**

(Syn. *C. medica* Linn. var. *acida* Watt.)

(Family: Rutaceae)

Description : It is a shrub or small tree with greenish-grey bark. Leaves are coriaceous; leaflets are elliptic-oblong or ovate-lanceolate and actuse or obtuse. The flowers often are unisexual, 2.5 cm long, white and 5-10 in a raceme. The fruits are globular, ovoid or oblong, often mamillate at the apex; rind is thin and tightly attached, yellow when ripe; pulp yellow-green and usually acidic with pleasant smell.

Flowering is during March-April and fruiting in May-June.

Distribution : It is found in the tropical parts of India including valleys of the Himalayas and the Khasi hills. It is also cultivated in West Bengal, Punjab, Madhya Pradesh, Maharashtra, Karnataka, Andhra Pradesh, Tamil Nadu and Uttar Pradesh.

Parts used : Fruits and aerial parts of the plant are used.

Medicinal uses : Its fruits are considered antiscorbutic, antiseptic, appetizing, astringent, digestive and stomachic and are used in liver troubles and in vomitting. The juice of the fruits is used as a refrigerant drink in burning sensation and in allaying thrust. Besides, an ethanol extract of its aerial parts is known to act as central nervous system depressent and diuretic.

CORIANDER

***Coriandrum sativum* Linn.**

(Family : Apiaceae)

Description : It is an erect and glabrous annual herb with terete and striate stem. Lower leaves are palmatilobed-partite; middle ones pinnate and upperones linear-lanceolate. The umbels are terminal and axillary and 3-5-rayed. Involucres are absent or one. Fruits are 0.3 - 0.4 x 0.2 cm with undulate primary ribs.

Flowering and fruiting is during cold season.

Distribution : It is cultivated throughout the warmer parts of India as cold season crop.

Parts used : Fruits, leaves, seeds and whole plant are used.

Medicinal uses : The fruits are aromatic, carminative, diuretic, stomachic, refrigerant, aphrodisiac and stimulant and their decoction is given in flatulent colic and bleeding piles and the infusion is used as eye wash in conjunctivitis. Its leaves and the seeds are chewed to correct foul and a poultice of its seeds is applied on carbuncles and chronic ulcers. The watery paste of its seeds is used as a gargle for the cure of mouth and throat ulceration.

A strong decoction of entire herb with milk and sugar is given for bleeding piles. A poultice of the herb is applied as cooling in headache and its juice is used as a dressing to soothe the irritation and inflammation caused by marking nut.

CUMIN

***Cuminum cyminum* Linn.**

(Family : Apiaceae)

Description: It is an annual, glabrous, branched and creeping herb with striate and slender stem upto 15-40 cm tall. Leaves are 2-pinnate, short petioled or sessile; segments linear–filiform with white margined. Flowers are small, white or rose coloured in terminal or leaf - opposed compound umbels. The fruits are oblong, 0.5-0.6 cm long and setulose with short style.

Flowering is in January-February and fruiting during March-April.

Distribution: A natie of Egypt, now widely cultivated in several parts of the country excluding Assam and Bengal.

Parts used: Its fruits are used.

Medicinal uses: Its fruits are known to possess astringent, carminatie, stomachic and stimulant properties, and are used in dyspepsia and diarrhoea. Besides, these are also used as spice in cookery.

CUSCUTA

***Cuscuta reflexa* Roxb.**

(Family: Cuscutaceae)

Description : It is a leafless, climbing, yellowish-green and thread -like twining herb which germinates in soil but becomes parastic on the plant on which it meets with. Flowers are subracemose; bracts are small, fleshy and subquardate. The fruit is a globose capsule which is acute with black warts. The seeds are black.

Flowering is during October - December and fruiting in December-February.

Distribution : It is common as parasitic climber throughout the plains of India ascending the hills upto 2438 m.

Parts used : The whole plant is used.

Medicinal uses : The entire plant is known as purgative and is used internally in protected fevers; its infusion as a wash for sores. Its fruits are used in cough and fever. The seeds are demulcent, diaphoretic and tonic. A cold infusion of its seeds is used as carminative and depurative. Its stem-parts are purgative and their decoction is useful in bilious affections; their paste is also applied over skin diseases.

In Unani system of medicine, the seeds are considered germinative and anodyne and in powder form, these are used as antifertility drugs. Besides, the juice of the plant is useful in hook worm and in diphtheria and paste of the herb is used to cure dislocated joints, to check falling of hairs and also in treatment of swellings of testicles and in headache.

Its seeds are used as a substitute for that of *Cassytha filiformis*.

CYPERUS

Cyperus rotundus Linn.

(Family : Poaceae)

Description : It is an erect and perennial glabrous herb with woody subterranean stoloniferous rhizomes which are clothed with fibrous remains of leafsheaths. Stems are nodose at base, 3-gonous and 10-60 cm high. Leaves are basal and usually shorter than the stem and are linear, tapering in the upper part to a slender acuminate apex and 0.3-0.5 cm broad. Inflorescence is an umbel of more or less condensed spikes. The flowers are reddish-brown. The nuts are obovid, glabrous and 0.1 cm long.

Flowering and fruiting is during July-December.

Distribution : The plant occurs throughout India; commonly in waste grounds, gardens, and along roadsides in open spots upto an elevation of 1828 m.

Parts used : Tubers are used.

Medicinal uses : Its tubers are known as diuretic, emmenagogue, anthelmintic, diaphoretic, astringent and stimulant and are used in disorders of the stomach and irritation of the bowels. The root-paste is applied in healing wounds and sores etc. and also used in intestinal diseases. Besides, the root-paste is used as '*anjan*' (collyrium) in eye-diseases. An aqueous extract from its methyl alcohol extract is useful in conjuctivitits. Its bulbous roots scraped and pounded with green ginger and mixed with honey are also given in dysentery.

DANDELION

Taraxacum officinale Webber

(Family: Asteraceae)

Description : It is a perennial milky herb with a stout rootstock. Leaves are basal, sessile, oblanceolate or linear, entire to lyrate pinnatifid; lobes acute and denticulate. Floral heads are solitary on scapes. The achenes are obovoid, ribbed; beak as long as or longer than the body.

Flowering and fruiting is during March-Novermber.

Distribution : It is found throughout the Himalayas between 330-6000 m and in Mishmi hills.

Usable parts : The roots and the leaves of the plant are used medicinally.

Medicinal uses : The roots of the plant are described as aperient, diuretic and tonic and these are used as a remedy for chronic disorders of kidney and liver. About 25-50 gm decoction of the roots and *Podophyllum* is used in jaundice, hepatitis and in indigestion effectively. Besides, its leaves are also used for fomentation. Indigenous people, take 5-10 gm crushed roots or its root paste orally with one glass of water in case of urinary problems, liver disorders and in constipation.

Its leaves are used as a substitute and adulterant of Henebane (Dried leaves and flower tops of *Hyoscyamus niger*) and roots as a substitute or adulterant of coffee (Garg, 1992).

DARBHA

***Imperata cylindrica* (Linn.) P. Beauv.**

(Syn. *I. arunidnaceae* Cyrillo; *Lagurus cylindricus* Linn.)

(Family: Poaceae)

Description: It is an unbranched, glabrous and perennial grass with creeping rootstocks and erect culms upto 30-90 high. Leaves are erect, linear, 5.0-20.0 x 0.2 – 0.6 cm, glabrous, mainly at basal parts; sheath glabrous or hariy. Panicles are narrow, cylindric and silvery – woolly tomentose and 5.0-15.0 cm long; branches short. Spikelets are 2-nate, both pedicelled, 0.3 cm long; calus bearded with soft-white 0.1 cm long hairs. The grains are small and oblong.

Flowering and fruiting is almost throught the year.

Distribution: It is common along forest edges, grassy slopes and vacant lots in the hills asceding upto 2000 m; also in the warmer and temperate parts of the country.

Parts used: The roots and woolly hairs of the inflorescence are used.

Medicinal uses: The woolly hairs of its inflorescnes are used for staunching the wounds and for stuffing purposes. Its roots are known to have antifebrile, emollient and haemostatic properties and are as used tonic. Besides, fumigations of its wooly hair of inflorescences are used in piles.

DATURA

***Datura metal* Linn.**

(Syn. *D. fastuosa* Linn.; *D. fastuosa* Linn. var. *alba* (Nees) Cl.; *D. alba* Nees)

(Family : Solanaceae)

Description : It is an erect, perennial, coarse and minutely pubescent herb about 60-120 cm high. Stem is woody below and purplish towards tips. Leaves are large, entire, sinuate and 7.5-15.0 × 5.0-10.0 cm with unequal base. The flowers are erect and whitish purple. Fruits are globose or ellipsoid capsules which are nodding, spinous, 1.2-2.5 cm across and 4-valved or irregularly breaking up near the apex. Seeds are compressed, rugose and brown.

Flowering and fruiting is during April-June; sometimes during July-December.

Distribution : It is a native of Mexico, now naturalized and very common in waste places, along road-sides and railway lines and in scrub jungles throughout the tropical parts of India.

Parts used : The parts used are, seeds, leaves and the roots.

Medicinal uses : The seeds, leaves and roots are used in insanity, fever with catarrh, diarrhoea, cerebral complication, skin diseases and as antiseptic. An extract of its bruised leaves or seeds in oil is often very effective in allaying the pain in rheumatic swellings, boils and tumours. Its leaves are considered as anodyne, antiseptic, antispasmodic and narcotic and are smoked to cure

the cough. The roots are antidiarrhoeal, antipyretic and antiseptic and are used in toothache and for brushing the teeth. These are boiled in milk and are administered with clarified butter to treat insanity.

Besides, various parts of the plant are used in headache, otitis, media suppurative, sores, mumps, pain, dropsy, anasarca, madness, rheumatism, rigid thigh muscles, haemiplegia, epilepsy, convulsions, cramps, delirium, febris, pimples, small pox, venereal sores, syphilis, orchitis, epididymitis and hydrocele.

The juice of its leaves is considered as a good substitute of belladona.

DEVIL'S TREE

***Alstonia scholaris* (Linn.) R. Br.**

(Family: Apocynaceae)

Description : It is a medium-sized evergreen tree with grey bark, whorled branches and bitter milky juice. Leaves are in whorls of 5-7, coriaceous, 10.0-20.0 × 2.5-3.7 cm, obovate-oblong or oblong, and obtuse; main lateral nerves parallel. Flowers are greenish-white or greenish-yellow and fragrant and are borne in compact umbellate- corymbose cymes. Fruits are slender folicles, 10.0-12.0 cm long and 1.25 cm across and hanging in pendulous clusters. Seeds are 0.7 cm long, slender, flattened, peltatley attached and densely ciliate with long brown hairs all around.

Flowering is during October-December and fruiting in January-March.

Distribution : It is found in Sub-Himalyan tract, West Bengal, Bihar, Peninsular India and in the Andamanns also.

Parts used : The leaves, bark and wood are often used medicinally.

Medicinal uses: The decoction of its leaves is used in beriberi disease and in congestion of liver and the bruised leaves boiled in oil is given internally in dropsy. Their juice mixed with gingiber juice is prescribed after confinement and poultice is applied to ulcers. The bark is known as alterative, anthelmintic, antidysenteric, antimalarial, astringent and galactogogue and is used to cure gastro-intestinal troubles and as sedative and tonic. Its wood paste with water is applied in rheumatism and wounds. The bark-latex is used in tuberculosis; as antimicrobial, antipyretic and antimalarial; also applied in rheumatic pains, sores, toothache, tumours and ulcers and after mixing with oil is used as ear drops and in dental diseases. The stem-bark of the plant with the leaves of *Vitex negundo* is said to be used as poultice in bodyache and joints pains.

Besides, *Ditamine*, an uncrystallizable substance obtained from its bark is as efficaceous as quinine in malarial fever without disagreable secondary symptoms of that drug.

DHATAKI

Woodfordia fruticosa **(Linn.) Kurz.**

(Syn. *W. floribunda* Salisb; *Lythrum fruticosum* Linn.)

(Family: Lythraceae)

Description : It is a semi-deciduous undershrub or shrub with long and spreading branches. Stems are hairy at apices. Leaves are opposite, short petioled, lanceolate-oblong and rounded-subcordate at base and are grey-pubescent beneath. The flowers are scarlet, tubular on slender pedicels and dilated above and are borne in axillary clusters. The fruits are ellipsoid and membranous capsules, included in the calyx. The seeds are cuneate-obovate and smooth.

Flowering is during March-April and fruiting in June-July.

Distribution : It is found throughout India in high altitudes ascending to 1500 -2000 m, particularly in the Himalayas.

Parts used : Its flowers are used.

Medicinal uses : Its dried flowers are considered as astringent and are used in dysentery, menorrhagia, leucorrhoea, impaired hepatic functions and in piles. A powder of the dry flowers or their decoction is applied over foul ulcers and wounds.

The flowers alone with sesamum oil forms a good liniment, which is used for burns and scalds; also as a source of inoculum, for microbial fermentation to prepare different asavas.

DRAKSHA

Vitis vinifera Linn.

(Family: Vitaceae)

Description : It is a large woody climber with bifid tendrils. Leaves are glabours above, clothed beneath with grey deciduous tomentum, suborbicular, cordate and more or less deeply 5-lobed. The flowers are pentamerous and green and are borne in umbel-like cymes, which form large pyramidal compound panicles. The fruits are subglobose berries with 1-5 seeds. But the fruits rarely come to perfection due to heavy rainfall, which usually takes place before these have properly ripened.

Flowering is during April - May and fruiting in June - July.

Distribution : It is a native of West Asia and Mediterranean region, and is cultivated in many parts of India specially in North-West regions.

Parts used : Grapes (fruits), juice, sap, leaves, dried fruits and ashes of its wood are used.

Medicinal uses : The grapes are known for their demulcent, laxative, refrigerant, stomachic, diuretic and cooling properties and are considered very useful in chronic bronchitis, heart - diseases, Bright's disease and gout. The juice of unripe futits is considered astringent and is used in throat affections. It is stated that strained grape juice, one teaspoonful is given to children for constipation during teething and to prevent convulsions due to constipation. The juice is also good for thrust in children and that of sour grapes is useful for bruises and sprains. The sap of its young branches is used as a remedy for skin diseases. The leaves are astringent and are used in diarrhoea.

Its dried fruits, known as '*munakka*' (raisins) are cooling, demulcent, sweet, laxative and stomachic. These are useful in thirst attendant on fevers; heat of body, cough, hoarseness, and consumption and in wasting diseases. Chakradatta advised, raisins, sugar, honey and powdered chebulic myrobalans in equal parts to be taken after washing out the stomach with vomitting for acid dyspepsia and Sharangdhara recommended a linctus, prepared by taking of raisins, emblic myrobalans, dates, long pepper and black pepper in equal parts and rubbing them together with honey and ghee, to be used as demulcent and expectorant.

Besides, the ashes of its wood are recommended as a preventive of stone in the bladder, cold swellings of the testes and in piles.

DURVA

***Cynodon dactylon* (Linn.) Pers.**

(Family: Poaceae)

Description : It is a perennial and creeping herb with underground rhizomes. Culms are decumbent-ascending and nodes are glabrous. Leaves are linear-subulate and scabrid on the upper surface and margin. Ligule is a minute, scarious, erose and ciliate rim. The sheaths are compressed, keeled, and glabrous except hairy throat. Spikes are 2-4 and 1.5-3.0 × 0.1-0.2 cm. Spikelets are 0.2 × 0.1 cm. Grains are oblong and free within the glumes.

Flowering is during July-September and fruiting in October-December.

Distribution : It is found throughout India, ascending upto 2438 m in the Himalayas.

Parts used : Whole plant in the form of panchang is used.

Medicinal uses : A decoction of its roots is used as diuretic and in dropsy and in secondary syphilis and the infusion to stop the bleeding from piles. The roots after crushing and mixing with curds are used in chronic gleet. Besides, the juice of plant is said to be astringent and is used externally to fresh cuts and wounds and internally as diuretic, it is used in dropsy and anasarca, hysteria, epilepsy, insanity, in chronic diarrhoea and dysentery.

A decoction of its rhizomes is used internally as diuretic, refresher, antinflammatory for digestive tract and as urinary antiseptic by the native people. About 100 gm juice of the plant is taken daily to control blood pressure locally. Its leaves wetted-with morning dew are rubbed on warts to cure them. Besides, the bruised grass is also used as a dressing for fresh wounds.

EMETIC NUT

Catunaregam spinosa **(Thunb.) Tiruv.**

(Syn. *Gardinia spinosa* Thunb.; *Randia dumetorum* (Retz.) Poir; *R. brandisii* Gamble; *Xeromphis spinosa* (Thunb) Keay).

(Family: Rubiaceae)

Description : It is a small tree or rigid shrub armed with strong straight nearly opposite decussate, 1.3 - 3.0 cm long spines. Leaves are 3.2 - 5 5 x 2.0 - 3.2 cm, obovate, obtuse, wrinkled, shining above with cuneate base; stipules ovate and acuminate. Flowers are solitary or rarely 2-3 on short peduncles and are greenish yellow or white. Berries, the fruits are yellowish, globose or broadly ovoid, smooth or obscurely longitudinally ribbed and crowned by large calyx-limb. Seeds are numerous, compressed and are embedded in pulp.

Flowering is during March-June and fruiting later.

Distribution: It is found in sub Himlayan tract from the Kashmir eastwards, ascending in Sikkim upto 1400 m, south ward extends to Chittagong and Peninsular India.

Parts used: Fruits and bark are used.

Medicinal uses: In ayurveda, its fruits are considered aphrodisiac, bitter, carminative, emetic, alexiteric and antipyretic and are used to cure abscess, inflammations, tumours, skin diseases and ulcers. While in Unani system of medicine, these are used in chronic bronchitis, pain of muscles, paralysis, leprosy, boils, and eruptions of the skin and in the diseases of brain, asthma and leucoderma. The pulp of its fruits is applied on tongue and incidental ailments of children during teething and is also used as anthelminitc and abortifacient and in dysentery. Besides, its bark is known to possess astringent property and is externally applied in bone ache during fever and as anodyne in rheumatism.

It is also used as a substitute of Ipecacuanha.

EPHEDRA

Ephedra gerardiana Wall. ex Stapf

(Family: Ephedraceae)

Description: It is a densely tufted shrub upto 30-120 cm high with green, ascending branches and grey bark. Leaves are scale like, connate into 2 lobed sheaths and are yellow or brownish. Male spikes are ovate, solitary or 2-3 together; staminal column exserted. Female spikes are red, ofthen succulent; bracts 2-3 pairs. The seeds are black.

Cone formation starts and matures in July – September.

Distribuion: It is known to occur in drier regions of temperate and alpine Himalayas from Kashmir to Sikkim between 2400-5500 m.

Parts used: The fruits, roots and the shoots are used medicinally.

Medicinal uses: Its fruits are eaten and the extract of roots and that of shoots is given in blood pressure and their decocotion as a remedy in rheumatism and syphilis. Besides, their paste is applied on joint pain.

ELECAMPANE

Inula racemosa Hook. f.

(Family: Brassicaceae)

Description : It is a tall and stout herb reaching a height upto 0.3-1.5 m. Leaves are leathery, rough above, densely hairy beneath and crenate; basal leaves are 20.0-45.0 x 12.5-20.0 cm, long stalked and elliptic-lance-shaped and stem leaves oblong and often lobed at the base. Floral heads are many, large and 3.5-5.0 cm across in racemes. The fruits are 0.4 cm long, slender and hairless achenes.

Flowering and fruiting is during September-October.

Distribution : It is found in temperate and alpine western Himalayas between 1700-4500 m, and in Kashmir between 1700-2500 m.

Usable parts: The roots are used medicinally.

Medicinal uses : In Unani system of medicine, the roots of the plant are used to cure pains of the heart, spleen, liver and joints and in hemicrania, eruptions, inflammations, ear pain, cough and boils. The roots of the plant are also used as expectorant and as resolvent in indurations. Its seeds possess aphrodisiac and bitter properties and are useful in strenghening the hair and in preventing them to fall.

Its roots are adulterated with that of *Kuth* (*Saussurea lappa*) and *Digitalis* (Garg, 1992).

EUCALYPTUS

***Eucalyptus citriodora* Hook.**
(Syn. *E. muculata* Hook. var. *citriodora* Bail.)
(Family: Myrtaceae)

Description : It is a tall tree with smooth and shining stem. Leaves are ramal and cauline, simple, alternate, exstipulate, lanceolate or falcate, entire, acute and gland-dotted. Flowers are white, hermaphordite, pedicellate, small, scented and ebracteate and are borne in panicles. The fruits is a capsule.

Flowering and fruiting is during winter season.

Distribution : It is an exotic species, adopted well in subtropical regions in India.

Parts used : Leaves, essential oil and kino gum are generally used.

Medicinal uses : Its leaf-tea is added to bath water and joints soaked to relieve pain. An essential oil, obtained from the plant is used as antimicrobial, insect repellant and insecticidal and is also applied to muscle spasm

Besides, the gum like substance, known as kino obtained from the plant, is used in medicines for cold effects and astringent.

FENNEL

***Foeniculum vulgare* (Linn.) Miler**

(Syn. *Anethum foeniculum* Linn.)

(Family: Apiaceae)

Description: It is an annual or perennial, erect and glabrous herb with striate, fistular and about 2 m high stem. Leaves are 3-4- pinnate; segments filfiform, to 4.0 cm long; sheath white and margined with a cup-shaped top. The flowers are small, yellow in compound umbels. Rays are 10-50 on 5.0-10.0 cm long peduncles and bracteoles are absent. The fruits are oblong – ovoid and glabrous, upto 0.4-0.6 cm long.

Flowering is in February – April and fruiting during May – June.

Distribution : It is widely cultivated throughout the country.

Parts used: Leaves, roots, seed – oil. fruits and the flowers are used.

Medicinal uses: Its leaves are used as diuretic and the roots as purgative. The oil obtained from its seeds is used as vermicide. Its fruits are used as spice and carminative. Besides, its flowers after boiling are given to infants during teething.

FENUGREEK

***Trigonella foenum-graecum* Linn.**

(Family: Fabaceae)

Description : It is an erect, simple or branched and hairy annual herb about 30-60 cm tall. Leaves are pinnate and trifoliolate; leaflets are 0.7-4.0 x 0.4-1.5 cm, obovate, rounded-truncate-emarginate, glabrous and faintly serrate at the top. The flowers are yellowish. Pods, the fruits are straight or slightly curved, beaked and 3.0-15.0 cm long. Seeds are 10-20, oblong with a deep groove across one corner, greenish-brown and 0.2-0.5 x 0.2-0.3 cm.

Flowering is during January - February and fruiting in March-April.

Distribution : It is wild in Kashmir, Punjab and the upper Gangetic plains; also cultivated in many parts of India.

Parts used : The seeds, leaves and whole plant are used.

Medicinal uses : The seeds of the plant are considered carminative, tonic and aphrodisiac and their infusion is given to smallpox patients as a cooling drink. These are eaten boiled or roasted, and as a vegetable in dyspepsia, diarrhoea, especially of a lying-in mother, colic, flatulance, dysentery, rheumatism, dropsy, enlargement of the liver and spleen and chronic cough. A decoction of the roasted seeds is prescribed in disorders of the throat and chest. The gruel of its seeds is given with milk and sugar as a lactagogue and the powder of the seeds one teaspoonful daily is prescribed in scrofula, anaemia, gout, diabetes and debitity. A poultice of the seeds is applied to reduce swellings and inflammatory affections and their paste as a cosmetic to keep the skin soft and clean. Besides its seeds are soaked in water, to get their mucilage which is locally used over boils, carbuncles and abscesses.

Its leaves are used externally as well as internally for their cooling properties. As aperient, they are used to relieve indigestion and bilious disorders. Their paste is applied over swellings and burns. The pessary made from the herb or of lint saturated with its decoction is used for the treatement of leucorrhoea; and the herb-poultice to reduce swellings.

Its seed gum, known as Fenugreek gum is used as a substitute for Guar gum, obtained from *Cyamposis tetragonoloba*.

FLAXSEED

***Linum usitatissium* Linn.**

(Family: Linaceae)

Description: It is an annual, erect and glabrous herb upto 80 cm high. Stem is usually solitary, corymbosely branched above and striate. Leaves are linear to linear – lanceolate or ovate, glabrous and 3-nerved. Flowers are blue, usually solitary, axillary or in clusters. Capsules, the fruits are globose, 5 – celled and apiculate. Seeds are compressed, ovoid-oblong and dark brown.

Flowering is in February – April and fruiting during March-July.

Distribution: It is cultivated throughout India upto 2000 m.

Parts used: Seeds, flowers, leaves and bark are used.

Medicinal uses: In ayruveda, the seeds of the plant are described as aphrodisiac, bitter, hot, oily and sweet which remove biliousness, backache and inflammation, heal ulcers, also used to cure leprosy and urinary discharges, but lead to impotency. Whereas, in Unani system, these are known for aphrodisiac, bad taste, emenagogal and galactagogal properties, which cure, cough and also used in kidney problems. An oil prepared form its seeds, commonly known as *Alsi-ka-tel,* is used to remove biliousness and bad blood; also useful for internal wounds and ringworms. Its crushed seeds are also applied externally to accelerate suppuration of abscess, boils and carbuncles. Besides, the flowers are used as cardiac and nervine tonic and leaves and bark in gonorrhoea.

GAMBHARI

***Gmelina arborea* Linn.**

(Family: Verbenaceae)

Description : It is an unarmed large deciduous tree about

20 m high and pubescent with some-what corky bark. Leaves are large, tawny tomentose underneath when young, cordate, ovate, acuminate and 10.0-20.0 x 7.5-15.0 cm. The flowers are yellow tinged with brown in terminal and axillary racemiform cymes. The fruits are ovoid or pyriform, smooth and 1.7-2.5 cm long drupes and are orange-yellow when ripe. Seeds are oblong.

Flowering is during February-April and fruiting during April-July.

Distribution : It is found along road-sides and in the forests throughout India.

Parts used : Fruits, leaves and roots are usable.

Medicinal uses: The fruits are refrigerant and their decoction is given in fever and bilious affections. Its leaves are demulcent and their juice is useful in cough, gonorrhoea, foetid discharge and maggot in ulcers. The paste of its leaves is applied on head to relieve headache. The roots are bitter, tonic, demulcent, laxative, refrigerant and stomachic and their decoction is given in anasarca, fever and indigestion. Its root-bark improves thirst and relieves abdominal pain. Besides, its other parts are used in swellings of throat, fever, dropsy, spleen trouble, pain, colic, rheumatism, convulsions, delirium, small-pox, syphilis, sores, urticaria, dyspepsia, cholera, phthisis, bronchitis, asthma, diarrhoea, intoxication, haemorrhage, septicaemia, gravel and rinder-pest.

GARLIC

Allium sativum Linn.

(Family: Liliaceae)

Description : The plant is 30-60 cm high with soft stems. Leaves are flat and scape is slender. The spathes is long-beaked and its heads bear bulbils and flowers. Flowers are white. The bulb consists of smaller bulbs called cloves, which are 5-12 in numbers.

Flowering and fruting is during winter.

Distribution : It is cultivated in various parts of the country and is grown during September - October in the plains and February - March in hills.

Parts used : Its bulbs and the oil are useful.

Medicinal uses : This forms an important drugs In Ayurveda, and has been effective drug for rheumatism and catarrhal affections. As an antiseptic, its use has long been recognized. In the late war, it was widely employed in the control of suppuration in wounds. The raw juice is expressed, diluted with water and put on swabs of sterilized Sphagnum moss, which are applied to the wound. Where this treatment has been given, it has been proved that there have been no septic results and the lives of thousands of men have been saved by its use. In olden days, it was employed in ointment and lotion.

An infusion of its bruised bulbs if given before and after every meal, has been considered good in epilepsy. The juice of garlic and milk of garlic made by boiling the bruised bulbs in milk is used as vermifuge. It shows antibacterial, antinflammable, anticanceral and pesticidal properties. The raw garlic is used to decrease glucose, total cholesterol, phospholipids, triglycerides etc. in healthy persons. It is also useful in dyspepsia and cryptococccal meningitis in man. It is also applied as resolvant to indolent tumours. Internally, it is given in nervous diseases, headache etc. with salt. Its regular use kills harmful intestinal bacteria. Its liniment is useful in infantile convulsions and other spasmodic affections and in gout and sciatica. The juice is applied to bruises and sprains and is also used to relieve earache and to allay pain in otorrhoea i.e., the state of discharge from the external auditory meatus.

Externally, the juice of garlic is used in leprosy and after frieying in mustard or coconut oil, the garlic is applied on maggot-infested wounds, sores and scabies. The garlic or its impure oil would apear to produce an irritant type of poisoning if it is taken in excess. Cases have been seen where its use internally has proved fatal to children. On account of the volatile nature of the essential oil of this plant, it may enter the blood through the alimentary canal as well as from the respiratory tract. The plant produces a depressing effect upon the heart shows the rate and lessens the contractiblity of the myocardium but care should be taken in using garlic juice, as it in purity is irritant to skin.

GENTIAN

***Gentiana kurroo* Royle**

(Family: Gentianaceae)

Description: It is a perennial herb with thick root stock and decumbent and tufted stem, reaching a height of 12.5-30.0 cm. Leaves are oblong; radical rosulate, 7.5-12.5 x 6.0-12.0 cm and stem leaves are narrow and about 2.5 cm long. Flowers are blue dotted with white and are borne solitary or racemose. Capsules, the fruits are oblong.

Flowering is during August-September and fruiting later.

Distribution : It is found in Kashmir and North Western Himalayas between 1700 – 3400 m.

Usable parts : Entire plant and roots of the plant are used medicinally.

Medicinal uses : In Unani system of medicine, this is known for its bitter taste and for emmenagogue and tonic properties and is used successfully to treat leucoderma and syphilis. Its roots are used as febrifuge, stomachic and tonic and in urinary affections. It is stated that its decoction of roots with equal amount of 'sunthi' and 'dikamali' or an infusion of its roots in cold water with addition of 0.2 gm camphor and shilajit and 5.0 gm honey is used as a remedy in debility after fevers, indigestion and loss of appetite; also in catarrh, syphilis, leprosy and other skin diseases. Besides, an infusion of its entire plant mixed with a little powder of long pepper is used to relieve in fevers accompanied with coughs and difficulty of breathing and a powder of roots mixed with honey is given in hiccup and to stop the vomiting.

It is used as a better substitute of yellow Gentian (*Gentiana lutea*) (Garg, 1992).

GINGER
***Zingiber officinale* Rosc.**
(Family: Zingiberaceae)

Description : It is a perennial and erect herb with horizontal jointed tuberous rhizomes. The stems are leafy, erect and about 15-150 cm long. Leaves are 10-30 cm long, lanceolate and glabrous beneath. The flowers are bisexual and are borne solitary in heads. The fruit is a capsule. Seeds are many, endospermic and arillate.

Flowering is in rainy season but less seen.

Distribution : It is widely cultivated in India up to an altitude of 1500 m.

Parts used : The rhizomes and their juice is used.

Medicinal uses : Its rhizomes are considered stimulant and carminative and are used as flavouring agent and in dyspepsia, flatulent, colic and vomitting. An infusion of the dry ginger with two teaspoonful of castor oil is recommended in painful affections of the bowels and stomach. It is stated that the ginger is chewed to stimulate the flow of saliva, to warm and tone the stomach, to relieve toothache and hoarseness of voice, to restore loss of voice, to relax the congested uvula and tonsils and the paralysed muscles of the tongue and faces. A paste of the ginger is considered local stimulant and rubefacient in headache, toothache and short sight due to deficient contractile power of the iris. The powder of ginger is rubbed on the extremities of the limbs, to check cold perspiration and to improve blood circulation in the collapse stage of cholera.

In Unani system of medicine, the ginger is considered carminative, digestive and aphrodisiac and is used to strengthen memory, to remove viscid matter and obstruction in the vessels, incontinence of urine, in nervous diseases and in balgham. For indigestion with want of appetite, equal parts of ginger-juice, lemon-juice and rock salt, well mixed together should be taken just before meals. Twenty grams of ginger-juice mixed together with seventy grams of cow's milk is boiled down to half its volume, then sugar candy powder is added to it and it is recommended to be taken at bed time in biliousness. Ten grams of ginger-juice and mango-juice, fine sugar and cow's ghee are well mixed and melted down to half the quantity, which is advised to be taken every morning and evening daily also in biliousness. The juice mixed with sugar candy is given twice daily in diabetes.

GOKSHURA

***Tribulus terrestris* Linn.**

(Family: Zygophyllaceae)

Description : It is a small prostate or decumbent and hairy or silky annual herb. Leaves are in unequal pairs, stipulate, opposite and abruptly pinnate; leaflets are in 4-7 pairs, oblong and mucronate. The flowers are yellow, 1.0-1.5 cm across, solitary and are axillary or leaf opposed. The fruits are globose and hairy 5-angled cocci with 2 long and 2 short spines. Seeds are obliquely pendulous.

Flowering and fruiting is during rainy season.

Distribution : It is found in waste places and dry habitats throughout the warmer regions of India ascending upto an altitude of 3000 m including West Rajasthan and Gujarat.

Parts used : The fruits, leaves, stems and roots are used.

Medicinal uses: Its fruits are known as cooling, diuretic, tonic and aphrodisiac and their decoction or infusion is used in painful micturition, kidney diseases, chronic cystitis, gonorrhoea, gout, gravel and in impotence. The dry fruits are powdered and are given in doses of 18 gm with sugar and black pepper in gleet, spermatorrhoea and impotence. Its leaves are used in affections of urinary calculi and as stomachic and the stems are used as astringent and in infusion form, are given interally in gonorrhoea. Besides, its roots are used as aperient, demulcent and as tonic.

GUDUCHI

***Tinospora cordifolia* (Willd.) Miers ex Hook.f. & Thoms. (Family: Menispermaceae)**

Description : It is a large, glabrous and climbing succulent shrub with rocky bark. Leaves are petioled, membranous, cordate with broad sinus and 5.0-10.0 cm long blade. The flowers are small, yellow and unisexual; male flowers are fascicled and females are usually solitary. The fruits are ovoid drupes, succulent, lustrous and red when ripe. Seeds are curved.

Flowering is during summer and fruiting in winter.

Distribution : It is found throughout the tropical India, ascending upto an altitude of 300 m.

Parts used : Leaves, stem, roots and fruits are used.

Medicinal uses : The leaves of the plant are prescribed in fevers and the stem is used as bitter, stomachic and antipyretic. An infusion of its stem-powder is used as alterative and aphrodisiac and stem-juice is given in fever and mixed with honey in jaundice and decoction alone for rheumatic fever and vomitting due to excessive bile secretion. Its decoction mixed with the fruits of *Piper longum* and honey is used in fever associated with cough in the doses of 0.35-1.05 gm per day and in combination with the stem of *Piper longum* and honey is used to control heart palpitation due to flatulency and with combination of sweet oil, is administered in elephantiasis. A kind of starch, known as '*Giloe ka sat*' is prepared from the aqueous extract of dry stem which is used as tonic and also as antidiarrhoeal, antidysentric and antacid substance in the doses of 0.7-2.0 gm per day.

Its roots are considered as a powerful emetic and are used for visceral obstruction. The watery extract of the same is used in leprosy. Its pulverized fruits are considered good tonic and are used in jaundice and rheumatism. The fresh plant is considered more efficacious than the dried ones and its watery extract known as '*Indian quinine*' is used as febribuge. Besides, various parts of the plant are used in general debility, dyspepsia, fever and urinary diseases.

GUGGUL

Commiphora wightii (Arnott) Bhandari

(Syn. *C. mukul* (Hook. ex Stocks) Engl.; *Balsmodendron wightii* Arnott; *B. roxburghii* Stocks; *B. mukul* Hook. ex Stocks)

(Family: Burseraceae)

Description : It is a small tree or more usually a stunted bush with spinescent branches. Leaves are usually unifoliate, alternate or crowded at the end of short branches, cuneate-obovate, rhomboidal or oval, acute, deeply serrate and smooth and shining. Flowers are small, nearly sessile, few together and unisexual; male with short and barren ovary and females with short stamens and imperfect anthers. The drupes are red and ovate-acuminate containing 2-celled stones, rarely 4-valved.

Flowering is during March-April and fruiting later.

Distribution : It is reported to found in the arid and rocky zones in some parts of South-west and North - western regions of India including Mysore and Rajasthan.

Parts used medicinally: Gum, obtained from the plant is used medicinally.

Medicinal uses : The gum, obtained from this plant commercially known as Indian bdellium, is known as alterative, antiseptic, anti-inflammatory, antispasmodic, antisuppurative, aphrodisiac, aperient, appetizing, ecbolic, emmenagogue and expectorant and is used in amenorrhoea, anaemia, encometritis, leucorrhoea, menorrhagia, nervous diseases, rheumatism, scrofulous affections and cutaneous diseases, specially applied in bad wounds and indolent ulcer and is recommended in the treatment of urinary diseases, obesity, in marasmus of children and rheumatoid arthritis. The fumes of burnt gum are also inhaled in chronic bronchitis, chronic nasal catarrh, laryngitis, and tuberculosis. In indolent ulcer, it is applied as a plaster after mixing with limejuice or Coconut oil and a lotion, prepared after mixing 80 gm of its tincture (20 percent in 90 percent of alcohol) in 280 gm of water, is used as a gargle in pyrrhoea, weak tonsilitis and pharyngitis and ulcerated throat.

The gum obtained from this tree is uses as a substitute or adulterant to Harbol myrrh (*Commiphora myrrha*).

GURMAR

***Gymnema sylvestre* R. Br.**

(Famliy: Asclepiadaceae)

Description : It is a large, stout, much branched and woody climber with densely appressed hairy branchlets. Leaves are 3.2-5.0 x 1.3-3.0 cm, rarely pubescent above, thinly coriaceous and elliptic or obovate-acute. Flowers are yellow, small in crowded umbelliform cymes; corolla sub-rotate with thick lobes and fleshy coronal processes on the throat. The follicles are 6.0-7.5 x 0.7-0.8 cm, slender and glabrous; one follicle often suppressed. Seeds are about 1.2 cm long, narrowly obovoid-oblong and flat with a broad thin wing and pale brown in colour.

Flowering is during July-August and fruiting in October - December.

Distribution : It is commonly occurred in the hills of Bihar, Orissa, Madhya Pradesh and Deccan Peninsula.

Parts used : Whole plant, seeds, roots and the leaves are used.

Medicinal uses : *Sushruta* has described this plant as a destroyer of glycosuria and other urinary disorders. On account of its abolishing property to sugar, it has been given the name '*Gurmar*' and it has been proved that it neutralizes the excess of sugar present in the body in diabetes mellitus. In ayurveda, the plant is described as acrid, bitter, alterative, anthelmintic, alexiteric and tonic and is used in eye complaints, to cure corneal opacity, heart diseases, piles, leucorrhoea and biliousness.

Its fruits are used in bronchitis, heart diseases and urinary discharges and the seeds as emetic and as a remedy for colds. The roots are used as astringent, emetic, expectorant, refrigerant, stomachic and tonic. Its leaves are hypoglycaemic and are used in cough, fever and in the management of maturity onset diabetes. Besides, these are mixed with castor oil and are applied externally to swollen glands and enlarged spleen and in powder form are used as diuretic and stimulant.

HARENU

***Vitex agnus castus* Linn.**

(Family: Verbenaceae)

Description: It is a shrub or tree with obtusely quardrangular and tomentose branches, which pass into a wide panicle. Leaves are long – petiolate and digitately 5- rarely 7-foliate; leaflets slightly tomentose above and green, below canescent, lancolate, acumnate, attenuate at the base and petiolulate and subentire. The flowers are liliac, in compact, subsessile, forming long-spiked cymes. The fruits are spherical, obtuse and slightly logner than the calyx.

Flwoering and fruiting is during July-October.

Distribution: It is known to be distributed in the hilly parts of the country.

Parts used: Its seeds are used.

Medicinal uses: Its seeds in the ayurveda, are described as abrotifacient, bitter, diuretic, heating, pungent and stomachic and are used in *kapha* and *vata* diseases, pruritus, itching, burning sensations, thrist and to improve the taste. While in Unani system of medicine, these are known for their astringent and bitter properties and are used to purify the brain and liver, and also used in inflammations, pains, dropsy and the enlargement of the spleen.

In tranditional medicine, the plant is used for pains due to chills. one who is suffering from cold takes a bath in water in which the leaves of the plant are boiled. Besides, the plant is also used as a cure for eye diseases as well as for stomach-ache.

HARITAKI

***Terminalia chebula* Retz.**

(Family: Combretaceae)

Description : It is a large deciduous tree with dark-brown bark; young branchlets, leaf-buds and leaves are long and soft and with shining rust coloured, sometimes silvery hairy. Leaves are mostly sub-oppossite, distant, 7.5-15.0 cm long, ovate or oblong-ovate, acuminate and deciduous in the cold season. The flowers are dull white or yellowish with offensive smell and bisexual and are borne in spikes from the upper axils and in small terminal panicles. The fruits are 2.5-5.0 cm long, obovoid, ellipsoid or ovoid glàbrous and more or less 5-ribbed when dry. The nuts are hard and with a rough grooved surface.

Flowering is during April-June and fruiting in January-March.

Distribution : It is abundantly found in Northern India from Kangra to Bengal and South wards to the Deccan tablelands at 304-914 m and upto 1828 m in Travancore; higher forests of the Mumbai ghats, Satpuras, Belgaum and Kanara.

Parts used : The fruits, bark, gum and leaves are used.

Medicinal uses : The fruits of the plant are known as laxative, astringent, alterative and stomachic and their cold infusion is used as a gargle in stomatitis and in chronic ulcers, carious teeth, in cough, asthma and urinary diseases. Finely powdered fruits are used in bleeding and ulcerations of the gums. Internally, fruits are efficaceous in chronic diarrhoea, dysentery and flatulence. Its fruit extract is used as wash in watering eyes and fruit paste in burns. its bark is used as diuretic and cardiotonic and the gum obtained from the plant, is eaten as tonic and also used in colitis.

HOLY BASIL

***Ocimum sanctum* Linn.**

(Family: Lamiaceae)

Description : It is an erect and much branched herb with about 30-90 cm height and sometimes woody at the base. The stems and branches are clothed with soft hairs. Leaves are ovate or elliptic-oblong, entire or subserrate and hairy on both the surfaces. Flowers are closely whorled in racemes. The nutlets are 4, dry, small, reddish brown, ellipsoid and smooth.

Flowering and fruiting is almost througout the year, chiefly during winter.

Distribution : It is cultivated throughout India and often runs wild.

Parts used : Whole plant, its roots, seeds, leaves and flowers are usable.

Medicinal uses : The entire plant is considered expectorant, stomachic, diuretic, antiseptic and cardiac stimulant and its decoction is used in catarrh, croup and bronchitis. Its root-decoction is given in malarial fevers as a diaphoretic. Leaves are stimulant, diaphoretic, antiperiodic and expectorant and are used again in catarrh and bronchitis, ringworm and other cutaneous diseases. Its leaves are also reported to possess antifertility and abortifacient activites. An infusion of its leaves is used as stomachic in gastric disorders of children and in hepatic affections and their juice is dropped into ear as a remedy in earache; also used as demulcent and in genito-urinary disorders. Besides, its flowers with honey, ginger and onion juice are used in cough as expectorant.

INDIAN ACONITE

***Aconitum ferox* Wall. ex. Ser.**

Description : It is a perennial herb with tuberous roots. Leaves are scattered, orbicular - cordate to reniform; palmately 5-lobed with pubescent blade and petiole. The peducles are straight bearing flowers on both sides. The flowers are dirty blue and are borne in a dense terminal raceme, about 10 - 25 cm long and helmet-vaulted with a short sharp beak. Follicles, the fruits, are oblong with long and obpyramidal to obovoid seeds.

Flowering is in July-August and fruiting during October-December.

Distribution : It is found to grow wild in alpine Himalayas and in Kashmir upto 3600 m.

Parts used : Its underground stems and roots of the plant are used.

Medicinal uses : A liniment of its underground stems and of roots in small doses of 0.023 - 0.018 gm is used in nasal catarrh, uvula hypertrophy, sore throat, gibbous, paralysis and in chronic fever, while in larger doses it acts as a narcotic, powerful poison and sedative. Internally, the tincture of its roots (1 in 8 of alcohol) in the doses of 2-5 drops is used in combination with other drugs for the treatment of fever and rheumatism and also as a remedy for cough and asthma.

Its roots are cardiac stimulant, hypoglycaemic, diaphoretic and antiphologistic and the powder or liniment prepared from its roots is spreaded over the skin in case, of arthritis and scabies.

ISABGHUL

***Plantago ovata* Forsk.**

(Family : Plantaginaceae)

Description: It is a stemless or nearly stemless softly hairy or woolly annual herb. Leaves are 7.5-23.0 cm long, scarcely reaching 0.6 cm broad, narrowly linear or filiform, finely acuminate, entire or distantly toothed, attenuated at the base and usally 3-nerved. Scapes are longer or shorter than the leaves and are glabrous or pubescent. Flowers are in ovoid or cylindric spikes which are 1.3-3.8 cm long; bracts 0.4 cm long and about as broad as long, broadly ovate or suborbicular, concave, membranous except the narrow midrib and glabrous. Capsules, the fruits are 0.8-1.0 cm long, ellipsoid and obtuse; the upper half coming off as a blunt conical lid, membranous and glabrous. Seeds are 0.3 cm long, ovoid-oblong, boat-shaped and smooth and yellowish brown.

Flowering is during April-May and fruting in October-November.

Distribution: It is found in the plains of Punjab and its low hills.

Parts used: Its seeds are used.

Medicinal uses: Its seeds in ayurveda, are described as acrid, astringent, mucilaginous and sweet to the bowels. These are also used as tonic and in *kapha* diseases, biliousness, dysentery and leprosy. Whereas in Unani system of medicine, these are described as cooling and demulcent and are useful in inflammatory and bilious dearrangements of the digestive system; applied as poulitice to rheumatic and gouty swellings and also good in dysentery and irritiation of the intestinal tract. Its decoction is used in cough and chronic diarrhea also. As its seeds yield a good deal of mucilage and form a cooling demulcent drink, hence are prescribed in cases where emollients are requied. A slight degee of astringency and some tonic property may be imparted to the seeds by application of a moderate degree of heat and it is said that this remedy cures the chornic diarrhoea of children on the failure of other medicines.

A poultice of its cruhsed seeds with vineagar and oil is made and is applied on rheumatic and gouty swellings. With the mucilage a cooling lotion for the head is also made. About 50-75 gm of moistened mucilage with hot water and mixed with sugar are given in dysentery and irriation of the intestinal canal to produce an easy stool. Besides, the roasted seeds are useful in irritations of the bowels in children and in dysentery. Because of the demulcent and diuretic properties, its seeds are given with water of tender coconuts in the diseases of gastro – intestinal and genito-urinary tracts.

JAMBU

***Syzygium cumini* (Linn.) Skeels**

(Syn. *Eugenia jambolana* Lamk.; *Myrtus cumini* Linn.)

(Family: Myrtacae)

Description : It is a large evergreen tree with light grey bark. Leaves are 7.5-15.0 × 3.7-6.2 cm, coriaceous, shining, entire, oval-oblong or lanceolate-oblong, long-acuminate, tough and smooth; lateral nerves are numerous, parallel and confluent near the margins. The flowers are tetramerous, small, greenish and sub-sessile and are arranged in broad trichotomous panicles. The fruits are oblong-obovoid or subglobose berries, pink and turning black when ripe and are smooth and shining.

Flowering is in March-May and fruiting during May-July.

Distribution : It is found almost throughout India ascending upto an altitude of 1800 m.

Parts used : The fruits, seeds, leaves and bark are used.

Medicinal uses : Its fruits are used as astringent and in bilious diarrhoea and their juice as carminative, diuretic and stomachic; also beneficially used in chronic diarrhoea and spleen enlargement. The powder of the dried stone of its fruits is used in diabetes. The most ancient direct evidence of its being used in diabetes is in *Dhanwantri nighantu*, where it is mentioned that the Jambu seeds are effective in madhumeha (diabetes). Its seeds are used as hypoglycaemic and also to allay the thirst in diabetes.

The leaf-juice is used in dysentery. The bark is astringent and its decoction in combination with cardamon and cinnamon is useful in chronic diarrhoea and dysentery; also used as a gargle in sore throat and spongy gums. Their fresh juice is given with goat's milk in diarrhoea to children. The powder of its bark is used as gargle and as washes in leucorrhoea, ringworm and skin diseases. Besides, the vinegar of its ripe fruits is used in stomachache and in spleen enlargement.

JASMINE

***Jasminium grandiflorum* Linn.**

(Syn. *J. officinale* Linn. var. *grandiflorum* (Linn.) Stokes; *J. officinale* Linn. fa. *grandiflorum* (Linn.) Kobuski)

(Family: Oleaceae)

Description : It is a large scandent and glabrous shrub with striate branches. Leaves are opposite and imparipinnate; leaflets are 7-11, rhomboid-oblong, the lowest larger than uppermost pair. The flowers are fragrant, white and tinged with purple outside and are borne in divaricate cymes. The fruits are didymous and ovoid berries. Seeds are erect and exalbuminous.

Flowering and fruiting is during March-August.

Distribution : It is found wild in the Western Himalayas upto 2133 m; extensively cultivated in gardens throughout India.

Parts used : The flowers, roots and leaves are usable.

Medicinal uses : The flowers of the plant are considered cooling and are used externally in headache, skin-diseases and in weak eyes. *Mahomedan* writers mentioned that its flowers are used as a plaster to loins, genitals and pubes as an aphrodisiac. An oil of its flowers is applied as cooling agent externally and the roots are used in ringworm. Leaves are astringent and they are chewed as a treatment for ulcerations or eruptions in the mouth. The fresh juice of its leaves is applied to corns between toes. A bland oil prepared with the juice of its leaves is poured into the ear in otorrhoea.

JATAMANSI

***Nardostachys grandiflora* DC.**

(*N. jatamansi* DC.; *Valeriana jatamansi* auct non. Jones)

(Family: Valerianaceae)

Description : It is a perennial herb with woody rhizomatous root stocks covered with fibres from the petioles of withered leaves. Stem is about 10-60 cm long, more or less pubescent upwards and often glabrate below. Radical leaves are 15.0 - 20.0 x 2.0 - 2.5 cm, glabrous or slightly pubescent, narrowed into the petiole and cauline leaves 1 or 2 paired, 2.5-7.5 cm long, sessile and oblong or obovate. Floral heads are usually 1,3 or 5; corolla-tube about 0.6 cm long sometimes hairy within. The fruits are about 0.4 cm long, covered with white hairs and crowned by calyx teeth.

Flowering is during February-May and fruiting is in May-June.

Distribution : It is distributed in alpine Himalayas between 3352-4572 m, extending eastwards from Kumaon to Sikkim upto 5600 m.

Parts used: The roots of the plant are used.

Medicinal uses : In ayurvedic system of medicine, the roots of the plant have been using since a long time and are described to cure 'tridosha', 'kapha' and biliousness of the blood, burning sensation, erysipelas and various skin diseases. While in Unani system, these are said to be used to promote the growth and blackness of the hair and also to increase the appetite. Its roots are aromatic, antiseptic, bitter, stimulant and tonic and are used for the treatment of epilepsy, hysteria and convulsive affections. An infusion of its fresh roots in the doses of 25-50 gm three times daily is recommended in spasmodic, hysterical affections, palpitation of heart, nervous headache, chorea and flatulance. Besides, a powder of its root is also said to be useful in menopause disturbances, hystero-epilepsy and similar nervous and convulsive ailments.

The roots and aromatic rhizomes of the plant are used as a good substitute of Valerian drug, obtained from *Valeriana officinalis* and adulterant with rhizomes of *Cymbopogon shoemamthus* (Garg, 1992).

JIMSON WEED

***Datura stramonium* Linn.**

(Syn. *D. stramonium* var. *tatula* (Linn.) Cl.)

(Family: Solanaceae)

Description : It is an erect, coarse and glabrous or farinose-puberulous annual herb about 60-120 cm high. Leaves are stalked, 15.0-17.0 cm long, ovate, deeply toothed or sinuate and pale-green. Flowers are large and purplish or violet coloured. Fruits are ellipsoid, 4.0-7.0 cm long and spinous capsules. Seeds are many, compressed and rugose.

Flowering and fruiting is during July - December.

Distribution : It is found in the Himalayas from Kashmir to Sikkim upto 2743 m.

Parts used : Generally, the fruits, seeds, flowers and leaves are used.

Medicinal uses : The fruits fo the plant are known as sedative and intoxicating and their juice is applied to scalp for curing dandruff and loss of hairs. Its leaves and seeds are considered antiseptic, anodyne and narcotic and the leaves alone are applied to sores and fish-bites and are smoked like cigarettes to give narcotic effect. An ointment made from its leaf-paste is applied in the treatment of haemorrhoids. Besides, the juice of its flowers is used for earache.

JIVANTI

***Flickingeria macraei* (Lindl.) Bennet**

(Syn. *Desmotrichum fimbriatum* auct. non Blume)

(Family: Orchidaceae)

Description: It is a rhizomatous, creeping and annulate plant which gives off pendulous, smooth and polished stems of 60-90 cm length and bears at irregular intervals narrowly fusiform somewhat compressed shining pseudobulbs of 5.0-6.5 cm length. Leaf terminal is from the top of the pseudobulbs and is soltirary,

10.0-20.0 x 2.2-5.0 cm, linear – oblong and obtuse with numerous parallel slender veins. Flwoers are white, 2.0-2.5 cm across, borne 1 - 3 from near the base of leaf and remain open for a few hours only.

Flowering and fruiting is during August-October.

Distrbution: It is found in Western Ghats of Mumbai and Chennai, Sikkim and Khasia hills.

Parts used: The entire plant is used.

Medicinal uses: In ayurveda, the plant is described as alterative, astringent, cooling and sweet with a flavour and asphrodisiac and expectorant. It is used in asthma, bronchitis, throat problems, consumptions, fevers, burning sensations and biliousness and the diseases of the eye and the blood. Besides, its fruits are used as aphrodisiac and eaten for its sweet tastes.

KAKOLI

***Polygonatum verticilatum* (Linn.) Allioni**

(Syn. *Convallaria verticillata* Linn.)

(Family: Liliaceae)

Description: This is an annual – perennial, tall and erect herb upto 80-150 cm high with angled or grooved stem. Leaves are sessile, in whorls of 4-8, linear or naroowly lanceolate, 8.0-15.0 x 0.5 – 3.0 cm, acuminate or acute. Flowers are white in terminal whorls of leafy racemes. The fruits are globose, 0.5 cm across and purple black when ripe.

Flowering and fruiting is during June – September.

Distribution : It is known to found in monatne to alpine Himalayas from Kashmir to North east states and in Sikkim.

Parts used: The roots are the part, used medicinally.

Medicinal uses: Its roots are eaten raw of after cooking and their powder is given internally in gastric complaints. Besides, their paste is applied on wounds.

KANTAKARI

***Solanum surattense* Burm.f.**

(Syn. *S. xanthocarpum* Sch. & Wendl.; *S. mccanni* Sant.).

(Famliy: Solancaeae)

Description : It is an annual - perennial, prickly and diffuse herb. Stems are aculeate with 0.5-2.5 cm long straight prickles and glabrous except stellate - hairy young parts. Leaves are ovate or elliptic, sinuate or subpinnatified and glabrascent with many straight spines. The flowers are in 2-6-flowered cymose inflorescence. The fruits are globose and glabrous berries, about 1.5 cm long and yellow when ripe. Seeds are 0.2 x 0.1 cm and glabrous.

Flowering and fruiting is during March-June.

Distribution : It is found commonly in waste places and along road-sides throughout India.

Parts used : Whole plant is used medicinally.

Medicinal uses : The whole plant is known for its alterative, antiasthmatic, aperient, astringent, digestive, febrifuge, bitter and pungent properties and is used in bronchitis, cough, dropsy and constipation. A decoction of the plant is given in gonorrhoea and to promote conception. Its fruits, flowers and stems are bitter and carminative and are prescribed in ignipetiditis associated with vesicular and watery eruptions. The buds and flower juice is used in watery eyes and the fine powder of its fruits with honey is used for chronic coughs of the children and also in sore throat.

It is also stated that the vapours of its burning seeds are used as an expectorant in asthma, coughs and in toothache. Leaves are considered anodyne and their juice with black pepper is prescribed in rheumatism. The roots are expectorant, diuretic, antiasthmatic and antiemetic and are used for cough and pain of the chest. Its roots are beaten up and mixed with wine and are given to check vomiting and the decoction of the roots with that of Giloya (*Tinospora cordifolia*) is given in fever and cough.

KAPIKACCHU

***Mucuna pruriens* (Linn.) DC.**

(Syn. *M. prurita* Hook.; *Dolichos pruriens* Linn.; *Stizolobium pruriens* (Linn.) Medicus)

(Family: Fabaceae)

Description : It is an annual herbaceous twiner. Leaves are grey-silky below and 3-foliate; leaflets are ovate - oblong or ovate - rhomboid, unequal at base and 12.0-15.0 × 6.0-7.0 cm. The flowers are dark violet in pendulous racemes. Pods, the fruits are curved, turgid, longitudinally ribbed, 5.0-8.0 cm long and clothed with grey bristles. Seeds are 4-6 and ovoid.

Flowering is during September- October and fruiting in December -March.

Distribution : It occurs almost throughout India and in Andamann and Nicobar islands.

Parts used : Its pods, seeds, roots, and leaves are used.

Medicinal uses : The pods (fruits) are anthelmintic and considered most active against *Tenia caunina* and *T. paraphistonum*. The seeds are aphrodisiac and nervine tonic and also used in scorpion-stings. It is experimentally shown that an aqueous extract of its seed powder has the power to increase sexual activity. Its roots are diuretic and nervine tonic and their decoction is given in urinary problems and delirium in fevers beside, the strong infusion mixed with honey in cholera. A paste of its powdered roots is also applied to the body in dropsy.

A paste of its leaves with water is used to heal the ulcers. The hairs after prolonged heating are used in form of an infusion in cases of gall and liver disorders. An ointment in oil is also prepared from its root-paste, which is used in elephantasis, as a local stimulant and mild vesicant.

KAPITTHA

***Limonia elephantum* (Correa) Panigrahi**

(Syn. *L. acidissima* Linn.; *Feronia limonia* (Linn.) Swingle; *F. elephantum* Correa; *Schinus limonia* Linn.)

(Family : Rutaceae)

Description : It is a large spinous, deciduous and glabrous tree with white or ash-coloured corky bark. Leaves are alrernate, imparipinnate with axillary, strong and straight spines; leaflets are opposite, 3-9, obovate and cuneate with winged petiole. The flowers are polygamous and are borne in terminal or lateral, loose panicles or racemes. The fruits are large berries, 4.0 -7.0 cm in diameter, globose, 1-celled and many seeded. The seeds are embedded in edible pulp and are oblong and compressed.

Flowering is during January-April and fruiting in winter.

Distribution : It is mostly cultivated in dry regions of India and sometimes grows wild.

Parts used : Fruits, leaves, bark and seeds are usable.

Medicinal uses : Its ripe fruits are used as astringent, stomachic, stimulating and appetizing and the unripe ones in scurvy and sore throat and their pulp is applied externally as a remedy for bites of venomous insects and reptiles. Its leaves are aromatic and carminative and the bark beneficially used in liver diseases. Besides, its seeds are used to check infectious diseases like cholera etc.

According to Ambasta (1986), the gum of the plant ressembles with the gum arabic in properties and may be used as a substitute for that.

KARANJ

Caesalpinia bonduc **(Linn.) Roxb.**

(Syn. *C. crista* Linn.; *C. bonducella* (Linn.) Fleming; *Guilandina bonduc* Linn.)

(Family : Fabaceae)

Description : It is a large scandent shrub with small and yellow branches and is covered with downy prickles. Leaves are about 30 cm long and bipinnate; leaflets are 12-16, elongated, upper part thick, 2.0-2.5 x 1.0-1.5 cm, oblong or elliptic and obtuse. The peduncles are long and bear dense flowers at the top, which are yellow in colour. Pods, the fruits are shortly stalked, prickly wingless, swollen in the middle and slightly flat. Seeds are 2-3, lead coloured, 2.5 cm long and bean shaped.

Flowering is during July-September and fruiting in December-January.

General distribution : It is found throughout the hotter parts of India particularly along the sea coast and upto 830 m. Common in West Bengal and South India. Also cultivated as hedge plant in the villages.

Parts used : The seeds, leaves, roots and bark are used.

Medicinal uses : The seeds are antiperiodic, tonic and febrifuge and in powder form they are used in fever, asthma and colic in the doses of 0.7-2.0 gm with equal parts of black pepper and externally in inflammation. The oil of the seeds is emollient and efficacious for stopping discharges from ear and other skin diseases. This oil is also used as embrocation to remove freckles from the face. Its tender leaves are used for disorders of liver and after boiling with castor oil or butter fat are applied externally on painful and swollen testicles. Its leaves and bark both, are used as emmenagogue, anthelmentic and febrifuge. Besides, a decoction of its root is said to be useful in calculus and with honey is used for leucorrhoea.

KASA

***Saccharum spontaneum* Linn.**

(Family: Poaceae)

Description : It is a perennial gregarious grass with glabrous and erect culms. Leaves are linear-filiform, glaucous beneath, often reduced to midrib, scabrid on the margin and 0.1-0.4 cm broad. The sheaths are auriculate and glabrous except hairy throat. Panicle is silvery white, upto 45 cm long. Joints and pedicels are ciliate and 0.2-0.3 cm long. Sessile spikelets are linear-lanceolate.

Flowering and fruiting is during September-December.

Distribution : It is found throughout India in the warmer parts ascending upto 1828 m in the Himalayas.

Parts used : Its roots are used.

Medicinal uses : The roots are diuretic and their decoction with that of Gokshru and mishri is given to remove urinary bladder calculi; as laxative and aphrodisiac. The extract of its roots alongwith the aerial parts is given in burning sensation, phthisis, blood diseases, vesical calculi, bilousness and haemorrhagic diathesis.

KASMARD

***Cassia occidentalis* Linn.**

(Family: Fabaceae)

Description : It is a diffuse undershrub or herb with 60-120 cm height. The stem is angular, striated with reddish purple and glabrous except short gland-hairy young parts. Leaves are paripinnate with foetid smell. Peduncle is small bearing a few yellow flowers having reddish ringe. Pods, the fruits are laterally compressed, slightly upcurved, appressed-short hairy, 12.0-15.0 × 0.8 - 1.0 cm and dehiscent. Seeds are many.

Flowering and fruiting is throughout the year, chiefly during July - December.

Distribution : It is found scattered from the Himalayas to South India.

Parts used : The whole plant is used.

Medicinal uses : The whole plant is said to be febrifuge, purgative, diuretic and tonic. Its leaves and seeds are used as purgative. The root is diuretic, purgative and antiperiodic and is said to be used in snake-bite. The seeds and leaves are used externally in skin diseases and as antiperiodic. Its root juice is used in ringworm. Its leaves are pounded and made into a paste which is applied to fresh wounds to bring their healing by first intention. Besides, the seeds are used externally in the treatment of scabies.

Its seed gum is used as a substitute for Guar gum obtained from *Cyamopsis tetragonoloba* (Farooqi, 1995).

KATHAL

***Artocarpus heterophyllus* Lamk.**

(Syn. *A. integrifolia* auct. mult non Linn. f.)

(Family: Moraceae)

Description : It is a large evergreen tree about 10-15 m in height. The stem is cylindrical and straight and is covered with slightly rough or smooth bark with latex. The wood is moderately hard; sapwood is pale and heartwood is bright yellow which becomes darken on exposure. Leaves are alternate, evergreen, entire, simple, thick, elliptic to obovate-elliptic, lower surface rough with 5.25 × 3.5-12.0 cm sized; stipules leave scar on the branches. Inflorescence is axillary, solitary, cauliflorus and ramiflorus on short leafy shoot, where male flowers occur above the female flowers on the inner side of receptacle. The flowers are small, unisexual and monoecious or dioecious. Fruit is a syncarp some what cylindric which is borne on the main branches and on the trunk, 30-100 × 15-30 cm, yellow, drying to brown with a strong sweet aroma, covered with closely set, firm obtuse and tapering minutely hispid processes. The fruit contains numerous seeds; each enclosed in a yellowish juicy sheath. Seeds are 2.5 cm long, kidney shaped or rectangular.

Flowering is in winter and fruiting in rainy season.

Distribution : This tree is indigenous to India, and is cultivated throughout the hotter parts of the country mainly in Kerala, Bihar and South India.

Parts used : The fruits, seeds, leaves, latex, bark and roots are used.

Medicinal uses : Its unripe fruits are known as acrid, carminative and tonic and the ripe ones as cooling and fattening and are useful in biliousness. Its seeds are used as diuretic and the leaf-ash in healing ulcers. The young leaves and the shoots of the plant with '*gur*' are used as lactagogue for women. Its tender leaves are used in skin diseases and are supposed to be antidote to snake poison. The latex of the plant is applied to glandular swellings and abscesses to promote the suppuration. Its roots are useful in skin diseases, asthma and diarrhoea. The decoction of its bark is given in diarrhoea. Besides, various parts of the plant are used in toothche, caries, stomach complaints, sores, smallpox, carbuncle, sterility and postnatal complaints in women.

KATUKA

Picrorhiza kurroa Royle ex Benth.

(Family: Scrophulariaceae)

Description : This is a low hairy herb with perennial and bitter rootstocks upto 15-25 cm long. Leaves are sub-radical, spathulate, serrate and 5.0-10.0 cm long with narrow base into a winged sheathing petiole. Flowering stems or scapes are ascending, stout and longer than the leaves. Flowers are borne in many – flowered spikes. Sepals are 0.6 cm long and ciliate. Capsules, the fruits are ovoid and about 1.2 cm long.

Flowering is during May-July and fruiting in July – August.

Distribution: It is found in alpine Himalayas from Kashmir to Sikkim upto 3000-5000 m.

Parts used: Its roots are used.

Medicinal uses: In ayurveda, its roots are described as antelminitc, antipyretic, bitter, cardiotonic, cooling, laxative and stomachic, which promote appetite and cure '*kapha*' and are used in biliousness, bilious fevers, urinary discharge, hiccough, burning sensation, leucoderma and jaundice. In small doses, powder of its roots acts as anthelmintic and laxative, while in larger doses, as cathartic and is also used in dropsy. It is combined with liquorices and is given effectively in heart diseases and hiccup.

In the treatment of eczema, 250 gm *panchang* of the plant is boiled in 1 liter of water and cooled; then a cotton cloth is soaked into it and squeezed on the affected parts 3-4 times daily for 20 days. Simultaneously, butter is rubbed with the help of fingers on a bronze plate for 30 minute which is applied as an ointment. Besides, the roots are ground, then fried in ghee and after cooling, they are applied on rheumatic joints and powder of the roots is taken orally with water.

KOKILAKSHA

***Hygrophila auriculata* (Sch.) Heine**

(Syn. *H. spinosa* T. Ander.; *Asteracantha longifolia* (Linn.) Nees; *Barleria auriculata* Sch.)

(Family: Acanthaceae)

Description : It is a stout herb usually with unbranched and subquadrangular erect stems upto 0.6-1.5 m height. Leaves are sparsely hispid on both sides, tapering at base and sessile in verticals of 6 at a node; 2 outer leaves of whorl are 1.8 x 3.5 cm, oblong - lanceolate or oblanceolate and 4 inner 3.8 cm long; each of 6 leaves with straight sharp yellow spine in its axils. Flowers are purple-blue in a whorl of 8 in 4 pairs at each node. Capsules, the fruits are 0.8 cm long, linear - oblong and pointed with 4-8 seeds.

Flowering and fruiting is during March-May.

Distribution : It occurs wild in moist places throughout India; chiefly in Darbhanga (Bihar).

Parts used : Leaves, seeds and roots are used.

Medicinal uses : The leaves of the plant in ayurveda, are known to possess aphrodisiac, bitter and hyptonic properties and are used in diarrhoea, dysentery, thirst, urinary calculi, inflammations, biliousness, constipation and anuria. While in Unani system of medicine, these are applied in gleet, lumbago and pain of joints. Its seeds are acrid, aphrodisiac, bitter, cooling and tasty and with milk and sugar are given in spermatorrhoea and gonorrhoea. Besides, leaves, roots and seeds are used as diuretic and employed for jaundice, dropsy, anasarca and diseases of urino-genital tract. A confection of its seeds containing a large number of aphrodisiac, demulcent, nutrient and aromatic stimulant substances is used in impotence, seminal and other debilities beside, the powder with honey and ghee to be used in asthma.

KUSHA

***Desmostachya bipinnata* Stapf.**

(Syn. *Eragrostis cynosuroides* Beauv.)

(Family: Poaceae)

Description : It is a tufted and perennial grass with a thick rootstock. Culms are erect and nodes are glabrous. Leaves are linear, narrowed into a fliform tip and 0.1-0.3 cm broad and Sheaths are glabrous with hairy throat. The panicles are 45.0 x 1.0-2.0 cm. Spikes are crowded and 1.5 × 0.3 cm. The spikelets are purple brown, biseriate and 3-4 flowered. Grains are 0.05-0.06 cm long, obliquely ovoid, trigonous and laterally compressed.

Flowering is during August - November and fruiting later in cold season.

Distribution : It occurs throughout India in hot and dry parts.

Parts used : Roots and culms are used.

Medicinal uses : Its roots are bitter, sweet, cooling, diuretic, emollient, galactagogue and astringent and are used in asthma, jaundice, vitated conditions of '*pitta*' and hyperdipsia. Besides, the culms are diuretic and stimulant and are used in diarrhoea, dysentery, leucorrhoea, skin diseases, stones, menorrhagia and thirst.

KUTAJ

Holarrhena antidysenterica (Linn.) Wall.

(Family: Apocynaceae)

Description : It is a small decidous tree with rough brown bark which exfoliates in irregular flakes. Leaves are elliptic, oblong and ovate or ovate-oblong and their nerves are 10-14 paired and strong arched. The flowers are white and slightly scented. The fruits are of 2 distinct and divaricate follicles and are slender, parallel, terete, coriaceous and usually with long white spots. Seeds are numerous, 0.8 cm long, linear and glabrous.

Flowering is during April-Juiy and fruiting in August-October.

Distribution : It is found in tropical parts of India and abundantly in the Sub-Himalayan tracts: also planted on road-sides.

Parts used : The seeds, leaves, bark, roots and fruits are used.

Medicinal uses : The seeds and bark are considered anthelmintic, antidysenteric, astringent, bitter, febrifuge and stomachic. The bark alone is used is dysentery and after being dried and ground, is rubbed over the body in dropsy and the seeds as antiperiodic and carminative; and seed-decoction is used in chronic dysentery and bleeding piles. Its seeds are used in pessaries also for promoting conception. The powder of its seeds mixed with honey is given in chronic chest affection, asthma and in colic pain. Its Leaves are used in chronic bronchitis and are also applied to boils and ulcers. An oil for external application is made by mixing the decoction of its bark, a number of astringent and aromatic substances in small quantities and sesamum oil which is used for various diseases. Its fruits are said to be applied in snakebite to allay swelling and irritation also.

Besides, various parts of the plant are used in anaemia, colic pain, diarrhoea, haematuria, menorrhagia, obstetric conditions, spermatorrhoea and splenomegaly.

LAJWANTI

***Mimosa pudica* Linn.**

(Family: Fabaceae)

Description : It is a diffuse or spreading under shrub, about 50-80 cm high. Its stems and branches are densely clothed with prickles. Leaves are bipinnate and collapse on touching; pinnae are 2-4 which are digitately arranged with 10-20 pairs of leaflets. The flowers are as soft as cotton, in pinkish globose heads; peduncle slender about 5.0 cm long. Pods, the fruits are flat, small, 1.2-1.8 cm long and membranous with densely prickly sutures. Seeds are 3-5.

Flowering is during August - September and fruiting in November-December.

Distribution : It is a native of tropical America, now got naturalized and found throughout the tropical and subtropical parts of India. Common in waste places where the climate is moist and warm.

Parts used : The leaves, roots and stem are used.

Medicinal uses : The leaves of the plant are used in sinus, sores, piles and fistula and their paste is applied to hydrocele and glandular swellings. A decoction of its roots is usefully given in gravel and other urinary complaints. The juice of its leaves is used for dressing in sinus and also for sores and piles. A hot decoction of its leaves is used for hip bath for relieving pains. It is gathered at special times and its administration is accompanied by a certain ceremony. In the first week, all billous diseases and fevers are cured, in the second, piles jaundice etc. and in the third, leprosy, scabies and pox.

Besides, a paste made of its roots along with that of *Withania somnifera* is applied over breast to make the nipples hard and attractive by women.

Its seed gum known as, Lajwanti gum is used as a substitute for Guar gum, obtained from *Cyamopsis tetragonoloba*.

LANGULI

Gloriosa superba Linn.

(Family: Liliaceae)

Description : It is a climbing glabrous herb with leafy tendrils and fleshy cylindric tubers. Leaves are sessile, opposite or alternate or verticillate, ovate-lanceolate with cordate base, narrowed into a coiled tendril at apex, glabrous and 10.0-15.0× 2.0-5.0 cm. Flowers are axillary, solitary and forming a terminal corymb. Capsules, the fruits, are oblong and about 4.7 cm long.

Flowering and fruiting is during June-October.

Distribution : It occurs throughout India. ascending upto 1650 m in the Himalayas.

Parts used : Root tubers and leaves are used.

Medicinal uses : The root tubers of this herb are known to have tonic, antiperiodic, cholagogue, alterative and purgative properties and a white flour prepared from its root tubers is given with honey in gonorrhoea and alone in leprosy, colic and intestinal worms. For promoting labour pain, a paste of its root tubers is applied over the supra-pubic region and the vagina. A warm poultice of the root tubers is also used in rheumatism and neuralgic pains. Besides, the juice of its leaves is also used for killing lice in the hair.

The colchicine obtained from the plant can be used as a substitute for *Colchicum autumnale*.

LEMON GRASS

***Cymbopogon citratus* (DC.) Stapf.**

(Syn. *Andropogon citratus* DC.)

(Family: Poaceae)

Description : It is a tall and tufted perennial grass with sparingly branched rhizomes. The culms are upto 1.8 m long, 7-8-noded and simple below the panicle. Leaf-blade is linear, long-attenuated towards base and tapering upwards, 90.0 x 1.6-2.0 cm, firm, glaucous green, glabrous, smooth and more or less rough upwards and along the margins. The ligules are short, scarious and rounded or truncate. Sheaths are terete, 10-30 cm long, subcoriaceous, glabrous and smooth and more or less cinnamon-coloured or russet inside and sheath of the culms tight and pubescent or velvety at the nodes. Spatheate panicle is decompound to subdecompound and loose. Peduncles are 0.6-1.0 cm long and glabrous. Racemes are binate and finally spreading at right angles or epinastically deflexed. Lower glume is usually shallowly concave in the lower half. Pedicelled spikelets are male or neuter. Grains are oblong.

Flowering and fruiting is during July-December.

Distribution : It is grown in the gardens throughout India.

Parts used : Whole plant, its leaves and oil obtained from the grass are used.

Medicinal uses : The grass is pungent, bitter, hot, appetizer, alexipharmic, anaphordisiac, anthelmintic and laxative and is used in epilepsy, bronchitis and leprosy. An infusion of the grass is taken as refreshing beverage. Its leaves are used in elephantiasis and their juice is applied in headache. An oil obtained from the plant is used as antimicrobial, central nervous system depressant, analgesic and antipyretic; this is also used in flatulent and spasmodic affections of the bowels and in gastric irritablity.

LIQUORICE

***Glycrrhiza glabra* Linn.**

(Family: Fabaceae)

Description: It is a tall, erect and perennial plant upto 50 – 100 cm high or more. Leaves are 4-7 pairs, oblong to elliptical – lanceolate, acute or obtuse. The racemes are loose and shorter than the leaves or a little longer. Flwoers are 1.0 cm long. Pods, the fruits are oblong to linear, 1.0-3.0 cm long, flattened, straightish, more or less densely echinate glandular and many seeded.

The plant is generally propagated by crown or rooted cuttings of underground stems.

Distribution: It is found distributed in sub – Himālayan tracts in India.

Parts used: Its roots and leaves are used.

Medicinal uses: In ayurveda, its roots are described as alexeteric, alterative, aphrodisiac, bitter, diuretic, galalctagogue, refrigenrant, sweet and tonic·and they are used in the diseases of eye and ear, to remove biliousness, to improve taste and to lessen thrist, in hiccough, vomiting and in fatigue. These are also used to improve the voice and to cure *vata* diseases. Whereas in Unani system of medicine, these are knwon for their demulcnent, diuretic, emmenagogue and sweetish properties and are used to relive in ashma, thirst, cought, vomiting, bronchitis and abdomenical colic. Its roots are chewed as pleasant and mixed with other drugs are used for dearangemnts of the blood. Besides, its leaves are used for scalds of the head and in foul perspiration of the armpits.

LODHRA

***Symplocos racemosa* Roxb.**

(family : Symplocaceae)

Description: It is an evergreen shrub or small tree upto 6 m high with more or less pilose young branches. Leaves are elliptic-oblong or elliptic – lanceolate, 7.0-15.0 x 2.0-4.5 cm, acute or obtuse, serrualte towards apex and rounded of cuneate at the base; lateral nerves 5-9 pairs. Flowers are white, fading yellow, 0.7-1.2 cm across, pedicielled in simple, axillary 7-15 flowered racemes. The fruits are 0.4-0.5 cm across, oblong and purplish black and glagrous with persistent calyx. Seeds are 1-3.

Flowering is during December – January and fruiting in April – June.

Distribution: It is found in submontane Himalayas to North east states upto 900 m, from the Terai of Kumaon to Assam.

Parts used : The bark is used medicinally.

Medicinal uses: Its bark is known to be astringent and cooling and is used in menorrhagia, bowel complaints, eye diseases and ulcers. Its decoction is used as a gargle for giving firmness to spongy and bleeding gums.

LONG PEPPER

***Piper longum* Linn.**

(Family : Piperaceae)

Description : The plant is a slender, aromatic and climbing herb. Stems are creeping, jointed and become attached to other plants. Leaves are 5.0-9.0 × 3.0-5.0 cm, ovate, cordate, shorthy acuminate, glabrous and membranous; the lower are long petioled and upper sessile. The spikes are pedunculate and upright; male larger and slender and female 1.3-2.5 cm long and 0.4-0.5 cm in diameter. The fruits are very small and ovoid and sunk in solid fleshy spike which is 2.5-3.8 cm, erect, blackish green and shining.

Flowering is during rainy season and flruiting in autumn.

Distribution : The plant is found distributed in hotter parts of India from Central Himalayas to Asaam, Khasi and Mikir hills, lower hills of West Bengal and evergreen forest of Western ghats from Konkan to Kerala; also recorded from Car Nicobar islands.

Parts used : Fruits and roots are used.

Medicinal uses : Its unripe fruits are used as alterative and tonic and mature ones in the diseases of respiratory tracts, bronchitis, asthma and cough. These are also applied on sprains and muscular pains, and are used as carminative, as sedative in insomnia and epilepsy, as general tonic, as cholagogue, in bile and gall bladder obstruction, as emennagogue, abortifacient and anthelmintic. Its roots are said to be used as antidote to snakebites.

It is an important ingredient in the preparation of medicated oil, used externally in sciatica and paraplegia. A mixture of long pepper, its roots, black pepper and ginger in equal parts is a useful preparation for colic, flatulence, cough, coryza and hoarseness. Long pepper in combination with black pepper is used in the preparation of irritating snuff, which is used in coma and drowsinoss. In the form of a powder, it is suspended in warm water and is given to women after parturition to check piles and fever. As vermifuge, it is prescribed for colic in children. The *pipla mul* in combination with borax and baiberang in equal doses is used as contraceptive.

LOTUS

Nelumbo nucifera **Gaertn.**

(Syn. *Nelumbium speciosum* Willd.)

(Family : Nelumboaceae)

Description : It is an attractive perennial herb with creeping rhizomes. Leaves are orbicular, glaucous, floating, peltate and 60-90 cm in diameter; petiole is very long and smooth or prickly. Flowers are solitary, bisexual, regular, large, rosy, white or rarely yellow and 10.2-25.4 cm across. Fruits are torus, spongy, top-shaped and 5.0-10.0 cm in diameter. Seeds are elongated, spherical, smooth, black and exalbuminous.

Flowering is during summer-autumn and fruiting in winter season.

Distribution : It is found throughout the warmer parts of India in ponds; also cultivated often for its sweet-scented flowers.

Parts used : Leaves, rhizomes, flowers, seeds and filaments are used.

Medicinal uses : The juice of its tender leaves mixed with sugar is given in elephantiasis. Powdered rhizomes are prescribed for piles as demulcent and also beneficial in dysentery and chronic dyspepsia. Externally, these are used as a paste in skin affections and ringworm. It is reported that its rhizome extract possesses antipyretic activity also. Its flowers are cooling and astringent and are used in cholera, diarrhoea, fever and liver diseases and their decoction is used as cardiac tonic. Lotus-honey is useful in opthalmia. The seeds are anthelmintic and are given to children as a diuretic and refrigerant and also used in skin diseases and leprosy. Its flowers are also considered as antidote to poisons. Besides, the powder of its fliamants is found beneficial in burning sensation of the body and piles. These are mixed with butter and sugar, prescribed in piles to stop bleeding and in menorrhagia.

MADHUKA

***Madhuca longifolia* (Koen.) Mac Bride**

(Syn. *M. indica* Gmel.; *M. latifolia* (Roxb.) Mac Bride; *Bassia longifolia* Koen.; *B. latifolia* Roxb.)

(Family: Sapotaceae)

Description : It is a large decidous tree with grey or

blackish bark with shallow wrinkles and vertical crakes and about 17 m height. Young branches, leaves and petioles are pubescent or tomentose. Leaves are clustered at the ends of branches, 12.5-17.5 x 7.5-10.0 cm, elliptic or oblong-elliptic and shortly acuminate with cuneate base. The flowers are many, at the ends of the branches and are borne on drooping pedicels. The fruits are ovoid, fleshy amd green berries and about 2.5-5.0 cm long. Seeds are 1-4.

Flowering is during April-May and fruiting in June-July.

Distribution : It occurs in the plains and lower hills of India upto 1200 m. Common throughout West Bengal, Bihar, Madhya Pradesh, Orissa, Punjab and Uttar Pradesh.

Parts used : Seeds, bark, flowers, roots and fruits are used.

Medicinal uses : The seeds of the plant are used as laxative in piles and consipation. The gummy juice of the seeds is applied in rheumatism and skin-affections and the oil derived from its seeds is also used in skin-diseases. The residual cake 'mowrah meal', obtained after the extraction of the oil from the seeds is said to be used as fish poison and as a worm-killer for lawns. The decoction of its bark is useful in itching and ulceration and the bark alone is used as astringent, emollient, hypoglycaemic and tonic and its powder is used in bleeding gums, stomachache, tonsilitis and diabetes. The flowers are considered demulcent, tonic and cooling and are used in coughs, colds and bronchitis. The fomentation with dried flowers produces relief in orchitis and with milk, they are administered in impotence due to general debility. The roots of the plant are also said to be applied on ulcers. Besides, the fruits of the plant are eaten raw or cooked.

MAHABALA

***Sida rhombifolia* Linn.**

(Family: Malvaceae)

Description : It is an erect, much - branched and glabrate to stellate-hairy, annual or perennial herbs. Leaves are lanceolate to rhomboid, acute, cuneate or rounded at base and glabrous above and hoary or grey pubesent beneath. The flowers are yellow and small and are borne axillary, solitary or in pairs. Fruits are small capsules, 0.35-0.4 cm across and stellate-hairy in the upper part. Seeds are 1-2, smooth and black.

Flowering is during rainy season and fruiting in winter.

Distribution : It is found throughout India, particularly in moist regions ascending upto 1800 m in the Himalayas.

Parts used : Whole plant, its leaves, stem and the roots are used.

Medicinal uses : The whole plant is used in pulmonary tuberculosis and rheumatism. Its leaves are pounded and are applied on swellings. The stem is mucilaginous and both externally and internally is used as demulcent and emollient. Its roots are considered valuable in the treatment of rheumatism and their paste in milk with honey is given to relieve pain of leucorrhoea.

Besides, its leaves are used as a substitute for tea.

MAKARADHWAJ

***Rubia cordifolia* Linn.**

(Family: Rubiaceae)

Description : It is a climbing perennial herb with stout and smooth branches. Leaves are in whorls of 3-4, ovate or ovate-oblong to lanceolate with a cordate or rounded base, acute or acuminate with short - bristly margins, glabrous except prickly nerves beneath and 2.0 - 10.0 x 1.5 - 5.0 cm. Flowers are greenish yellow in cymes arranged in axillary inflorescences which are combined into a many-flowered and widely branched panicle. The fruits are bluish black and glabrous with single seed and 0.4 - 0.6 cm in diameter.

Flowering is during July - September and fruiting in November - December.

Distribution : It is known to found in hilly districts throughout India.

Parts used : Its roots are usable.

Medicinal uses : The roots of this plant are considered alterative, astringent and tonic and are applied in eye sores, paralysis, liver complaints, enlargement of spleen, rheumatism, leucorrhoea, leucoderma and dysentery. *Hakims* prescribe it much in paralytic affections, jaundice, and obstruction of the urinary tracts and in amenorrhoea. An infusion of its roots is prescribed as a drink to women after delivery to procure copious flow of lochia. Besides, a paste made of its roots with honey is applied externally on freckles and discolouration of the skin; also in external inflammation, ulcers and various skin diseases as pityriasis and vesicular etc.

MALABAR NUT

***Justicia adhatoda* Linn.**

(Syn. *Adhatoda vasica* Nees; *A zeylanica* Med.)

(Family: Acanthaceae)

Description : It is a dense, evergreen and erect undershrub or shrub attaining a height upto 1.2 - 2.5 m. Stem is densely appressed - pubescent on young parts. Leaves are ovate - lanceolate to oblong with cuneate often decurrent base, acuminate, glabrous except hairy nerves beneath, subentire - crenulate and 5.0 - 15.0 x 3.0- 8.0 cm; petiole is 0.5 - 3.0 cm long. The flowers are white and are borne in 3.0-15.0 cm long peduncled spikes. Capsules, the fruits are 2.0 cm long, short hairy and 4-seeded.

Flowering is during December-April and fruiting in February-May.

Distribution : It is found throughout in the sub-Himalayan tracts upto 1219 m.

Parts used : Leaves, roots and flowers are used.

Medicinal uses : The leaves are considered antiseptic

and are used in cough, chronic bronchitis, asthma and phthisis. These are also used in rheumatism and as insecticidal. A crude extract of its leaves is more useful for respiratory ailments as it exhibits uterine stimulation and bronchoconstrictor as the undesirable effects. Its leaves are also used in homeopathy for colds, coryza, coughs, pneumonia, spitting of blood, fever, jaundice, chixilly, catarrh, whooping coughs and bronchitis. The roots are antiseptic and expectorant and are used in cough, asthma and phithisis and are also given in intermittent fever. Besides, its flowers are used as antiseptic.

MASHA

***Vigna mungo* (Linn.) Heeper**

(Syn. *Phaseolus mungo* (Linn.) Mant.)

(Family: Fabaceae)

Description: This is an annual suberect or decumbent - ascending hairy herb. Leaves are trifoliolate and stipellate. The flowers are small and yellow and are borne in dense racemes. Bracts are lanceolate and bracteoles linear and small. Pods, the fruits are erect, hairy and long with 10-15 seeds. The seeds are black or brown dotted with black.

Flowering and fruiting is during cold season.

Distribution : It is cultivated throughout India.

Parts used : Its seeds and roots are used.

Medicinal uses : Its seeds are known for their demulcent, cooling, aphrodisiac, lactagogue and nervine tonic properties and internally, these are used in gastric catarrh, dysentery, diarrhoea, cystitis, paralysis, piles, rheumatism and affections of the liver and of nervous system in the form of a decoction. Externally, their poulitice is applied in gastritis, dysentery and rheumatism. Its seeds are parched and eaten in urinary complaints. Besides, the roots are used as narcotic and as a remedy for aching bones and their poultice for abscesses and inflammations.

Its seeds are reported to contain traces of a cyanogenetic

glycoside and an unidentified substance, which reduces blood sugar level hence, eaten by diabetic persons.

MEDA

***Roscoea alpina* Royle**

(Syn. *R. intermedia* Gagi: *R. longifolia Ibaker*)

Description: It is a small, glabrous and erect herb with tuber-roots. Stem is with membranous bracts below and leafy above upto 10-15 cm high. Leaves are 2-4, sessile, narrow, elliptic-lanceolate, 5.0-12.0 x 1.0-2.0 cm and acute with sheating base. Flowers are several, dark-purple, appearing one at a time with small and persistent bracts. Capsules, the fruits are globose. Seed is enclosed within red aril.

Flowering and fruiting is during July-September.

Distribution: It is seen distributed in hilly parts of the country between 1000-2700 m.

Usable parts: Entire plant is used.

Medicinal uses: It is one of the constituents of 'Ashtavarga' of ayurveda. An extract of entire plant is used as a tonic. Besides, dried powder of its leaves is applied on cuts and wounds.

Its another species ***R. purpurea* Smith** (Syn. *R. purpurea* var. *exilis* sensu Baker; *R. purupurea* var. *procera* (Wall.) Baker), commonly called '*Kakoli*' is found distributed in open grassy slopes in montane zones of the country upto 2400 m. Its tuberous roots are used as general tonic. In small quantities, its tuberous roots are collected and sold under the '*Ashtavaga*' drug with *R. alpina* roots in the market.

MUSTARD

***Brassica campestris* Linn. var *sarson* Prain**

(Family: Brassicaceae)

Description : The plant is an erect and glaucous annual

herb upto 10-90 cm high. Basal leaves are lyrate-pinnatified, dentate and broad; upper leaves are small and dentate. The flowers are yellow coloured. Pedicels are 0.6-1.5 cm long during anthesis and 1.0-2.5 cm long in fruiting. Pods, the fruits are upto 7.0 cm long and patent or erectopatent. Seeds are many, yellow coloured, 0.2 cm across and round.

Flowering and fruiting is during January - March.

Distribution : It is cultivated throughout the plains of India.

Parts used : Its roots, leaves, seeds and oil from the seeds are used.

Medicinal uses : The roots and leaves are used as stomachic. Its seeds mixed with hot water form an efficient counter irritant poulitice. Besides, the oil obtained from its seeds, combined with camphor forms an efficaceous embrocation which is used in dengu fever with great benefit and also rubbed on the chest in bronchitis and in spleen enlargement.

Its oil is adulterated commonly with that of *Argemone maxicana.*

NAGAKESAR

***Mesua ferrea* Linn.**

(Family: Clusiaceae)

Description: It is a medium - sized or large evergreen tree with short trunk and dark red heartwood; often buttressed at the base. Leaves are 5.0 - 15.0 x 3.5 - 4.5 cm, coriaceous and lanceolate; upper side shining and lower covered with a white waxy powder. Flowers are white, large and solitary or in clusters and fragrant. The fruits are ovoid, 2.5-5.0 cm long with persistent calyx. Seeds are 1-4, shining and dark brown with oily and fleshy cotyledons.

Flowering is in February - April and fruiting during September - October.

Distribution: It is found in the mountains of Eastern Himalayas and East Bengal, Assam and Eastern and Western Ghats as well as in Andaman, ascending upto 1500 m.

Parts used: Flowers, seeds, fruits, bark and leaves are the parts, used medicinally.

Medicinal uses: The flowers of this plant are considered astringent, stomachic and expectorant and they along with its stamens form a major drug *Nagapushpa* and *Nagkesar* in indigenous system of medicine. These are used in cough and their paste made in ghee is applied in bleeding piles and burning of the feet and buds in dysentery. The seed oil is used in rheumatism and cutaneous affections. The unripe fruits of the plant are considered aromatic and sudofiric, whereas ripe ones are astringent and are used in gastric troubles. The bark of the plant is aromatic and astringent and its decoction combined with ginger is used as sudorific. Besides, the leaves as poultice, are applied on forehead in severe colds.

NAGBALA

***Sida cordata* (Burm.f.) Borssum**

(Syn. *S. multicaulis* Cav.; *S. humilis* Cav.; *S. humilis* var. *veronicaefolia* (Lamk.) Masters; *S. veronicaefolia* Lamk.; *Melochia cordata* Burm.f.)

(Family: Malvaceae)

Description : It is a prostrate or decumbent-ascending and some-what hairy herb. Leaves are ovate-cordate, acuminate, serrate with alternate and short teeth and glabrate or thinly stellate-hairy. The flowers are yellow and axillary and solitary or borne in pairs or in small cymes. Fruits are subglobose and 0.35 - 0.38 cm in diameter. Seeds are brown.

Flowering and fruiting is almost throughout the year.

Distribution : The plant is found in the hotter parts of India upto 1500 m.

Parts used : Whole plant is used.

Medicinal uses : The flowers and unripe fruits of the herb with sugar are given for burning sensation in micturition. The juice of leaves is given in diarrhoea during pregnancy and as a poultice, leaves are also applied to cuts and bruises. Its root-bark is used in leucorrhoea, micturition and gonorrhoea. Besides, the whole plant is considered cooling, astringent and tonic and it is used in fevers and urinary complaints and its decoction is given internally to prevent joint swellings in arthritis.

NEEM

***Azadirachta indica* A. Juss.**

(Syn. *Melia azadirachta* Linn.)

(Family: Meliaceae)

Description : It is a large and handsome tree upto 18 m high with almost a straight trunk. Leaves are imparipinnate, crowded at the ends of branches, 22.0-40.0 cm long and glabrous; leaflets are 5-15, opposite, subopposite or alternate, lanceolate or ovate-lanceolate, acuminate, serrate or dentate and glabrous. The flowers are scented and are borne in numerous axillary panicles and pedicels which are shorter than the leaves. The fruits are one seeded drupes, oblong and greenish-yellow when ripe.

Flowering is in February-April and fruiting during June-August.

Distribution : The plant is commonly cultivated in various parts of India and also grows wild in Sub-Himalayan tract and forests of other areas.

Parts used : Fruits, seeds, flowers, twigs, bark and gum are the parts used.

Medicinal uses : Its fruits are antiperiodic, anthelmintic, astringent, emollient, purgative and tonic and are used in piles and urinary diseases; also to cure rheumatic pains. The seeds are poisonous in large doses to man and some animals producing gastro-intestinal irritation and severe purgation. The oil obtained from its seeds, is considered antiseptic and is used in eczema and leprosy. The kernel oil known as *Oil of Margosa* or *Neem oil* possesses antifertility, antifungal, antimicrobial and antiseptic properties and is useful in chronic skin diseases, leprosy and ulcers. Warm oil is used to relief in ear, dental and gum troubles. Hair oil, containing neem oil is used to prevent baldness and greying of the hairs. The oil is also stated as an effective oral antifertility agent, but its effect decreases as the pregnancy advances.

Its flowers are used as stomachic, tonic and purgative and constitue indigenous drug, *'Amber mezhugu'* which is useful against rheumatism. An indigenous preparation of its flowers with *Piper nigrum* is used as anthelmintic. Its leaves are antifungal, antiperiodic, antiseptic and antiviral and are applied in the form of poultice, in boils, abscesses, adenitis, eczema and ulcers. A hot infusion of its leaves is anodyne for formating brusies, sprains and swollen glands. The tender leaves with *Piper nigrum* are used for intestinal helminthiasis. Leaves are also used as one of the constituents of compound for diabetic patients. Aqueous extract of the leaves alongwith the leaves of *Zizyphus jujuba* is used against hair falling. Its twigs are widely used as toothbrush for its antipyorrhoel property and as carminative and digestive. The bark is considered antiemetic, antiperiodic, anthelmintic, astringent, hypoglycaemic and as tonic and is used in anorexia, colic, liver disorders, malaria and sprue and also as a good remedy for pyresis. The sap obtained from its stem-tip is beneficial in consumption, atonic dyspepsia, debility and skin diseases and also as refrigerant nutritive and tonic.

The gum obtained from the plant is considered as proteolytic, demulcent, stimulant and tonic and it used in catarrh and splenic enlargement. Besides, the ashes of its leaves are taken with water to remove urinary calculi and their extract to stop vomitting. The bark of the plant alongwith that of *Ficus religiosa, F. virens, F. racemosa* and *F. bengalensis* constitutes 'panchavalkala' which is used for gargle in salivation, as a wash for ulcers and as a injection in leucorrhoea.

NIRGUNDI

Vitex negundo Linn.

(Family : Verbenaceae)

Description : It is a deciduous shrub with thin grey bark. The branchlets, undersides of leaves and inflorescence are hoary with short grey pubescence. Leaves are 3-5-foliolate; leaflets are lanceolate, 2.5-12.5 x 0.7-3.3 cm, the lowest pair is smallest sessile or subsessile, the middle pair, if present, more or less distinctly petiolulate and the odd leaflet is largest with a 0.7-1.5 cm long petiolule, entire or crenate, glabrate, dark-green above and palegreenish-tomentose beneath. The flowers are small and bluish purple and are borne in lateral cymes forming an elongated terminal thyrsus and often componnd at the base. The fruits are succulent and black when ripe. Seeds are obovate or oblong.

Flowering is during June-August and fruiting in cold sesson.

Distribution : It is found in the scrub – jungles and road–sides in the warmer parts of the country.

Parts used : Leaves, roots, bark, fruits, seeds, flowers and whole plant are usable.

Medicinal uses : Its leaves are known to be used as vermifuge, aromatic, tonic, alterative anodyne, antiparasitic, discutient, antiinflammatory and antirheumatic. The rheumatic patients are advised to have bath in water boiled with its leaves. A smoke of its dried leaves is taken in headache and catarrh. The decoction of the leaves with long pepper is advised to be taken in catarrh fever with heaviness of head and dullness of hearing and also as bath in the puerperal state of women. The juice of its leaves is used for removing foetid discharges and worms from ulcers and with cow's urine, is administered in the doses of 25 gm every morning in the enlargement of spleen. Its leaves are considered very efficacious in dispelling inflammatory swellings of the joints from rheumatism and of the testes from suppressed gonorrhoea or gonorrhoeal epididymitis and orchitis and also over sprained limbs, contusions and leech bites. For the purposes, its fresh leaves are put into an earthen pot heated over a fire and applied as hot as can be tolarated without pain or the bruised leaves as poultice to the affected part.

Its roots are anodyne, diuretic, febrifuge, expectorant and tonic and are used in boils, colic, dyspepsia, leprosy and as anthelmintic and also as demulcent in piles and dysentery. The root-bark tincture is used in rheumatism and irritable bladder. The fruits are used as cephalic, nervine tonic and emennagogue and dried ones as vermifuge. Its seeds are cooling and are used in leprosy caused by *Mycobacterium tuberculosis* and other cutaneous diseases. The flowers are known as astringent, cardiotonic and cooling and are prescribed in cholera, fever, diarrhoea, liver complaints and haemorrhage of the digestive system. Besides, a compound oil is prepared from the juice of the plant and eleven other substances in different properties is thought to be specific for syphilis and other venereal diseases.

NISHOTH

***Operculina turpethum* Silva**

(Family: Convolvulaceae)

Description: It is a perennial plant with milky juice and long, slender and fleshy roots and very long, twining and much twisted stem. Leaves are 5.0-10.0 x 1.3-7.0 cm, ovate or oblong, rarely slightly lobulate, subacute, mucronate, more or less pubescent on the both sides expecially when young, and minutely reticulately veined with cordate or truncate base; petioles 2.5 cm long and pubescent. The flowers are pinkish in are few-flowerd cymes with stout and 2.5-5.0 cm long peduclces. Capsules, the fruits are 0.8-1.3 cm across, globose and enclosed in the enalrged. birttle and very imbricate sepals and are faintly pubescent or glabrous.

Flowering and fruiting is during March-December.

Distribution: It is known to occur throghuout the country upto 1000 m; sometimes cultivated.

Parts used: Its roots are used.

Medicinal uses: In ayurveda, its roots are descrived as anthelmintic, antipyrietic, alexteric, bitter, heating, purgative and sweet with sharp taste, and are used in ascities, leucoderma, itch, ulcers, constipation, piles, erysipelas, tumours, jaundice, consumption, ophtalmia, and in the diseases of heart and liver. Its black variety is a powerful drastic, and is used in loss of consciuousness, burning sensation and the intoxication and the white variety is moderately mild cathartic which is useful in bilious fevers, inflammations and the diseses of abdomen. About two scruples of its roots are rubbed into a pulp with water, and is taken with the addtion of rock salt and ginger or sugar and black pepper as purgative.

In traditional medicine, its flowers are applied to the head in hemcrania.

NUTMEG

Myristica fragrans

(Family: Myristicaceae)

Description: It is a lofty tree with slender branches. Leaves are coriaceous, 7.5-8.8 cm long, elliptic-oblong or elliptic - lanceolate, acuminate and sometimes oblancolate with caudate tips and pale yellow – brown or paler with red brown nerves beneath; petiole 0.6-1.3 cm long. The flowers are bracteolate and 0.6 cm long, ellipsoid or urceolate and nodding; male are in lax slender and super – axillary racemes. The fruits are sub-globose or pyriform and ovoid, about 3.8-5.0 cm long.

Flowering and fruiting is during rainy season.

Distribution: A native of Eastern Moluccas, is cultivated in certain places, chiefly in botanical gardens, where the climate is sufficiently hot and moist.

Parts used: Its fruits, seeds and nuts are used.

Medicinal uses: Its fruits in the ayurveda, are known as anthelmintic, aphrodisiac, astringent, bitter hot and pungent and are used to improve appetite, taste and voice; also in *kapha, vata* diseases, bronchitis, vomting, thirst and the diseases of heart and urinary discharges. The oil obtained from its fruits is known as carminative and stimulant and is used in diarrhoea, convulsions, pains, ulcers and to improve the appetite. The mace has a bitter and pungent taste and anthelmintic and alexiteric properties and is used in bronchitis, asthma, thrist and to improve the appetite.

Whereas, in Unani system, the nuts and the mace are aphrodisiac, digestive, dirutetic, hypnotic, lactagogue and stimulant and are used in choleraic diarrhoeas, diseases of the liver and spleen, headache, palsy and in eye problems. Besides, its seeds are knwon as carminative and stomachic and are used in flatulence, nausea, and vomiting and in larger doses as narcotic.

NUXVOMICA

Strychnos nux-vomica Linn.

(Family: Loganiacaeae)

Description : It is an evergreen and glabrous tree; often with short sharp strong axillary spines and thin grey, smooth or rough bark and reaching a height upto 30 m. Leaves are ovate, 5-nerved, glabrous, shining with obtuse base and 7.5-15.0 x 4.5-7.5 cm. Flowers are greenish - white in terminal pubescent, pedunculate, corymbose cymes. Berries, the fruits are globose, about 2.5-5.0 cm in diameter, slightly rough but shining and yellow when ripe. Seeds are usually many, discoid and about 1.2 cm across.

Flowering is during March-April and fruiting in winter.

Distribution : It is found throughout the tropical parts of India, including Bihar, Orissa, West Bengal and Uttar Pradesh ascending upto 1350 m.

Medicinal uses : In ayurveda, the fruits of the plant are said to be acrid, appetizer, bitter, pungent and tonic and are used to cure leucoderma, *'vata'* and *'kapha'* diseases, blood diseases, anaemia, piles, jaundice and urinary dischargement and in Unani system, these are described as aphrodisiac, bitter, diuretic, emmenagogue and tonic and are used to cure pain and weakness of joints, lumbago, piles and paralysis. Its root bark is ground into a fine paste with limejuice and made into pills, which are given efficaciously given in cholera.

Its leaf-paste is applied to sloughing ulcers and wounds; especially in cases when maggots are formed. The wood is also used in cases of dyspepsia. Besides, its seeds are described as tonic, antidiarrhoeal, antidysenteric, antispasmodic, emetic, febrifuge, stimulant and tonic and these are used in cholera, diabetes, emotional disorders, hysteria, epilepsy, intermittent fever, gout, rheumatism, hydrophobia, impotence, insomia, paralytic and neuralgic affections, prolapse of rectum, retention or nocturnal incontinence of urine and spermatorrhoea. In *Ilajul-gurba*, a paste made of the equal parts of seeds of nux-vomica, seeds of *Momordica charantia, red ochre, siah jira* and roots of *Bismari-ki-jhad,* is prescribed to be applied in tympanitis (Nadkarni, 1954). An oil obtained by heating its fresh seeds is also applied externally in chronic rheumatism, palsy and relaxation of the muscles and tendrons.

It is also used as antidote to alcoholism and opium poisoning.

NYAGRODHA

***Ficus bengalensis* Linn.**

(Family: Moraceae)

Description : It is a large evergreen tree upto 30 m height and extending laterally by sending down aerial roots. Aerial roots are many and sometimes develop into accessory trunks and assist the lateral spread of the tree indefinitely. The bark is light grey-white, smooth and about 1.25 cm in thickness. Leaves are coriaceous, 10.0-20.0 x 5.0-12.0 cm, ovate-elliptic with subcordate or rounded base. Male flowers are many near the mouth of the receptacle: sepals 4; gall flowers: perianth as in male and fertile flowers: perianth shorter than in male, style elongate; male and female flowers are in same receptacle. Fruits are sessile in pairs, puberulous, sub-globose, 1.3-2.0 cm across and red when ripe.

Flowering is during summer and fruiting during rainy season.

Distribution : It occurs throughout the plains and forest tracts of India; also planted in avenues for shades. Epiphytic when young and develops from seeds dropped by birds on walls or on other trees.

Parts used : Generally seeds, latex and the bark are used.

Medicinal uses : Its seeds are used as cooling and tonic. Leaves as poultice are applied to abscesses and tender leaves' paste with honey is considered beneficial in '*raktapitta*'. The milky juice obtained from its branches is applied externally for pains, in rheumatism and lumbago, sores and ulcers and soles of the feet when cracked or inflamed. The latex of the plant is also used in toothache and mixed with the sesamum oil is applied on burns and in genital diseases. The root fibres are used in gonorrhoea and tender ends of hanging roots as antiemetic. A paste of its roots is applied to scalp to grow hair long and for menorrhagia. An infusion of the bark is considered to be a good tonic, effective in diabetes, dysentery, gonorrhoea and in seminal weakness. The bark with black pepper is used in snakebites. Aqueous extract of its bark and that of leaves is used as a depressant on uterine and cardiac muscles; also on cholinergic-blocking of smooth and skeltal muscle.

According to Bhandari (1993), its bark along with the bark of *F. virens, F. religiosa, F. racemosa* and *Azadirachta indica*, pass by the name *Panchaval kala*, is used for gargle in salivation, as a wash for ulcers and as a injection in leucorrhoea.

PARPATA

***Fumaria indica* Pugsley**

(Syn. *F. parviflora* auct. non Lamk.)

(Family: Fumariaceae)

Description : It is a pale - green, diffuse and much branched herb upto 60 cm high. Leaves are divided into thin and flat segments. The racemes are 2.5 - 5.0 cm long and lax-flowered. The flowers are white, pink or purplish. The fruits are globose, rugose when dry and each with one seed.

Flowering and fruiting is during winter season.

Distribution : This is found almost throughout India as a weed of cultivation; commonly seen on road sides at hill-stations upto 3132 m.

Parts used : Whole plant is used.

Medicinal uses : The entire plant is known to possess diuretic, anthelmintic and blood purifier properties and is used in dyspepsia, scrofulous skin and liver complaints. Its seeds are useful in body pains. Besides, an infusion of its leaves and of stems is given as febrifuge and alterative.

The plant is used as a substitute for *Oldenlandia corymbosa*.

PASHAN BHEDA

***Bergenia ciliata* (Haworth) Sternburg**

(Syn. *Megasea ciliata* Haworth; *Saxifraga ciliata* Royle; *S. ligulata* var. *ciliata* (Royle) C.B. Clarke)

(Family: Saxifragaceae)

Description: It is a perennial herb with thick and rhizomatous rootstocks and short stem. Leaves are radical, shortly stalked, broadly ovate or sub-orbicular with both surfaces and margins covered with red-brown erectopatent hairs. Flowers are pinkish, 1.2-1.5 cm across on slender, one sided, spreading cymose-panicles. Capsules, the fruits are sub-globose with long persistent styles and surrounded by erect calyx lobes. Seeds are smooth and elongated.

Flowering is during February-April and fruiting in May-June.

Distribution: It is reported from temperate Himalayas from Kashmir between 3300 – 4000 m to Sikkim between 3000-4700 m.

Usable parts: The roots are used.

Medicinal uses : In ayurveda, its roots are known for their acrid, bitter, cooling and laxative properties which are used in '*tridosha*', in piles, tumours, strangury, calculi, urinary discharges, heart diseases, enlargement of spleen, ulcers and dysentery. While in Unani system, these are known as alexiteric, astringent, diuretic, tonic and styptic and are useful in hydrophobia, spleenic enlargement, menorrhagia and biliousness. After bruising, these are applied to boils and in ophthalmia.

In case of constipation, its root-paste is taken with lukewarm water and in dysentery, 10 gm with fresh water twice daily for 5 days. While in cases of stones, its roots with the seeds of *Tephrosia candida* (Roxb.) DC., are gound and in the doses of 10 gm are given twice daily for 15 days. For painful and slow urination, 5-10 gm of its root powder is given with cold water and root-paste is applied on naval of the patient.

PATALA

***Stereospermum chelonoides* (Linn. f.) DC.**

(Syn. *Bignonia chelonoides* Linn. f.; *B. suaveolens* Roxb.; *Stereospermum suaveolens* (Roxb.) DC.)

(Family: Bignoniaceae)

Description : It is a large deciduous tree about 9-18 m high with dark-grey bark which is exfoliating in large flat scales. Leaves are opposite, about 30-60 cm long and paripinnate; leaflets are 5-9 or more commonly 7, 7.5-15.0 x 5.0 - 7.5 cm, elliptic, acute or acuminate, entire and coriaceous. The flowers are dark purple, pubescent and fragrant in viscid trichotomous panicles. The fruits are loculicidally 2-valved capsules, about 30.0-60.0 x 1.2 - 2.7 cm, 4-ribbed and dark grey with white specks. Seeds are 3.0 - 3.7 x 0.8 cm with 2 oblong and lateral wings.

Flowering is in May-June and fruiting during cold season.

Distribution : It is found distributed throughout drier parts in India.

Parts used : Its root-bark, seeds and flowers are used.

Medicinal uses : The root-bark of the plant is considered cooling, diuretic and tonic and its decoction is used to remove calculi. A paste of its seeds is applied on forehead in migrane and the flowers rubbed up with honey, are given to check hiccough and in a form of confection as an aphrodisiac.

Besides, ethanolic extract of the flowers shows activity against '*Ranikhet disease*' and anticancerous activity against human epidermoid carcinoma of the nasopharynx in tissue culture.

PATOLA

***Trichosanthes cucumerina* Linn.**

(Syn. *T. brevibracteata* Kundu; *T. pachyrrhachis* Kundu)

(Family: Cucurbitaceae)

Description : It is annual herb with twining and more or less pubescent stem. Tendrils are 3-fid. Leaves are reniform-suborbicular, 3-7-lobed or angular, denticulate, obtuse, glandular hairy and 5.0 - 20.0 cm across. The flowers are white and dioecious; male flowers: bracts absent or rare, pedicels jointed at the top and 1.0 - 2.0 cm long; female flowers: pedicels 1.5 - 2.0 cm long. The fruits are 2.5 - 7.5 cm long, beaked, ovoid and conical. Seeds are compressed and corrugate and are embeded in red pulp.

Flowering and fruting is during July - December.

Distribution : It is found distributed throughout India.

Parts used : Whole plant is used.

Medicinal uses : Its fruits are described as bitter and laxative and the ripe ones are cooked and eaten. The juice of its leaves is emetic and externally applied to the bald patches of its alopecia. The roots are purgative and tonic and their juice is used as cathartic. A decoction of its leaves and that of stem is used for bilious disroders, skin diseases and as emmenagogue. Besides, the seeds are used as antifebrile and anthelmintic agent and are given internally in the disorder of stomach.

The *Hakims* consider the whole plant as general and cardiac tonic, alterative and antifebrile. In obstinate cases of fever, an infusion of entire plant and coriander, infused for a night is recommended to be given in the morning and the evening with honey.

PEPPERMINT

***Mentha piperita* Linn.**

(Family: Lamiaceae)

Description: It is a perennial, glabrous and stong scented herb. Leaves are petioled, 2.5-10.cm long, ovate or oblong-lanceolate with acute or obtuse base and coarsely serrate, smooth above and rarely sparingly hairy on the nerves below; upper smaller, sometimes bracteiform. Whorls are in terminal spikes, which are cylindric, interrupted below. Pedicels and flowers are glabrous or very sparingly hispid.

Flowering in August-September and fruiting during September-October.

Distribution: It is cultivated throughout the country in the gardens.

Parts used: The oil obtained from the plant, and its leaves are used.

Medicinal uses: The oil obtained from the plant is a well known medicine for its antiseptic, stimulant and carminative properties. Besides, its fresh leaves are bruised and are applied in local pains and headache and the hot infusion is taken as tea to soothe stomach ache and to allay the sickness and stay colicky diarrhoea.

PINUS

***Pinus roxburghii* Sarg.**

(Syn. *P. longifolia* Roxb.)

(Family: Pinaceae)

Description : It is a large tree with symmetrical branches high up on the trunk and forming a round head of light foliage and reaching upto 30 m in height. Normally, it is evergreen but becomes completely or partially deciduous in dry season. The bark is dark grey and deeply fissured. Leaves are 20-30 cm long, arranged in clusters of three, finely toothed and light green. Male flowers are arranged in form of cones, which are 1.5 cm long. Female cones are 10.0-20.0 x 7.5-12.0 cm, ovoid and are solitary or 2-5 together and woody. Seeds without wings are 0.7-1.3 x 0.5-0.6 cm and winged; wings are membranous and long.

Cone formation is started in January, next year during June-July its cones become old and in next summer, burst and seeds are shed out. About 26 month are spared to complete the whole process.

Distribution : It is found in the Himalayas from Kashmir to Sikkim and in the Shiwalik hills at the altitude of 450-2400 m. Sometimes, rose in gardens as an ornamental plant.

Parts used : The wood, resin and oil are used.

Medicinal uses : Its wood is stimulant, diaphoretic and is useful in the burning of the body, cough, fainting and ulcerations. It is also said to be beneficial in snakebite and scorpion-stings. The oleoresin known as *gandhbiroza*, is considered to be anodyne and diuretic and is beneficial in coryza and oedema and is advised to be given in the doses of 1.8-5.4 gm four times daily in gonorrhoea. It is expectorant and useful in chronic bronchitis and is especially recommended in gangrene of lungs, also given as carminative in flatulent colic and to arrest minor haemorrhages in tooth sockets and nose. Externally, it used as a rubefacient in rheumatic affections and for deep-seated inflammations, especially of abdomen and as plaster is applied to buboes and abscesses for suppuration.

Its oil mixed with mustard oil is rubbed in rheumatic pain. Besides, its vapours relieve the spasm of whooping cough and asthma and internally, it is given in indigestion, loss of appetite and intestinal worms.

PLAKSHA

***Ficus virens* Ait.**

(Syn. *F. lacor* Buch.-Ham.; *F. infectoria* sensu Roxb.)

(Family: Moraceae)

Description : It is a large spreading tree about 12-15 m high with greenish-grey and smooth bark; sometimes, sending down a few aerial roots. Leaves are alternate, 7.5-12.0 cm long, oblong-ovate or ovate and shortly acuminate with subundulate or entire margins; petioles 3.5 - 5.0 cm long and channelled. The fruits are usually sessile in axillary pairs, sub-globose and white when ripe.

Flowering is in rainy season and fruiting during February-May.

Distribution : It occurs in Northern India, Madhya Pradesh and Peninsular India. Frequently, is planted as an avenue and ornamental tree and often epiphytic in early stages.

Parts used : The bark, leaves and fruits are used.

Medicinal uses : The bark of the plant along with the barks of *F. bengalensis*, *F. racemosa*, *F. religiosa* and *Azadirachta indica*, pass by the name, *panchaval kala,* which is used for gargle in salivation, as a wash for ulcers and as a injection in leucorrhoea. Pulverized bark mixed with honey is applied externally in the diseases of female generative organs. In chinese medicine, its bark is considered diaphoratic. Its leaves are considered as useful diet for those who suffer from *'raktapitta'* disease. The juice of its fruits is considered a cardiotonic and is also used to increase appetite. Besides, its fruits are used in bronchitis and scabies.

POMEGRANATE

***Punica granatum* Linn.**

(Family: Punicaceae)

Description : It is a glabrous and decidous shrub or small tree with dark grey bark. Leaves are opposite or suboposite, often fascicled on short petiole, oblong or obovate and are 2.5-6.0 cm long. The flowers are terminal or axillary, solitary, large and showy and orange-red coloured. The fruits are large, globose 5.0 - 8.0 cm across, crowned by somewhat tubular limb of the calyx and are indehiscent with red pulp and juicy. Seeds are angular with coriaceous testa.

Flowering is in April - May and fruiting during June - August.

Distribution : It is cultivated throughout India and also found wild in the Himalayas from 914 - 1828 m and in Salt range.

Parts used : Leaves, bark, fruits, seeds and flowers are used.

Medicinal uses : A paste of its green leaves is made, which is applied on eyes for conjunctivitis and their juice is given in dysentery. The bark of its roots and that of stems is considered astringent and anthelmintic and is especially used against tapeworm. Its fruit juice is cooling and refrigerant. A decoction of fruid-rind is useful in chronic dysentery and diarrhoea and the decoction with that of the bark of *Holarrhena antidysenterica* is effective remedy for dysentery. The pulp and seeds are stomachic and the seeds alone are also used as laxative.

Besides, its floral buds are used in bronchitis. These are dried and powdered to a snuff, which is applied to epitaxis and internally used as an effective remedy in infantile diarrhoea and dysentery.

PRASARINI

***Paedaria foetida* Linn.**

(Family: Rubiaceae)

Description: It is a glabous or puberulous shrub. Leaves are opposite, ovate or lanceolate, acute or cuspidate with broad or narrowed and thin base and 5.0-7.5 x 2.5-3.8 cm; nerves 4-5 pairs. Panicles are 15.0 cm long, peduncle 7.5 cm wide and spreading. The flowers are violet and shortly pedicelled in slender trichotmous often scorpioid cymes. The fruits are orbicular and about 1.0 cm across.

Flowering is during rainy season and fruiting in the last of winter.

Distribution: It is found in Central and Eastern Himalayas upto 1500 m extending the Kolkata and Malya Peninsula.

Parts used: The whole plant is used medicinally.

Medicinal uses: In ayurveda, the plant is described as aphrodisiac, biter, and tonic which is used to cure *vata* and *kapha* diseases, in inflammations, piles and fevers besides, night blindness and as laxative. Its two varities are known; one is edible variety and the other is bitter, the seeds of which are used in piles and leucoderma.

Its roots are used as emetic by the Hindus. A decoction of its leaves is taken as nutritive by the sick and convalescent. Besides, its fruits are used to blacken the teeth by the indegnous people in hilly areas and also in toothache.

PRISHNIPARNI

***Uraia picta* (Jacq.) Desv. ex DC.**

(Syn. *Hedysarum pictum* Jacq.)

(Family : Fabaceae)

Description : This is an erect and about 0.8-1.2 m

high shrubby perennial herb or under shrub. Leaves are 25.0 - 30.0 cm long and 1-3-foliate; leaflets 4-6, lanceolate or linear-oblong, mucronate and obtuse. Flowers are purple coloured and are borne in dense cylindrical racemes. The fruits are glabrous, pale lead-coloured or whitish with 3-6 joints. Seeds are reddish, reniform and 1-12.

Flowering is during rainy season and fruiting in winter.

Distribution : It is reported to be distributed throughout the country in grassy localities and scrub jungles in tropical zone upto 1200 m.

Usable parts : Fruits and roots of the plant are used.

Medicinal uses : Its fruits and roots are used for prolapse of anus of infants and fruits alone are applied in sore mouth. Besides, a decoction of its roots is also given in cough, chills and in fever.

PRIYANGU

***Callicarpa nudiflora* Hook. & A.**

(Syn. *C. acuminata* Roxb.; *C. reevesii* Wall. ex Schauer; *C. macrophylla* var. *sinensis* Cl.)

(Family: Verbenaceae)

Description : It is a shrub with straggling branches and thickly woolly tomentose extremities. Leaves are 10-18 cm long, ovate or ovate-lanceolate, acuminate, with rounded or cuneate base and glabrate above and tomentose. The flowers are small and pale coloured in a dense flowered and globose axillary compound cymes. The fruits are white with 4 one-celled pyrenes, which are spongy succulent outside when ripe and globose.

Flowering is during rainy season and fruiting in cold season.

Distribution : It is found in upper Gangetic plain, in Western Himalayas from Kashmir eastwards upto 1828 m and in West Bengal.

Parts used : The leaves and roots are used.

Medicinal uses : Its leaves after heating are applied on rheumatic joints. An oil obtained from its roots is used as aromatic and stomachic. The paste of its seeds is known to be used in stomatitis and leprosy and also as diuretic. Besides, the fruit-paste is used in the treatment of boils and blisters on tongue.

The other species ***Prunus mahaleb* Linn.** also known by the same name *Priyangu*, which is reported from the north-western parts of the country. Its leaves and stem are used as insecticides and also to remove bad odour due to perspiration and the fruits are known to possess bitter property with a stong pleasant smell and are used as tonic to the brain and the chest; also analgesic, emmenagogue and anthelmintic and aphrodisiac.

PSYLLIUM

***Plantago afra* Linn.**

(Syn. *P. psyllium* Linn.)

(Family: Plantaginaceae)

Description: It is an annual, erect, strict and glandular–pubescent herb with leafy and 10-20 cm long stem. Leaves are opposite, linear or linear – lanceolate, flat, obtuse and 2.5-6.5 cm long with fascicles in their axils, hence apperaing whorled. Peduncles are in the upper axils, scapes usually shorter than the leaves. Spikes are ovoid, 0.8-1.3 cm long; bracts acute.

Flowering is in May-June and fruiting during September-October.

Distribution : It is known to found wild in North west Punjab.

Parts used: The seeds are used.

Medicinal uses: Its seeds are popular aperient and are widely prescribed as a laxative in lieu of mineral aperient waters. They act after being soaked for some hours in cold water, by their mucilage and when swallowed, by virtue of laxative oil set free within the intestines.

PUNARNAVA

***Boerhavia diffusa* Linn.**
(Syn. *B. repens* Linn.)
(Family: Nyctaginaceae)

Description : It is a diffusely branched and creeping perennial herb. Root-stocks are fusiform, stout and woody. Stems are 60-90 cm long, slender, prostrate or ascending, swollen at the nodes, minutely hairy and sometimes viscid. Leaves are opposite, 1.2-2.5 cm long, ovate, oblong or suborbicular, green and glabrous above with rounded or sub cordate base and subundulate margins; petiole is as long as the blade. Flowers are pink, small or minute and not involucrate and are borne in small umbels which are arranged in axillary and terminal panicles. Fruits are 5-ribbed, 1.3 cm long, clavate, rounded and glandular.

Flowering and fruiting is during winter season.

Distribution : It is a common weed which is found throughout India, especially in West Bengal during rainy season and in cold places.

Parts used : Whole plant is used.

Medicinal uses : The decoction of entire plant is used in oedema and dropsy. Its roots are expectorant, diuretic and laxative and are used in oedema, jaundice, ascites, anasarca, strangury, gonorrhoea and internal inflammation. The roots and leaf- ashes are taken to cure night blindness. A poultice of entire herb mixed with palm kernel oil is applied to boils. Leaves of the plant are used in eye wounds, muscular pain, and dropsy and in gonorrhoea. These are also used to purify the blood and to hasten delivery and their paste is taken orally to check bleeding after delivery. Dry powder of its leaves mixed with mustard oil is used externally on itches and eczema. Besides, boiled leaves with rice, garlic and water are rubbed on body in rheumatism.

PUTIKARANJ

***Derris indica* (Lamk.) Bennet**

(Syn. *Galedupa indica* Lamk.; *Pongamia glabra* Vent.; *P. pinnata* (Linn.) Pierre)

(Family: Fabaceae)

Description : It is a moderate-sized glabrous tree with a short bole and spreading crown and soft greyish-green bark. Leaves are imparipinnate; leaflets are 5-7, elliptic or ovate and 5.0-17.5 cm long. The flowers are liliac or white, tinged with pink or violet and fragrant and are borne in axillary racemes. The fruits are woody, compressed, glabrous, indehiscent, elliptic to obliquely oblong and 4.0-7.5 x 1.7-3.5 cm. Seeds are 1-2, white, elliptic or reniform, wrinkled and 1.7-2.0 x 1.2 -1.8 cm with reddish-brown leathery testa.

Flowering and fruiting is during May-June.

Distribution : It is found throughout India upto 1200 m and in the Andamanns.

Parts used : The seeds, flowers, leaves, bark and roots are used.

Medicinal uses : The plant is known to be used both in ayurvedic and unani system of medicines. Its seeds are efficaceous in whooping coughs and irritation and their pulp is applied on leprosy. The seed oil is applied to skin diseases including herpes, scabies and sores. A mixture of its seed oil and zinc oxide (3.8 gm: 31.1 gm) is applied usefully in eczema. Sometimes, the oil has been used internally as a stomachic and cholagogue in cases of dyspepsia with sluggish liver. An embrocation made of equal parts of its oil with lemon juice forms an application in psoriasis, pityriasis and pruigo capitis. Its flowers are used as a remedy for diabetes. The leaf- juice is used in cough, flatulency, dyspepsia and diarrhoea. A paste of its leaves is applied internally in ulcers infested with worms. In leprosy, its leaves with that of *chitraka* are made into a powder, which is given with curd to cure the disease. The bark is used externally in bleeding piles and a decoction of the same is given is *beri-beri*. Besides, the juice of the roots by itself or with *Neem* or *Nirgundi* juice is effective to destroy worms of foul ulcers and fistulous sores and also for cleaning teeth and strengthening the gums.

RASNA

Pluchea lancolata C.B. Clarke

(Family: Asteraceae)

Description: It is an erect undershrub with terete, slender and softly, ashy-pubescent stem and branches. Leaves are sessile, very coraceous, 2.5-5.7 x 0.5-1.5 cm, oblong or oblanceolate, obtuse, apiculate, narrowed at base and finely ashy-pubescent on both the sides. Heads are in compound corymbs. Involucre is contracted at the mouth; outer bracts 2-3 seriate, oblong, very obtuse, pubescent and usually tinged with purple.

Flowering in during cold season and fruiting in hot season.

Distribution: It is found distributed in Punjab and Gangetic plains as far as Kanpur in the country.

Parts used: Medicinally, its leaves are used.

Medicinal uses: Its leaves are used as aperient and also as a substitute for senna.

RHUBARB ROOT

Rheum emodi Wall.

(Family: Polygonaceae)

Description: It is a rhizomatous stout herb with leafy stem and upto 1.5-.8 m high. Radical leaves are very large, often 60.0 cm in diameter, orbicular or broadly ovate and obtuse with cordate base and 5-7 nerved. Panicles are 0.6-0.9 m long, papillosely puberulous, fatigiately branched and leafy with erect strict branches. Flowers are dark purple in colour and 0.3 cm in diameter. The fruits are ovoid-oblong, 1.3 cm long, purple with cordate base and notched apex.

Flowering is in July-August and fruiting during September-October.

Distribution: It is found distributed in sub-alpine and alpine Himalayas between 3600 – 4000 m.

Parts used: Its rhizomatous roots are used.

Medicinal uses: Its roots are bitter, laxative and pungent and in ayurveda, are used in dysentery, loss of appetite and bad ulcers. Whereas, in Unani system of medicine, these are known to have bitter taste, emmenagogue and purgative properties and are used in biliousness, chronic bronchits, lumbago, heating of the brain, sore eyes, piles and asthma and bruises.

ROHITAKA

***Tecomella undulata* (Sm.) Seem**

(Syn. *Bignonia undulata* Sm.; *Tecoma undulata* G.Don)

(Family: Bignoniceae)

Description : It is a medium-sized tree with drooping branches. Leaves are 5.0-12.0 x 2.5-3.7 cm and narrowly oblong with undulate margins. The flowers are dark yellow in corymbose racemes and terminating into short lateral branches; pedicel is about 1.2 cm long. The fruits are slightly curved, glabrous and about 15-20 cm long. Seeds are discoid and winged.

Flowering is during April-May and fruiting later in June-July.

Distribution : It is known to grow wild in North and Western India including Himalayas.

Parts used : The bark is usable.

Medicinal uses : An extract of its bark is considered as relaxant and chloretic. Besides, the bark of its young branches is used as a remedy for syphilis and leucorrhoea.

SAFFRON

Crocos sativa Linn.

(Family: Iridaceae)

Description: It is a rootstock of sheathed corm which is closely reticulated. Leaves are radical, narrowly linear and chanelled with recurved margins. Basal spathes are embarcing the scape and 2-valved. Flowers are violet coloured and autumnal, appearing with the leaves. Perianth throat is bearded.

Flowering and fruting is during winter season.

Distribtuion: It is cultivated in Kashmir upto an elevation of 1700 m.

Parts used: Saffron, obtained from the dried stigmas and tops of the styles, and the leaves are used.

Medicinal uses: In ayurveda, saffron obtained from the plant is alexiteric, anthelmintic, bitter, fragrant, laxative, pungent and tonic which is used to improve the taste and in bronchitis, throat troubles, headache, hemicrania, vomiting and scabies; also in biliousness, skin diseases and the diseases of the brain. Its leaves are useful in fractures and the pain of the joint.

As a medicine, saffron is used in fevers, melancholia and enlargement of the liver. It also has stimulant and stomahic properties and is highly thought of as a remedy for catarrhal affections of children.

SANDALWOOD

Santalum album Linn.

(Family: Santalaceae)

Description : It is a small, evergreen, glabrous and semi-parasitic tree with slender branches attaining a height upto 18 m with dark grey or nearly black or reddish and rough bark. Sapwood is unscented and white but heartwood is scented and yellowish-brown or dark brown. Leaves are opposite, ovate or ovate-lanceolate, glabrous, 1.5-8.0 x 1.5-3.0 cm or larger and thin. The flowers are brownish purple, violet or straw-coloured, unscented and are borne in terminal and axillary paniculate cymes. The fruits are globose drupes, 1.2 cm across, purple black with hard ribbed endocarp. Seeds are ovoid or globose.

Flowering is during June-September and fruiting in November-February.

Distribution : It occurs from Vindhya mountains southward, particulary in Karnataka and Tamil Nadu and ascending upto 1200 m; also introduced in Rajasthan, Uttar Pradesh, Madhya Pradesh and Orissa, where it has become naturalized.

Parts used : The wood and wood oil are used.

Medicinal uses : Its wood ground up with water into a paste, which is applied to the temples in headache, fevers and local inflammations and to skin diseases to allay head and pruritus and also used as diaphoretic. A decoction of its wood mixed with that of dried ginger is used in haemorrhoids. The sandalwood oil and oil derived from its heartwood is considered as cooling, diuretic, diaphoretic and expectorant, which is used in symptomatic treatment of dysuria, gonorrhoeal urethritis and cystitis. The oil mixed with its double quantity of mustard oil is used for pimples on the nose.

An emulsion of the wood is used as a cooling application in erysipelas and prurigo. *Ilaj-ul-gurba* recommends a paste made of equal parts of sandal oil and borax with sufficient quantity of water as useful application in *pityriasis-versicolor* and similar affections.

Its oil is frequently adulterated by mixing Cedar wood oil or Castor oil in the market.

SAUSSUREA

***Saussurea lappa* Cl.**

(Family: Asteraceae)

Description: It is a tall, robust and perennial herb with erect and simple stem upto 1.2-2.0 m high. Leaves are membranous and irregularly toothed; basal ones very large, 0.6-1.2 m long, tranngular with a long lobately winged stalk, end lobe often 30 cm across; stem leaves are smaller, stalked or stalkless with 2 hard stem clasping lobes at the base. Floral heads are stalkess, hard, rounded and 2.5-3.8 cm in diameter, forming axiallry and terminal clusters. Bracts are many which surround the heads and are ovate-lanceolate, long pointed and rigid. The fruits are compressed and curved with narrowed tip and 1 rib on each face and about 1.0 cm long.

Flowering and fruiting is during winter.

Distribution: It is found distributed in Kashmir to Sikkim between 3300 – 5500 m.

Parts used : Its roots are used.

Medicinal uses: In ayurveda, its roots are described as aphrodisiac, alterative, bitter, hot, sweetens and pungent and known to cure *tridosha*. These are also used to improve the complexion, and to cure leucoderma, erysipelas, itching, ringworm and the diseases of the blood. In Unani system of medicine, its roots are of two kinds: the sweet and bitter and these are descrbed as alexipharmic, carminative, analgesic, anthelmintic, emmenagogue, aphrodisiac and tonic, which are used to stimulate the brain, to cure the diseases of blood, liver and the kidney. Besides, the roots are also used in chronic skin diseases and rheumatism. Its roots are known to have a remarkable effect in controlling bronchial asthma expecially those of the vago-tonic type.

SERPENTINA

***Rauvolfia serpentina* Benth. ex Kurz**

(Family: Apocynaceae)

Description : It is an erect and glabrous perennial suffruticose herb or undershrub. Leaves are in whorls of 3 or 4, rarely opposite, shining, green above and pale beneath, lanceolate or oblanceolate, acute or acuminate and narrowed into a short petiole. The flowers are white or pinkish and are borne in corymbose cymes. Drupes, the fruits are obliquely ovoid and purple black when ripe. The seeds are ovoid.

Flowering and fruiting is throughout the year but chiefly during April-May.

Distribution : It grows in waste places and in shady forest in different parts of India from Punjab eastwards to Sikkim and Assam; also in some parts of Central India and Western ghats.

Parts used : The leaves and roots are used.

Medicinal uses : The most common use of the plant mentioned in the literature is to cure snake - bite, but its efficacy could not be established in snake-bite. Actually, the root of the plant is a powerful sedative and whenever it was administered to victims of snake-bite, who became nervous, shocked, excited and often got hysterical fits, it calmed them. The sedative effect of the drug calms the victim and when the sedative action was over the victim returned to normal condition. Even today, in general treatment of snake-bite, a sedative is administered as a first aid. But, if the victim is bitten by a poisonous snake with a full fatal dose, the sedative action of root is ineffective and the victim dies. Earlier this fact was not realized and it was believed that the victim was cured due to administration of the root of this plant.

The root is hypnotic and sedative and their decoction is employed to increase uterine contractions and for expulsion of foetus in difficult cases and its extract is used in intestinal disorders. It is also supposed to be anthelmintic, febrifuge and bitter tonic. Its alkaloid extract induces bradycardia, hypotension and sedation and produces tranquillizing effect and is used in hydrophobia, neuropsychiatric disorders, psychosis and schizophrenia. Respirine, an indole alkaloid principle is sedative in action and is widely used in fevers. Besides, the juice of the leaves is applied for removal of opacities of the cornea of the eyes.

SHALPARNI

***Desmodium gangeticum* (Linn.) DC.**

(Syn. *Hedysarum gangeticum* Linn.)

(Family : Fabaceae)

Description : It is an erect or suberect undershrnb or herb about 60-120 cm in height with adpressed hairy branches. The stems are simple and straight. Leaves are 1-foliate and 7.5-15.0 x 0.8-1.5 cm; leaflets are entire, membranous or subcoriaceous and glabrescent above. Flowers are numerous and small in racemes which are 15-30 cm long. Pods, the fruits are in cluster of 6-8, glabrescent, sticky and 1.3-1.9 cm long.

Flowering is during June-August and fruiting in cold season.

Distribution : It is found in the lower Himalayan region upto 1600 m and throughout the plains of India.

Parts used : Its roots and the panchang (whole plant) are used.

Medicinal uses : The roots of this herb are astringent, tonic and diuretic and are used in diarrhoea, chronic fever, biliousness, cough, vomitting, asthma, snake-bite and scorpion-stings. Besides, the whole plant is known as febrifuge, digestive and bitter tonic and is used for hazy vision and in dysentery.

SHALLAKI

***Boswellia serrata* Roxb. ex Coleb.**

(Syn. *B. serrata* var. *glabra* Roxb.)

(Family: Burseraceae)

Description: It is a deciduous tree with pubescent branches and ash – coloured bark, which peels off in flakes. Leaves are crowded at the ends of branches and are alternate, 20.0-30.0 cm long and imparipinnate; leaflets in 5 pairs, suboppsite, sessile, lanceolate to linear, serrate and 2.5 - 7.0 x 0.6 – 1.5 cm with unequal sided tips and sometimes mucronate. Flowers are white, small in axillary or sub-terminal fascicled racemes. Capsules, the fruits are tardily dehiscent and tri-gonous.

Flowering is during March- April and fruiting in June - July.

Distribution: It is found in Bihar, Deccan Peninsula, Madhya Pradesh, Central India and Eastern states and North Gujarat.

Parts used: The gum resin obtained from its trunk and the bark is used.

Medicinal uses: The gum resin obtained from the trunk of the plant, is known as Indian oilbanum or *Salai guggul*, and it is the only non-coniferous source of turpentine and resin in India. It is known for its antiseptic, astringent, diaphoretic, diuretic, ecobolic, emennagogal and expectorant properties and is used in cutaneous and nervous diseases, cystic breast, chronic diarrhoea and dysentery, goiter, gout, piles, rheumatism, tumours and ulcers. This is also applied locally with benefits on buboes and the oil obtained from this resin, in gonorrhoea. The gum resin is the main constituent of an ointment for sores and with butter is used for syphilis. It is mixed with gum acacia and is used as a connective for foul breath.

Recently, it has been established that *salai guggul* is an effective antiperlipiadic and anti-antheroscleraic agent. Besides, the bark of the plant is used in diarrhoea, piles and skin diseases.

SHANKHPUSHPI

***Evolvulus alsinoides* Linn.**

(Family: Convolvulaceae)

Description : It is an erect-ascending or decumbent-ascending or prostrate herb with woody base. Leaves are linear-oblong or wide or wide - elliptic with acute or rounded base and 0.5 - 2.0 x 0.3 - 1.0 cm. Flowers are blue or rarely white, 1-3 together and peduncled. Capsules, the fruits are globose, 4-valved with usually 4 seeds. The seeds are glabrous and about 0.1 cm long.

Flowering and fruiting is during July - December.

Distribution : It is very common throughout the drier parts of India, ascending upto 1828 m.

Parts used : Whole plant and its leaves are used.

Medicinal uses : In ayurveda, the plant, is known for its alexiteric, alterative, anthelmintic, bitter, pungent and tonic properties and is used in bronchitis, biliousness, epilepsy and leucoderma. A decoction of the herb with *Ocimum sanctum* is prescribed in the doses of 50 -100 gm in fever associated with diarrhoea or indigestion and with oil is to promote hair growth. Besides, leaves of the plant are smoked in asthma and chronic bronchitis.

Another species *Crotolaria verrucosa* Linn. belonging to family Fabaceae,is also known by the same name *Shankhpushpi,* the juice of which leaves is used in scabies and impetigo both internally and externally; also considered effacious in diminishing the salivation.

SHATAVARI

***Asparagus racemosus* Willd.**

(Family: Liliaceae)

Description : It is a much branched perennial herb with a tuberous rootstock. Stems are triquetrous with 0.5-1.2 cm long patent or recurved spines. Cladodes are 2-3 and are arranged in a tuft and falcate. Racemes are 2.5-5.0 cm long and pedicels are jointed at the middle and slender below the joint. The flowers are white. Berries, the fruits are red or reddish violet and 1-3 seeded.

Flowering is in October-November and fruiting during cold season.

Distribution : The plant is found in tropical and subtropical parts of India and upto 1219 m in the Himalayas from Kashmir eastwards.

Parts used : Roots and bark of the stem are generally used.

Medicinal uses : The roots are known as refrigerant, demulcent, diuretic, aphrodisiac, antiseptic, alterative, antidiarrhoeal, antidysenteric and galactagogue and their decoction is given for fever and the extarct is considered antifungal. Its roots are also used as a stimulant and restorative. These are chiefly used as demulcent in veterinary medicine. Its bark is used as antibacterial and antifungal. Besides, the juice of entire herb with equal portion of cow's milk is used to remove the calculi.

SHIGRU

***Moringa conacanensis* Nimmo**

(Family: Moringaceae)

Description: It is a glabrous tree. Leaves are 2 (rarely 3-) pinnate, upto 45.0 cm long; primary pairs 5-6, distant, 10.0-20.0 cm long; the primary rachis thickened at the base, the secondary articulated and with a gland at the articulations; leaflets 4-6 pairs and an odd one, broadly elliptic or suorbicular, obtuse at both the ends and often retuse at the apex, of variable size, sometimes 2.0-3..3 x 1.2-2.5 cm, pale beneath, articulated with a slender petiolule of 0.2-0.8 cm long. Flowers are in lax divaricate thinly pubescent panicles reaching 45.0 cm long; pediciels 0.8-1.2 cm long, articulated with the flower; bracts minute and caducous. Capsules, the fruits are straight, acutely triquetrous and slightly constricted between the seds and 30.0-45.0 cm long with hard valves. Seeds are white or pale yellow and 3-angled and 3-winged.

Flowering is during January-March and fruiting in April-June.

Distribution: It is known to be distributed in the dry hills of the Konkan, Berar, North Circars and Deccan from Vishakhapatnam to Guntur, Kurnool and in Combatore.

Parts used: Its roots are used medicinally.

Medicinal uses: Its roots possess alterative, laxative, stomachic, tonic and sweet properties and are used efficiently in inflatmations, *vata* diseases and biliousness; also in asthma.

The roots of the plant are used as a substitute for *M. oleifera*.

SHINSHIPA

***Dalbergia sissoo* Roxb.**

(Family: Fabaceae)

Description : It is fairly a large deciduous tree with grey bark upto 15-18 m in height. The branches are downy, grey and spreading. Leaves are 3-5, alternate, imparipinnate, bifarious, roundish, acuminate and 3.5-6.0 x 3.0 - 5.4 cm. The flowers are sessile in axillary panicles, shorter than leaves and yellowish white. Pods, the fruits are 3.5-4.5 cm long, thin, strap shaped and pale grey. Seeds are 1-4, kidney shaped and flat.

Flowering is in summer and fruiting during winter.

Distribution: It occurs in the Western Himalayas upto 1500 m Sikkim to upper Assam; extensively planted along road sides in different parts of India.

Parts used: Leaves, bark, wood and roots are used.

Medicinal uses : Its leaves are considered bitter and stimulant and their decoction is used in gonorrhoea. The bark is alterative and dried bark is haemostatic and is effective in bleeding piles, menorrhagia and in varicose veins. Its wood is alterative and is used in leprosy, boils and eruptions and to allay vomitting. Besides, the roots are used as astringent.

The plant is also used in Unani system of medicine. The drug in Unani is called, *Shisham katel* and is used as counter-irritant, antisyphilitic and blood purifier. The mucilage of its leaves mixed with sweet oil is used in excoriations. Besides, raspings of the wood are boiled in water until these become half, then mixed with '*sharbat*' of shisham are advised to drink about for forty days in leprosy.

SHIRISHA

***Albizia lebbeck* (Linn.) Benth.**

(Family: Fabaceae)

Description : It is a large deciduous, erect and spreading tree, about 15-18 m high with dark grey bark which is irregularly cracked. Leaves are bipinnate with 8-18 leaflets; leaflets are 3.3-5.0 x 1.7-2.5 cm, shortly petioled, oblong, oblique, obtuse and glabrous or glabrescent. Inflorescence is in globose heads of greenish- yellow flowers. The flowers are shortly pedicelled and fragrant. Pods, the fruits are yellowish-brown, 15.0-25.0 x 3.7-4.3 cm, flat, thin, firm, straw coloured and 6-10 seeded with brown spots and depressions alternately on either side over the seeds.

Flowering is during rainy season and fruiting in winter.

Distribution: It is found distributed throughout India, ascending upto 1219 m in the Himalayas; also in Andamanns.

Parts used: Seeds, leaves, bark, pods and flowers are used.

Medicinal uses: Its seeds are known to show hypoglycaemic and anticancerous potential and are used as astringent and tonic. Its leaves are used as a remedy for night blindness. The powder of root bark is used to strenghthen the gums and is externally applied as plaster in leprous ulcers. An aqueous extract of its bark is used against conception in women and the fruit - extract as antiprotozoal, hypoglycaemic and anticancerous. Besides, the flowers are considered as a cooling medicine and are externally applied to boils, eruptions and swellings.

SHOBHANJANA

***Moringa oleifera* Lamk.**
(Syn. *M. pterygosperma* Gaertn.)
(Family: Moringaceae)

Description : It is fairly a large tree with thick corky bark upto 10 m in height. Leaves are usually tripinnate and 30.0 - 60.0 cm long; leaflets are elliptic and opposite and their glands are linear and hairy. The flowers are white, bisexual and irregular and are borne in large panicles. Capsules, the fruits are 20.0 - 50.0 cm long, triangular, ribbed and greenish. Seeds are 3 - cornered, winged and about 2.5 cm long.

Flowering is during February - April and fruting in May - June.

Distribution : It is indigenous to North West India and cultivated throughout India.

Parts used : Root, bark, leaves, flowers, fruits, gum and seed-oil are used.

Medicinal uses : Its roots are used as stimulant in paralysis and intermittent fever, as rubifacient in palsy and chronic rheumatism, as cardiac and circulatory tonic and in form of a compound spirit are useful in fainting giddiness, nervous debility, hysteria and flatulence. The root-juice is used internally in calculus affection in combination with milk and the decoction of roots is used as gargle in horseness and throat sore. The bark is abortifacient and root-bark is used as fomentation to relieve the spasm. Its bark-juice mixed with molasses is administered in headache.

The leaf-juice is useful in hicough and in higher doses is used as emetic; in combination with honey is applied to eyelids in eye diseases. Its flowers are used as diuretic, cholagogue and stimulant and the fruits are considered antipyretic and anthelmintic and are eaten. The gum of the plant is used for dental caries and mixed with sesamum oil is poured into ears for relief in otalgia. Besides, its seed oil in combination with equal parts of ground nut oil is applied locally to relieve the pain in rheumatism.

Its root-powder is used as a good substitute of mustard powder.

SHYONAKA

***Oroxylum indicum* Vent.**

(Family: Bignoniaceae)

Description : It is a small, deciduous and soft wooded tree with few branches and a small open crown. The bark is soft, light, brownish - grey and corky outside. Leaves are opposite, 3-pinnate near base, 2-pinnate about the middle and simply pinnate towards apex, very large upto 150 cm in length, with stout and cylindric rachis; leaflets are 2-4 paired, 6.0 - 12.0 cm long, ovate or elliptic, acuminate, entire and glabrous with a rounded or cordate base. The flowers are white or purplish and many in large and erect racemes. Capsules, the fruits are 30.0 - 90.0 x 5.0-8.0 cm, flat and straight. Seeds are many, 2.5-3.7 cm long and are surrounded by a broad transparent white papery wing.

Flowering is in June - July and fruiting during cold season.

Distribution: It is found throughout India except in the Western drier area ascending upto 1219 m in the Himalayas.

Parts used : The root - bark, stem-bark, fruits, seeds and leaves are usable.

Medicinal uses: The root-bark is astringent and tonic and is used in diarrhoea and also in dysentery and after boiling in oil, it is used in otorrhoea. A powder of its bark along with '*haldi*' is used to cure sore-backs of horses and the infusion in acute rheumatism and as bitter tonic. The tender fruits of the plant are used as refreshing and stomachic. Its seeds are used as purgative and the decoction of its leaves is said to be given in stomachache and rheumatism and externally leaf paste is applied in spleen enlargement.

SOAPNUT TREE

***Sapindus mukorossi* Gaertn.**

(Family: Sapindaceae)

Description : It is a small deciduous trees. Leaves are pinnate; leaflets are 10-16, shortly stalked, 5.0-15.0 cm long, lanceolate - oblong, alternate or subopposite, acuminate or obtuse and glabrous. Flowers are white or purple, 2.5 cm across and are borne in terminal panicles. The fruits are 1.7 cm across, subglobose, fleshy, glaucescent and saponaceous. Seeds are 0.8 - 1.2 cm in diameter, globose and black.

Flowering is in May - June and fruiting in cold season.

Distribution : It is cultivated throughout North West India, Bengal and Assam; also occurring wild in Dehradun and in the valleys of the Himalayas upto 1219 m.

Parts used : Fruits, roots, leaves and seeds are used.

Medicinal uses : Its fruits are considered expectorant and emetic and are used in salivation, chlorosis and epilepsy. The pulp of its fruits is rubbed in water until it soaks and then is strained and given through mouth to the people, those bitten by venomous reptiles and also to those suffering from severe diarrhoea or cholera. The pulp is given to relieve colic with sherbet and is also used as emetic in small doses and in larger doses as purgative. A few drops of a thick solution of the pulp are placed in the nose for relief of hemicrania, hysteria and epilepsy. A paste of its fruits with vinegar is used for reducing scrofulous swellings and also for killing the lice and that of fruits alone is externally applied to the bites of reptiles, scorpion and centipedes etc.

Its roots are also used as expectorant and in gout, rheumatism and paralysis. The fragrant leaves are used for baths in painful joints. The pessaries made of the kernel of its seeds are used to stimulate the uterus in child birth and in amenorrhoea. Besides, its seeds are pound up with water and introduced in mouth cut short the paroxysm of epilepsy.

TURMERIC

***Curcuma longa* Linn.**

(Syn. *C. domestica* (Medik) Val.)

(Family: Zingiberaceae)

Description : The plant is a perennial herb, about 90-120 cm tall with short stem and tufted leaves. Primary tubers are at the base of aerial stem and are ellipsoidal and bearing many rhizomes. The roots are fleshy with ellipsoidal tubers. Leaves are 25-40 x 10-15 cm linear, acuminate, ascending and pubescent beneath. The Infloresence is produced on short leafless peduncle, consists of cone-shaped collection of numerous ovate bracts and about 10-18 cm long and 5 cm broad. The flowers are pale-yellow and are borne in pairs in the axils. Seeds are black and shining with large, lacerate and white aril.

Flowering and fruiting is during winter.

Distribution : The plant is cultivated througthout India almost in all states, particularly in Mumbai, Bengal and Chennai.

Parts used : Its rhizomes and leaves are used.

Medicinal uses : The rhizomes of the plant are known as aromatic, stimulant, carminative, alterative, blood purifier, antiperiodic and tonic and these are externally applied to sprains and on wounds. Fresh juice of its rhizomes is considered anthelmintic and is used as antiparastic in many skin affections. Its decoction is used in purulent conjuctivitis. Leaves are used as an ingredient for stomachic preparations. An essential oil obtained from its leaves possesses antimicrobial activity against some bacteria.

Smearing of turmeric paste on the face and limbs during bath, clears the skin, blemishes and beautifies the face and also checks the growth of hairs on skin. In pemphigus and shingles, the part is first smeared with a thick coating of mustard oil and dusted with turmeric powder. This cured the disease within 2 to 4 days. In scorpion-stings, the smoke produced by sprinkling powdered turmeric over burnt charcoal gives relief when the affected part is exposed to the smoke for few minutes. Besides, the fumes of its burning roots are employed also in hysteric fits.

TUVERAK

***Hydnocarpus laurifolia* (Dennst.) Sleumer**

(Syn. *H. wighitana* Blume; *Munnicksia laurifolia* Dennst)

(Family: Flacourtiaceae)

Description : This is a tall evergreen and dioecious tree upto 15 m or more in height with fluted stem and rough brown bark. Leaves are 10.5-25.5 cm long, membraneous or thinly coriaceous, oblong, ovate or elliptic and somewhat serrate. Flowers are small, white about 1.2-2.5 cm in diameter and are borne solitary or in fascicles. The fruits are globlose, about 5.0-10.0 cm in diameter with 15-20 striate, subovoid and obtusely angular seeds.

Flowering is in January - May and fruiting almost throughout the year.

Distribution : It is met in tropical forests along the western ghats, the Konkan southwards and below the ghats in Kanara and Malabar in damp conditons, especially near water; common in Travancore upto 609 m.

Parts used : Seed-oil and Seeds are used.

Medicinal uses : Its seed oil, known as *'chaulmogra oil'* is used in leprosy and other skin diseases. About 15 drops gradually increased upto 30 drops of its seed - oil are recommended to be injected intra-muscularly or intravenously in the form of ethyl esters or salts of chaulmogric and hydnocarpic acids in leprosy and seed oil mixed with lime water is to be applied in sprains in rheumatic joints. A paste of its seeds mixed with sulphur, camphor, lime juice and seed oil of *Jatropha curcus* is applied externally in wounds and ulcers.

Besides, its seeds are used as a fish poison.

UDUMBARA

***Ficus racemosa* Linn.**

(Syn. *F. gloomerata* Roxb.)

(Family: Moraceae)

Description : It is a medium - sized or large tree with spreading branches and about 9.0 - 12.0 m height. The bark is smooth and reddish brown. Leaves are alternate, 10.0-17.5 cm long, ovate or obovate-oblong or oblong - lanceolate, glabrous above when full grown and 3-nerved. The fruits are borne in large clusters on short leafless branches derived from the trunk and main branches, subglobose, 2.5-5.0 across and red when ripe.

Flowering is during spring season and fruting in April - July.

Distribution : It occurs throughout India, along the sides of ravines and banks of streams. Also occurs on rocky slopes, sometimes gregariously; grows along road sides and in villages also.

Parts used : Leaves, fruits, latex, bark and roots are used.

Medicinal uses : A powder of its leaves mixed with honey is given in bilious affections and their decoction is used in bronchitis. The fruits are astringent, stomachic, carminative and are used in menorrhoea and haemoptysis. The roots and fruits are considered to have hypoglycaemic activity against diabetes. The juice of its roots is used in dysentery and that of fruits is given as a vehicle to medicine in diabetes and urinary complaints. The bark is astringent and is given to cattle when suffering from rinder - pest. Its milky juice is administrated in piles and diarrhoea and with sesamum oil in cancer.

Its bark along with that of *Ficus virens, F. religiosa, F. bengalensis* and *Azadirachta indica*, pass by the name *Panchaval kala*, used for gargle in salivation, as a wash for ulcers and as a injection in leucorrhoea.

VALERIAN

Valeriana jatamansii Jones

(Syn. *V. wallichi* DC.)

(Family: Valerianaceae)

Description : It is a slightly hairy perennial herb with thick and horizontal root stock. Basal leaves are 2.5 - 7.5 cm in diameter, long stalked, deeply cordate-obovate, usually toothed or sinuate and sharp pointed. Stem leaves are few, much smaller and entire or pinnate. Flowers are white or tinged with pink in terminal corymb; often unisexual. The fruits are hairy or nearly hairless.

Flowering is in June - July and fruiting during September-October.

Distribution : It is common in temperate Himalayas from Kashmir to Bhutan upto 3300 m and in Khasia hills between 1200-2000 m.

Parts used : The roots are used.

Medicinal uses: Valerian roots are very old drug, and in ayurveda, these are used for head problems, eye diseases, blood diseases and also in suppression of urine; and as laxative, astringent, carminative, emmenagogue and hypnotic in Unani system of medicine. The roots of the plant are considered as a good antiseptic, carminative and stimulant and these are successfully used in the treatment of chorea, epilepsy and hysteria.

Traditionally, its roots are used in sprains and contusions and a paste of entire plant with roots of *Hedychium spicatum* is applied on body before bath as a fragrant and refreshing agent. The rootstocks of the plant are used as a good substitute for other species viz., *V. jaeschekei* and *V. hardwickii*.

VANSHLOCHNA

***Bambusa arundinacea* Roxb.**

(Syn. *B. bamboos* Druce)

(Family: Poaceae)

Description : It is a tall, thorny bamoo with crowded culms arising from branching root stock. Culms-sheaths are rounded at apex and hairy with dark-brown hairs on the back and glabrous within. Leaves are linear or linear-lanceolate and glabrous or hairy beneath. The Inflorescence is an enormous panicle, often comprising of the whole culm. The spikelets are lanceolate and acute. Grains are ending in a short beak and are about 0.5-0.8 cm long.

Flowering is in summer and fruiting later during September-October.

Distribution : It is wild throughout the greater part of India, especially in the hill forests of Western and Southern India, ascending upto 914 m on the Nilgiris, also in Orissa, Assam and Eastern Bengal; also cultivated in the lower Himalayas and the valleys of the Ganga.

Parts used : Leaves, young shoots, stem, culms and banslochan (bamboo manna) are used.

Medicinal uses : Its leaves are used as emmenagogue and in haematemesis. A decoction of its leaves is given to induce lochia after childbirth and as anthelmintic, these are particularly useful for threadworms. The juice of its leaves with aromatics is given in blood vomiting and an infusion of the leaves is given internally for gonorrhoea. Its young shoots are stomachic and stimulant and are given in respiratory diseases and its pickled or cooked tender shoots aid digestion and are used as appetizer.

The young shoots of bamboo are used as poultice on the infected lesions and ulcers and are very efficacious in dislodgement of worm-infested wounds. A decoction of the joints of bamboo stem is used as emmenagogue and also as an abortifacient. Its decoction is applied to inflamed joints to get relief. Aerial parts including stem and leaves are used by Ayurvedic Physicians as blood purifier and in leucoderma and inflammatory conditions. These are burnt and applied locally to ringworm infection. The culms are used as expectorant, tonic, stimulant, and aphrodisiac, in blood tuberculosis, bronchitis and asthma. After mixing with lime, these are applied to cuts and wounds.

Banslochna or *tabashir* or bamboo manna, a crystalline secretion accumulate in the internodes of the female plant, is febrifuge, expectorant, tonic, aphrodisiac, demulcent and pectoral. It is given in hepatic fever, phthisis, asthma and paralytic complaints.

VETIVERT

Vetiveria zizanioides

(Syn. *Andropogon muricatus* Retz.)

(Family: Poaceae)

Description: It is a densely, tufted perennial grass with spongy roots. Culms are stout, upto over 1.8 m, usually sheathed all along. Leaf – sheaths are compressed. especially the lower which are sharply keeled and fan-like, imbricated, smooth and firm; ligules reduced to a scarious rim and blades are naroowly linear, acute, 30.0-90.0 x 4.2-10.6 cm, erect, rigid, firm or somewhat spongy and usually glabrous, rarely more or less hairy downwards on the face, and pale green with slender midribs. Panicle is oblong, over 30.0 cm long, usually contracted; rachis stout and smooth and whorls 6-10 with upto 20 rays. Racemes are upto 5.0 cm long or more and very slender; joints about as long as the sessile spikelets or sometimes distinctly exceeding them, smooth or more of less rough, minutely and enequally ciliolate at the tips. Sessile sikelets are linear – lanciolate to almost linear, acute or suacute, 0.4-0.5 cm long, yellowish, olive or violet brown or purplish to almost black. Pedicelled spikelets are sparingly aculeolate or almost smooth; upper floral glume is entire and acute.

Flowering and fruiting is during August-November.

Distribution: It is known to be distributed almost throughout the country.

Parts used: Medicinally, its roots are used.

Medicinal uses: In ayurveda, its roots are described as alexiteric, astringent, bitter and stomachic and are useful in burning sensations, bilious fevers, sweats, foul breath, thirst, strangury, ulcers and the diseases of the blood. Whereas, in Unani system of medicine, its roots are described as bitter and sporofic and are used in spermatorrhoea, headache and the diseases of the blood. An infusion of its roots is taken as febrifuge and the powder in bilious complaints; also as tonic. Besides, a pulverized paste of its roots in water acts as cooling external applicaton when applied locally.

VETRA

Salix caprea **Linn.**

(Family: Salicaceae)

Description: It is a small tree usually grown as a shrub for its sweet scented male flowers. Leaves are 5.0-10.0 cm ling, glabrous and more of less rugose above, more or less grey-tomentose beneath, crenate or nearly entire; stipules usually consipicous and subreniform. Flowers are appreared before the leaves. Male catkins are 2.5-3.8 cm long, sessile, stout and densely silky; stamens 2, filiform free and glabrous and side gland solitary. Female catkins are little shorter than the male, longer in fruits. Capsules, the fruits are downy and stiptate.

Flowering and fruiting is during February-March.

Distribution : It is cultivated in Rohilkhand and North West parts of the country.

Parts used : Its leaves, flowers, wood-ashes, gum and the fruits are used.

Medicinal uses: In Unani system of medicine. the plant is described as aphrodisiac. bitter and cooling. which is useful in pains and inflammation of the liver, thirst, biliousness and headache. The juice of its leaves is also possesses astringent, expectorant and laxative properties and is used in fevers, tremors in the limbs, muscular pains, opthalmia and the enlargement of the spleen. A distilled water obtained from its flowers is highly valued as a medicine being cordially, stimulant and aphrodisiac and is externally applied in headache and opthalmia. The ashes of the wood are useful in haemoptyisis and mixed with vinegar, applied to haemorrhoids. The gums and the juice of the plant is also used to increase the visual powers. Besides, its fruits are also used in biliousness and in inflammation of the eye due to injury.

VIDANAGA

***Embelia ribes* Burm. f.**

(Family: Myrsinaceae)

Description : It is a large scandent shrub with long, slender, flexible and terete stem with long internoded branches. Leaves are 5.0-9.0 x 2.0-3.5 cm, coriaceous, elliptic or elliptic - lanceolate, acuminate, entire, glabrous on both sides and shining above; petioles 0.6-1.6 cm long, more or less margined and glabrous. Flowers are yellow, pentamerous and small in lax panicled racemes. The fruits are globose, smooth, succulent, black when ripe and 0.3-0.4 cm in diameter.

Flowering is during July-August and fruiting in September-October.

Distribution : It is known to occur throughout India upto 1524 m.

Parts used : Fruits, roots and leaves are usable.

Medicinal uses : The fruits of the plant in ayurveda are known to possess anthelmintic, alexiteric, alterative, appetizing, carminative and laxative properties and these are used to cure ascites, bronchitis, mental diseases, dyspnea, urinary discharge, jaundice, hemicrania and the heart diseases. *Sushurta* recommends their use along with liquorice root for strengthening the body and preventing the effects of age. A decoction of its dried food is useful in fevers and diseases of the chest and skin. Besides, an infusion of its roots is also given in coughs and diarrhoea. Its young leaves cominbed with ginger are used as a gargle in sore throat, aphathe and indolent ulcers of the mouth.

The fruits of the plant resemble somewhat Black Pepper drupes and are used as an adulterant or substitute for them and also for the powder of *Piper cubeba.*

VIDARI

***Pueraria tuberosa* (Roxb. ex Willd.) DC.**

(Syn. *Heydsarum tuberosum* Roxb. ex Willd.)

(Family : Fabaceae)

Description: This is a deciduous and twining climber with underground root-tubers. Leaf – rachis is 8.0-22.0 cm long; leaflets broadly – ovate, 8.0-17.0 x 4.5 – 11.0 cm and acuminate apexed and glabrous above and pubescent beneath. Flowers are blue-purple, appear before leaves in simple, 1.0-1.2 cm long, terminal racemes; rarely in panicles. Pods, the fruits are 2.5-8.0 cm long, flat, linear, constricted between the seeds and clothed with silky-brown hairs. Seeds are 3-6.

Flowering is during March-April and fruiting in November–December.

Distribution: It is usually found climbing from Western Himalayas to Sikkim, upto 1200 m in Kumaon, lower hills of the Punjab, Mt. Abu and hilly tracts of Bengal and South India.

Parts used: Its tuberous roots are used.

Medicinal uses: The roots of the plant are used as demulcent and refrigerant. A cataplasm, prepared after peeling and bruising the roots, is rubbed on the body in fever and rheumatism. Besides, the roots are also used as emetic, lactagogue and tonic.

WHITE MUSELL

Aspcragus adscendens **Roxb.**

(Family : Liliaceae)

Description : It is a scrambling herb with white tuberous roots. Stems are tall, stout, suberect, terete, smooth, white and much-branched; branchlets are ascending, white, grooved and angled and spines stout, straight and 1.2-2.0 cm long. Flowers are white and 0.6-0.7 cm across and are borne in 3.0-5.0 cm long racemes. Pedicels are 1-2-nate, jointed above the base and 0.4 cm long. Berries, the fruits are ovoid, 0.6-0.7 cm across and 1-seeded.

Flowering is during September - October and fruiting in November - December.

Distribution : It is found in Western Himalayas and Punjab to Kumaon upto 1615 m.

Parts used : The roots of the plant are used medicinally.

Medicinal uses : Its roots are considered demulcent, galactagogue and tonic and these are used in diarrhoea, dysentery and general debility. These are boiled in milk and added with sugar, are given in spermatorrhoea, gleet and chronic leucorrhoea and also in general weakness.

Its roots are used as a substitute for Salep.

WINTERGREEN

Gaultheria fragrantissima **Wall.**

(Family: Ericaceae)

Description : This is a small, low and much branched shrub with orange-brown bark and pink twigs. Leaves are persistent, 3.5-6.0 cm long on short stout petioles, oblong-oval or oblong-lanceolate, obtuse, apiculate, serrate and glabrous. Flowers are small, many on short drooping pedicels with a pair of bractlets below the flowers and a bract at base and are closely placed in dense pubescent axillary racemes. Capsules, the fruits are small, pubescent and are completely enclosed in fleshy, ovoid and enlarged calyx.

Flowering is during June- July and fruiting later.

Distribution : It is distributed between 1828-2438 m in Khasia hills in Assam, Western Ghats, Nilgiris and in Travancore above 1500 m.

Parts used : Oil, obtained from its leaves is used medicinally.

Medicinal uses : The oil of *Gaultheria*, the genuine winter green oil is obtained from the leaves by distillation, which possesses aromatic, carminative and stimulant proprerties and is used in neuralgia and rhemumatism and also as antiseptic. It is in the doses of 6.0 ml, which is gradually increased, preferably in capsules is given successfully in acute rheumatism and sciatica and also applied externally.

YAVANI

Tracyspermum ammi (Linn.) Sprague

(Syn. *Ammi copticum* Linn.; *Carum copticum* (Linn.) Clarke; *Sison ammi* Linn.)

(Family: Apiaceae)

Description: It is an erect, glabrous or mintutely pubescent annual upto 0.3-0.9 m high. Leaves are rather distant, 2-3 pinnate, ultimate segments 1.3-2.5 cm, all linear. Bracts are usually many, linear, sometimes divided; bracteoles 3-5, small and linear. Rays are of umbel pubescent. Flowers are pure white. The fruits are 0.2 cm across, ovoid, muricate, subhispid and dorsally compressed.

Flowering and fruiting is during March-June.

Distribtuion: It is cultivated in the gardens throughout the country.

Parts used: Its seeds, fruits and roots are used.

Medicinal uses: The seeds of the plant are anthelmintic, appetizer, aphrodisiac, bitter, carminative, hot, laxative and pungent and in ayurveda, are used to cure ascites, abdominal tumours, and enlargement of the spleen, piles, vomiting and abdominal pains. Its fruits are also used as antiseptic, carminative, stimulant and tonic and also in diarrhea, dyspepsia, colic and flatulence. Besides, its roots are used as carminative and diuretic.

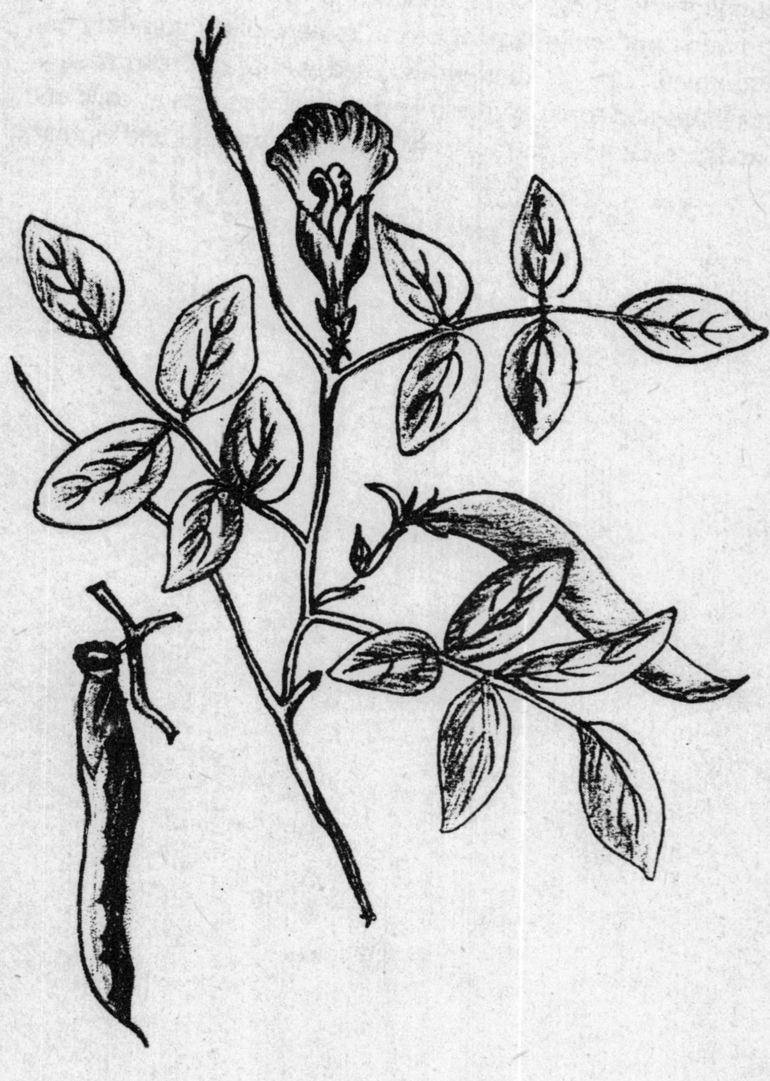

Fig. 1. Aprajita (*Clitoria ternatea*)

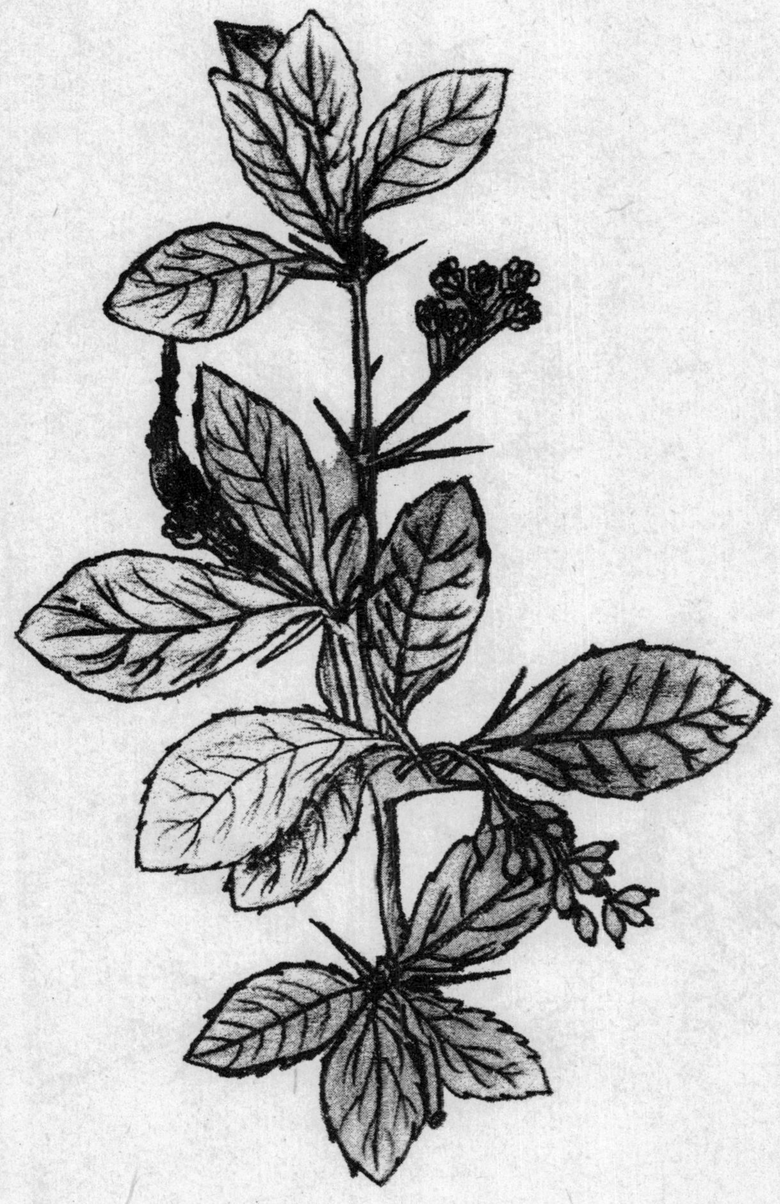

Fig. 2. Berberrry (*Berberis aristata*)

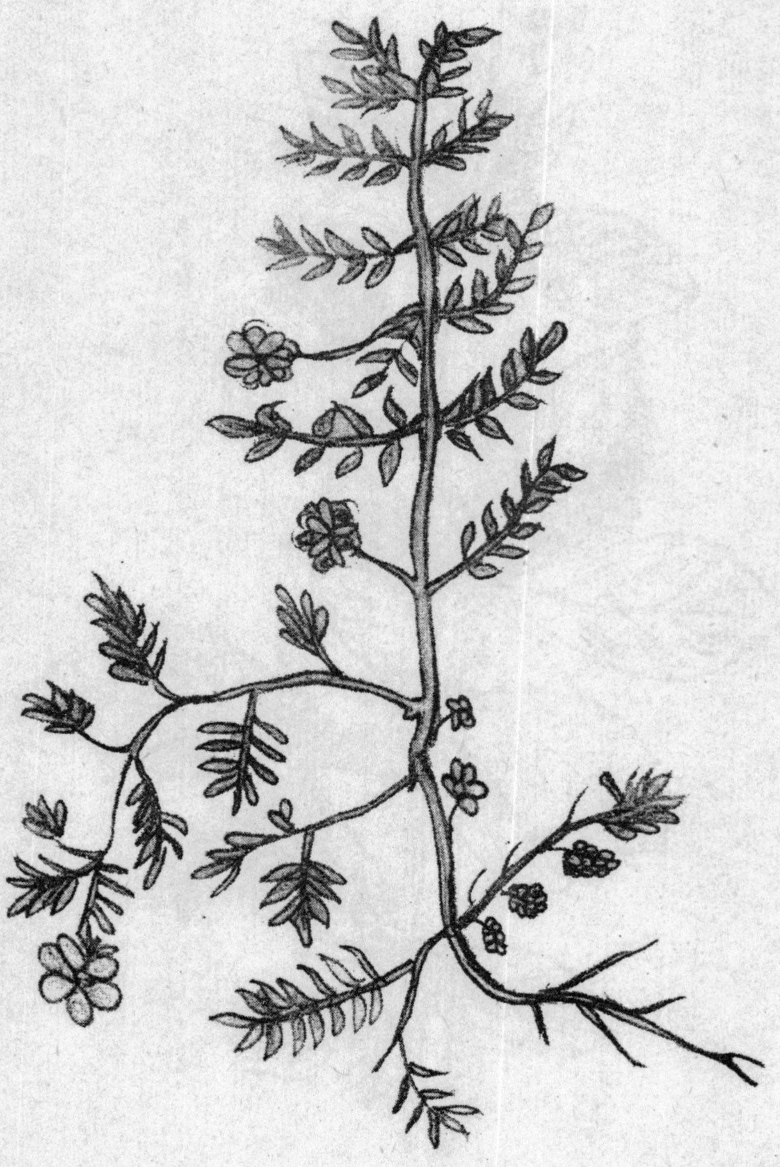

Fig. 3. Gokshura (*Tribulus terrestris*)

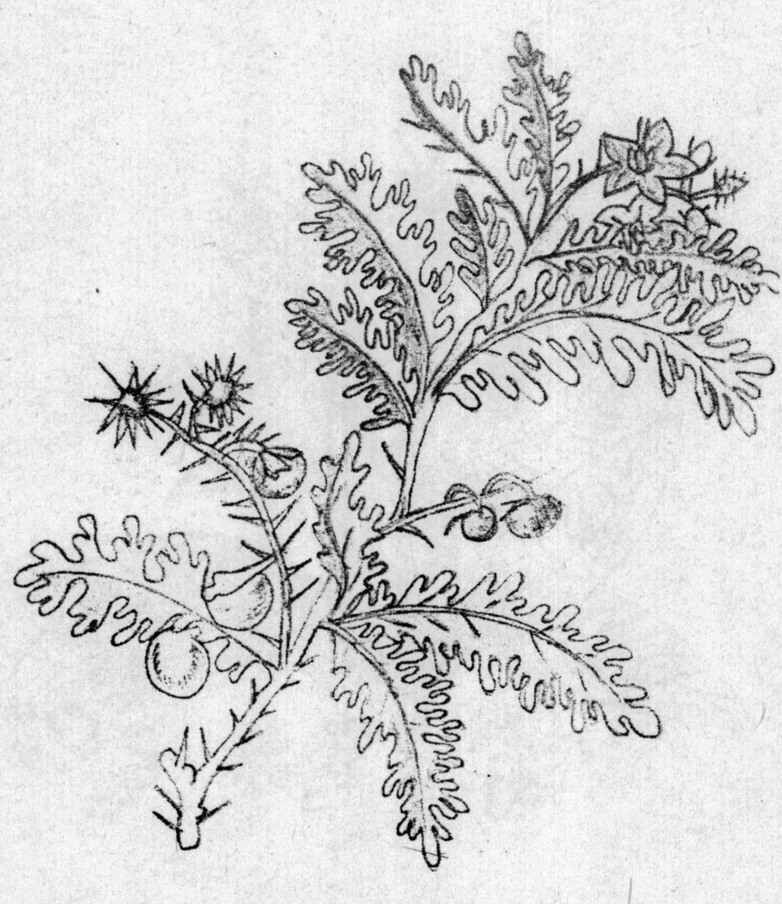

Fig. 4. Kantakari (*Solanum surattense*)

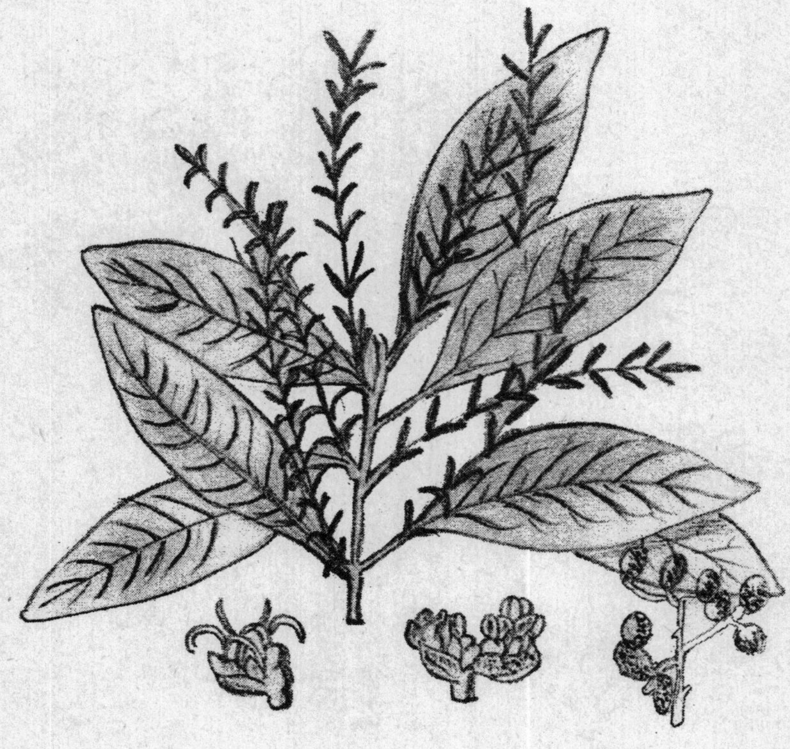

Fig. 5. Bayberry (*Mryica esculenta*)

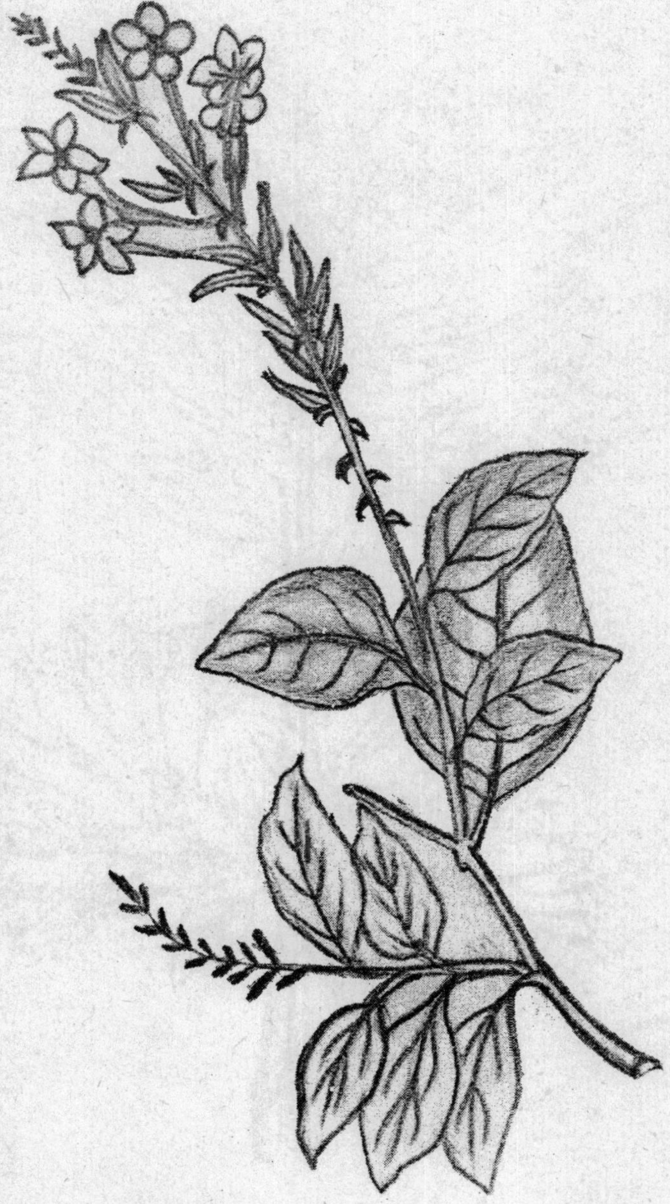

Fig. 6. Chitark (*Plumbago zeylanica*)

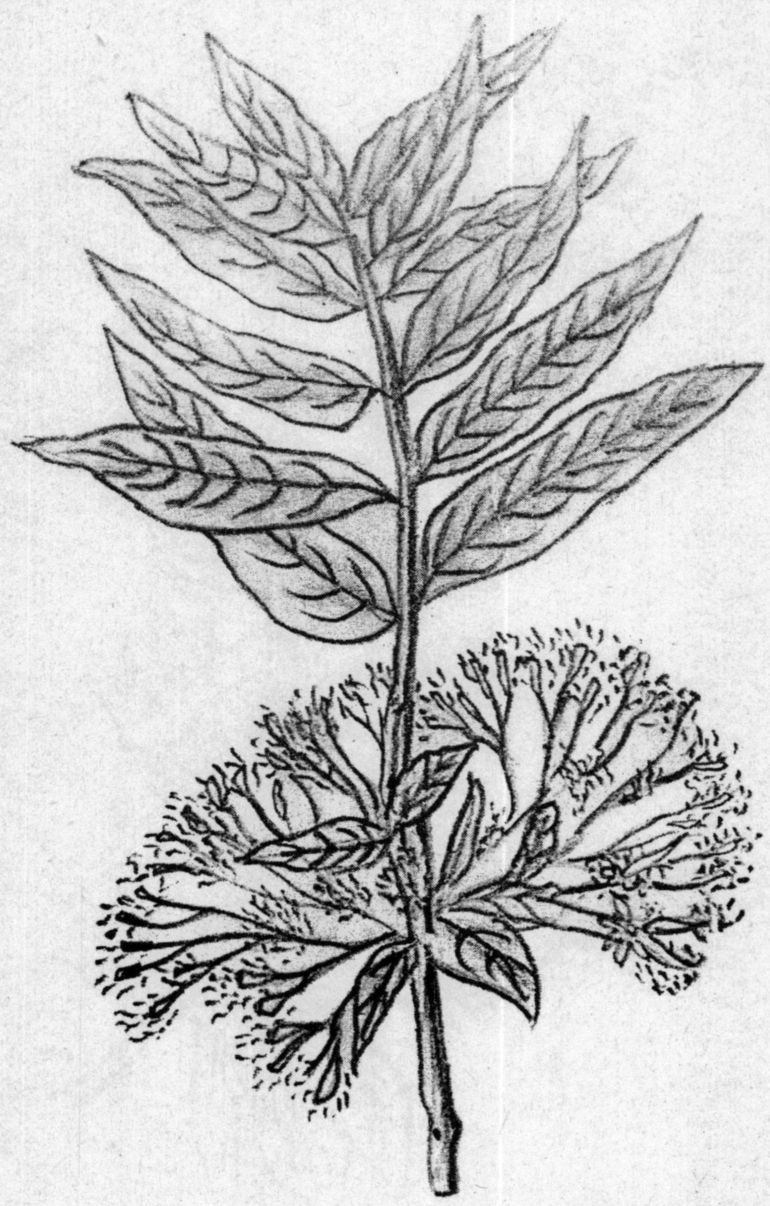

Fig. 7. Dhataki (*Woodfordia fruticosa*)

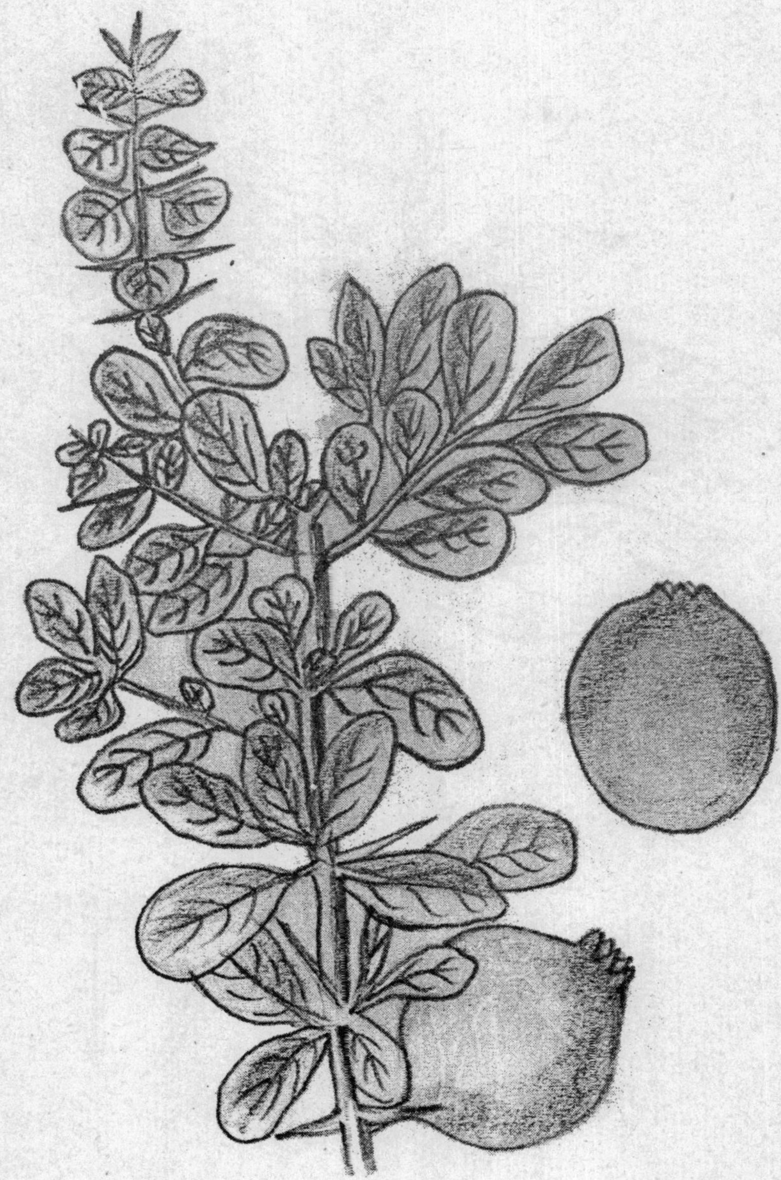

Fig. 8. Emetic nut (*Catunaregam spinosa*)

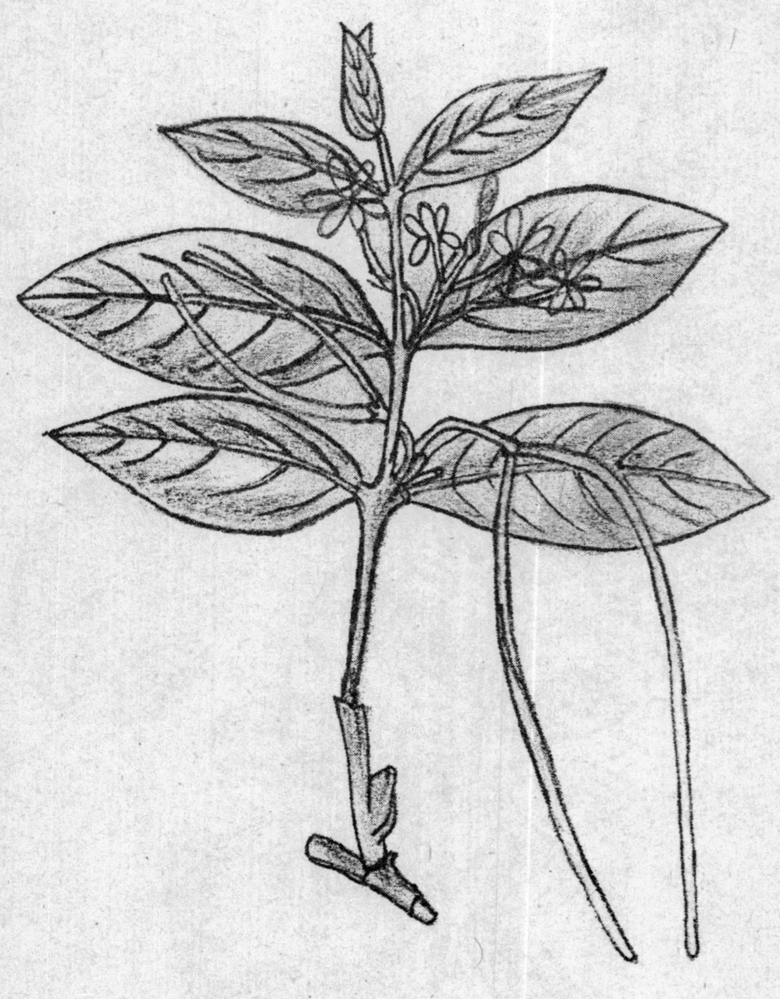

Fig. 9. Kutaj (*Holarrhena antidysenterica*)

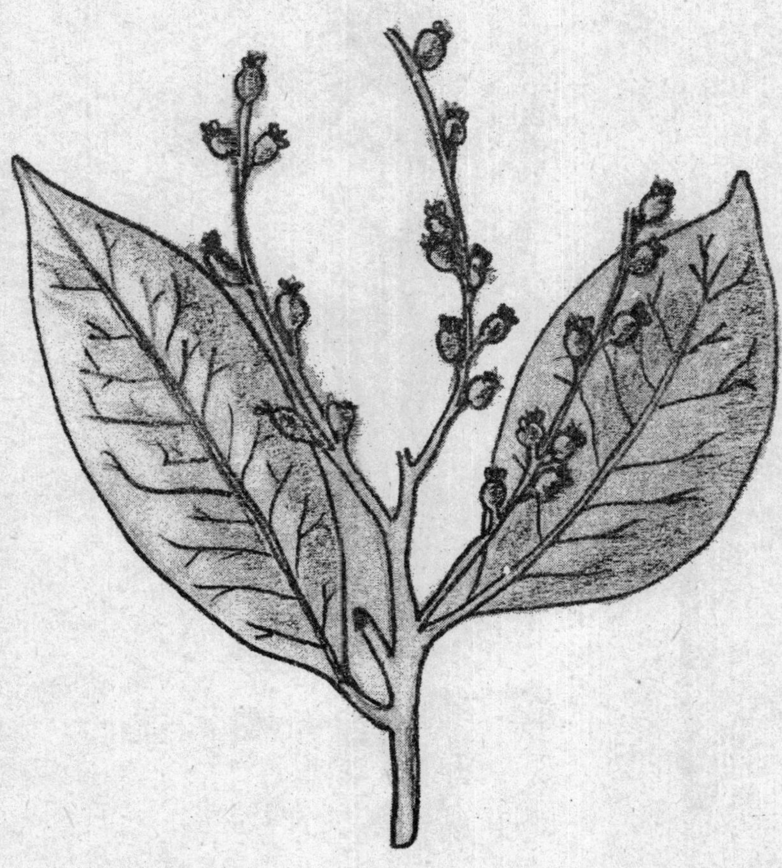

Fig. 10. Lodhra (*Symplocos racemosa*)

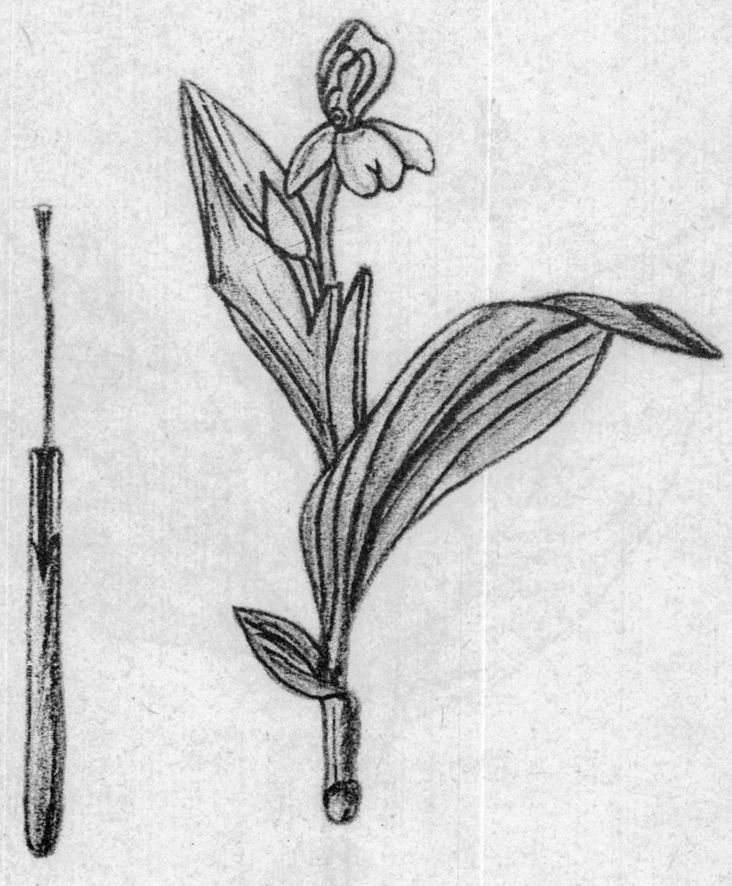

Fig. 11. Meda (*Roscoea alpina*)

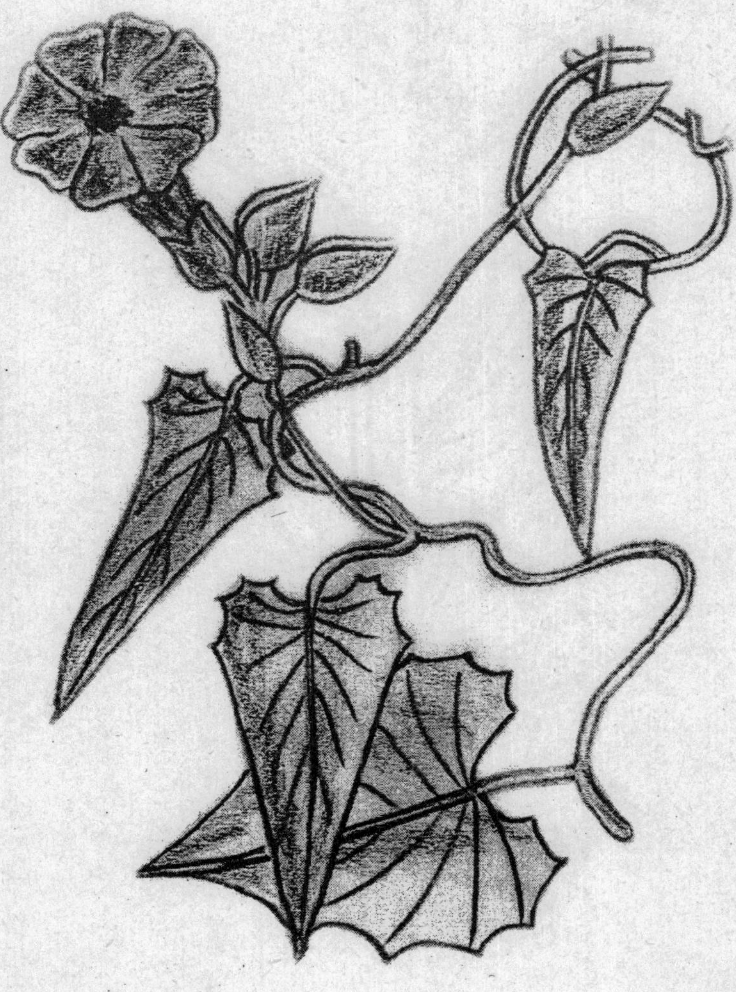

Fig. 12. Nishoth (*Operculina turpethum*)

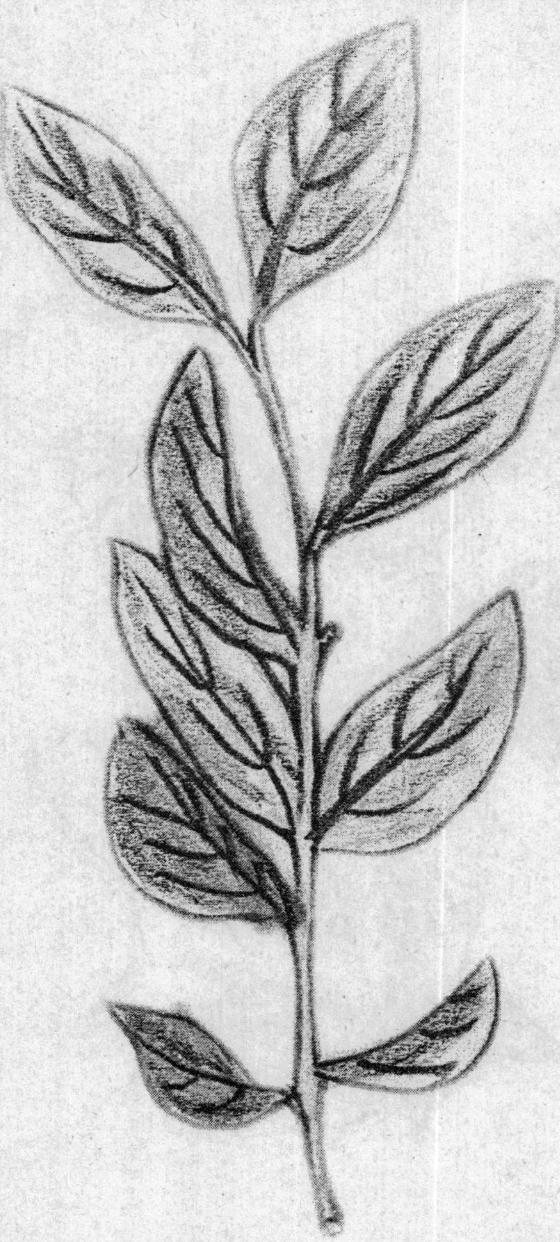

Fig. 13. Tuverak (*Hydnocarpus laurifolia*)

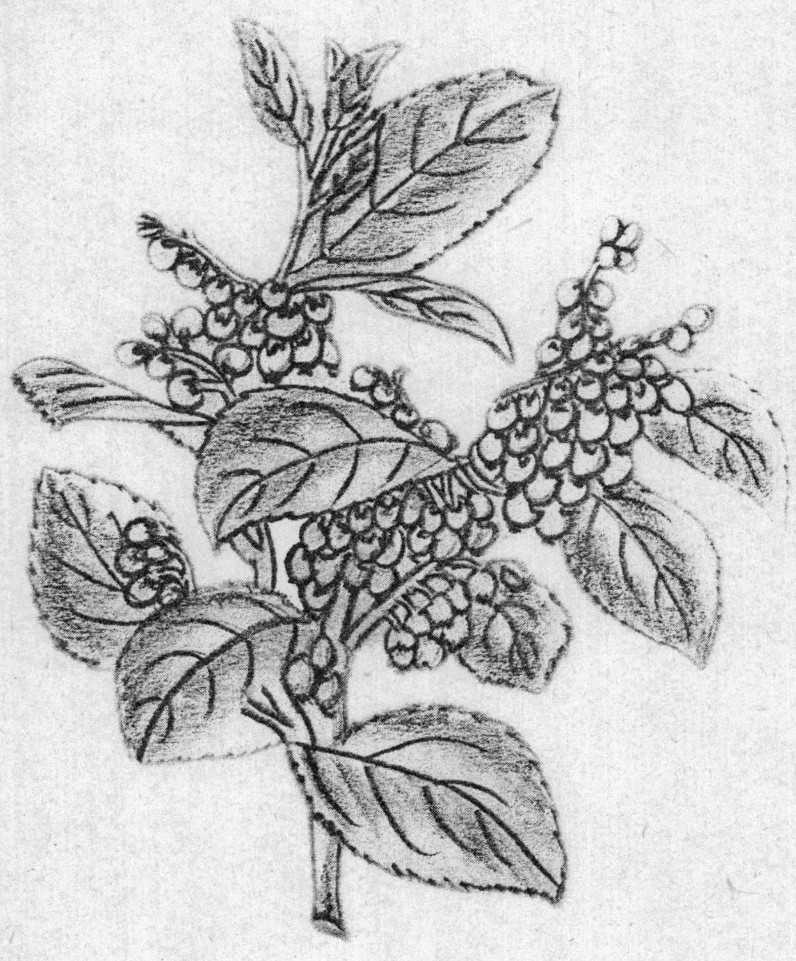

Fig. 14. Wintergreen (*Gaultheria fragrantissima*)

Part III
Remedies for Common Ailments

5
Remedies for Common Ailments

Herbal knowledge is continuing to grow as more people choose herbs as an alternative to pharmaceutical drugs. The following remedies are safe and effective treatments for a range of common ailments, but, like all medicines, they must be treated with respect. The suggestions given here are mostly quite straightforward. However, if you are unsure about what to do, always seek professional advice.

ESSENTIAL INFORMATION

Before using remedies read the following.

Dosage

- Except in Infants & Children, all dosages given are for adults.
- Never exceed the stated dose; doubling it will not make the medicine twice as effective.
- Before taking a remedy, check the cautions in the relevant herb entry.
- Do not take more than 2 internal remedies at any one time or more than 1 internal and 1 external remedy for the same complaint, unless specified. Alternative remedies using different herbs are divided by a leaf symbol. Where different forms of a remedy are given (e.g. take tincture or infusion), the first is preferable.

How long to take remedies

Take remedies until symptoms disappear. If there is no improvement within 2-3 weeks, if the condition worsens, or if in doubt, consult a professional practitioner.

Professional Advice

- Advice is given on when to seek professional guidance. Consult a professional if taking remedy for over 3 weeks.

Infants and Children

- Do not give babies under 6 months any internal herbal or other medicine without professional advice.
- Remedies elsewhere can be used for children under 12. Reduce doses as follows for Infants and Children.
    - 6-12 months old - 1/10 adult dose.
    - 1-6 years old - 1/3 adult dose.
    - 7-12 years old - ½ adult dose.

The Elderly

The elderly, due to a slower metabolism, may require less than the full adult dose. People over 70 should take 3/4 of the adult dose.

Pregnancy

- During the first 3 months of pregnancy, avoid all medicines, herbal or otherwise, unless absolutely essential.
- Avoid alcoholic tinctures in pregnancy.
- Though herbs in pregnancy are safe to use and many of the remedies elsewhere in this section are also safe, but always check the cautions for the remedy and in the relevant herb entry.
- Herbs in this section to avoid are : arbor vitae (*Thuja occidentalis*); black cohosh (*Cimicifuga racemosa*); buchu

(*Barosma betulina*); Chinese angelica (*Angelica sinensis*); Chinese rhubarb (*Rheum palmatum*); dan shen (*Salvia miltiorrhiza*); devil's claw (*Harpagophytum procumbens*); elecampane (*Inula helenium*); feverfew (*Tanacetum parthenium*); ginseng (*Panax ginseng*); juniper (*Juniperus communis*); liquorice (*Glycyrrhiza glabra*); motherwort (*Leonurus cardiaca*); myrrh (*Commiphora wighti*); pennyroyal (*Mentha pulegium*); prickly ash (*Zanthoxylum americanum*); senna (*Cassia senna*); shepherd's purse (*Capsella bursa-pastoris*); vervain (*Verbena officinalis*); white peony (*Paeonia lactiflora*); wild yam (*Dioscorea villosa*); wormwood (*Artemisia absinthium*); yarrow (*Achillea millefolium*); yellow dock (*Rumex crispus*).

- Avoid medicinal doses of angelica (*Angelica archangelica*), anise (*Pimpinella anisum*), cayenne (*Capsicum frutescens*), celery (*Apium graveolens*) and sage (*Salvia officinalis*). Cautions appear where relevant.
- Essential oils to avoid include German chamomile (*Chamomilla recutita*) and thyme (*Thymus vulgaris*).

Prescription Medicine

Some herbs interact with pharmaceutical drugs. If you are taking a prescribed drug, consult a professional practitioner before taking a herb and do not discontinue any medicine without their approval.

CONSULTING A HERBAL PRACTITIONER

Many common health problems, such as colds and indigestion, do not require a professional consultation and can be successfully treated using herbs at home. However, persistent or more serious ailments, such as stomach ulcers and shingles, require professional advice and treatment from a qualified herbal practitioner.

What Does Herbal Medicine Treat Best?

It is difficult to state exactly which ailments best respond to herbal medicine, since almost no research has been undertaken with this question in mind. Nevertheless, the experience of herbal practitioners and their patients suggests that many chronic and some acute illnesses readily improve with herbal medicine. Conditions that are commonly treated by herbalists include allergies, arthritis, chronic or frequent infections, circulatory problems, liver disease, menstrual and gynaecological problems, skin disorders, and stress-related complaints such as headaches, insomnia and palpitations.

Choosing A Herbalist

Herbal practitioners tend to treat ill health more effectively as they gain greater experience. Anyone with a serious illness, such as rheumatoid arthritis or cancer, should seek an experienced practitioner.

Nevertheless, herbalists newly launched into practice often bring a more flexible approach to treatment, having the time and enthusiasm for patients that may be lacking in their more senior counterparts. That said, a trusting relationship is as important as the treatment itself - always find a practitioner in whom you feel confident.

The Consultation

On visiting a herbalist you should be made to feel welcome, receiving an attentive and sympathetic ear. The first consultation takes about an hour, so there is ample time for the practitioner to gain a rounded view of your health problems and life as a whole.

You will probably be asked about family traits, diet, lifestyle, levels of stress and any particular anxieties that you may have. If appropriate, a physical examination will take place, and the practitioner will explain as far as possible what is wrong and how much improvement can be expected. Clinical tests may include urine analysis or measuring haemoglobin levels from a drop of blood.

The herbalist will then recommend appropriate treatment,

usually involving a herbal prescription, dietary advice and a suggested exercise regime. If you are already undergoing conventional treatment, the herbalist will advise you on its compatibility with herbal medicine and, if necessary, devise a programme to discontinue pharmaceutical medicines gradually,

Subsequent consultations generally last about 30 minutes and are likely to take place every 4 to 6 weeks for a period of 3 months. This, of course, may vary, depending on the nature of the treatment.

SELF-HELP

Lifestyle, diet and exercise advice is given in this section. In general, these suggestions do not provide a "quick fix" solution and need to be followed long-term to be effective. They should be used in addition to the recommended herbal remedy. By ensuring that your body has the right nutrition and level of fitness, you protect yourself against many ailments such as infections and circulatory problems as well as increasing your chances of a speedy and effective recovery.

OVER-THE-COUNTER REMEDIES

The number of shops and mail order companies selling ready-made preparations is growing. It is usually most convenient to buy tablets, essential oils, pessaries, ointments and perhaps tinctures, and to make your own infusions, decoctions and syrups. Belladonna plasters should be bought, not made.

Before buying a herbal medicine, always carefully read the list of contents on the label. Follow the instructions on the label and do not exceed the recommended dose. If buying preparations or dried herbs, use a reputable supplier and brand name. Many essential oils that are commercially produced use synthetic ingredients, which have little or no medicinal value.

GUIDE TO USE THE CONDITIONS AND ILLNESSES SECTION

Name and descriptions of condition.

Feeling and Emotions - possible thought and feeling patterns which may be causative at the psycho-physical interface (mind-body).

Cell Salts - simple homeopathic solutions using readily available simple cell salts.

Diet - Eating the Ayurvedic diet which is specific to your constitutional body type is generally beneficial. In certain conditions a specific diet or food is suggested (i.e., you are constitutionally a vata but in menopause extreme bleeding calls for a Pitta reducing diet).

Vitamins/Minerals - specific nutrients and amounts which have been beneficial for the conditions are suggested.

Essential Oils - a list of helpful essentials oils is given with body type effects. VP-means that these oils decrease (are good for) Vata and Pitta constitutions or conditions. K+ means that these oils increase (are not good for) Kapha symptoms or constitutions.

Herbs - a variety of herbs are suggested for assistance with the condition. You can use them singularly or make a blend. A specific recipe may be suggested but it can be altered due to herb availability and your personal tastes. Herbs are also marked as to effect. When choices are available, choose herbs which agree with your constitution or counter a particular condition's doshic aspect.

Cleanse - Always consult a health practitioner when doing a cleanse.

Alternative Therapy - Here alternative or complementary therapies are suggested which can be helpful. Understand you need not do any of the therapies and could be overwhelmed if you try to do everything. Go within and let your inner guidance decide what, of all your choices, to do.

Avoid - This category includes those things which might aggravate the condition.

Herbal Blends - This is a suggested blend of herbs to be used for up to three months. You can make your own blend from the list of suggested herbs.

Self-Care - This section describes special procedures to do at home. In next section, the weight of items to be taken for various receipts is given in oz. Here 1 oz is equivalent to 284 ml of today's weight

How to use the condition Section

V Means Vata.
P Means Pitta.
K Means Kapha.
(-) Means decreases.
(+) Means increases.
(=) Balancing to all body types.
(o) Neutral effect.

Example

VP-	Means this herb or essential oil will reduce Vata and Pitta.
K+	Means Kaphas should avoid as it will increase Kapha.
VPK =	Good for all doshas.
o	Neutral effect

After reading these herb recommendations for specific conditions, please don't imagine that you have ever made "wrong" choices in the past. All herbs contain nutrients and healing power. Intuition and the power of personal choice are powerful healers. However, experience has shown that by choosing herbs based on their Ayurvedic properties, one can experience better results.

ACNE

Acne is caused by a high Pitta condition, especially during the teen years. During times of development, the body goes through hormonal increase. Other factors include medication, allergic reaction, stress, poor diet, and the build up of Ama (toxicity). It can be triggered at various times of the menstrual cycle and during menopause. The first step is to look at the diet and begin to eliminate foods which could be aggravating the condition. The most common offenders are sugar, chocolate, dairy products, meat with hormones, fried foods, potato chips, salty foods, soda pop, and processed foods.

Vata Acne : The boils are dry and scaly with some patches of oil, yet the skin is dry.

Pitta Acne : Reddish pimples appear with yellowish discharge and inflammation (redness).

Kapha Acne : There is a fluid buildup with white discharge.

Feelings and Emotions : Not feeling good about the way you look.

Diet	*Vitamins & Minerals (Daily)*	*Essential Oils (Always dilute)*	*Herbs*	*Alternative Therapy*	*Avoid*
Ayurvedic	A: 50,000 IU before meals	Juniper : KV-P+	Turmeric : KV-Po	Facials	Sugar
diet for	E : 400 IU before meals	Sandalwood : PV-Ko	Sandalwood : PV-Ko	Steam	Chocolate
body type	B6-Pyrodoxine:	Jatamasi: KV-P+	Rose Petals : VPK =		Dairy
Elimination	50 mg. 2 x day	Tea Tree : VPK=	Gentian : PK-V+		Female Hormones
diet	Zinc: 90 mg.	Lemon: PV-Ko	Oat Straw: VP-K+		Iodine
High fibre	Multi-Mineral		Licorice : VP-K+		Inorganic Iodine
	Flaxseed or Evening		Burdock: PK-V+		B-12
			Red Clover: PK-V+		Commercial Soaps
	C: 3,000 mg.		Peppermint: PK-Vo		Soft Drinks
			Lemongrass: PK-Vo		

Herbal Brew

VATA		*PITTA*		*KAPHA*	
Turmeric	1 oz	Witch Hazel	1 oz	Echinacea	1 oz
Sandalwood	2 oz	Dandelion	2 oz	Myrrh	1 oz
Rose Petals	1 oz	Burdock	2 oz	Red Clover	2 oz
Amalaki	1 oz	Red Clover	1 oz	Lemongrass	2 oz
Gentian	1 oz	Peppermint	1 oz	Lemon Balm	1 oz
Oat Straw	2 oz	Lemongrass	2 oz	Guggul	1 oz
Liquorice	1 oz				

Vata Acne		*Vata-Pitta Acne*	
Sandalwood	2 oz	Use : 1/4 teaspoon of Sandalwood powder	Mix all dry ingredients and lemon juice into a paste.
Turmeric	1 oz	1/4-teaspoon turmeric powder	Apply to your face.
Chamomile	2 oz	1/3 of a lemon (juice)	Dry. Wash well.
Ginger	1 oz		Apply aloe vera gel.
			Wash.

Recipes for Acne

Ayurveda clays, Bentonite clays, fresh clays :

1/2 teaspoon of clay	1 Tablespoon lemon juice
Mix well to create a paste.	Apply and let dry.
Wash.	*Note : Do not use apple cider vinegar even though some brands of clay call for it.*

In the morning, wash face with chana flour (garbanzo flour) :

Mix enough flour to make a watery paste.

1 drop of Sandalwood essential oil.

For Kapha : Use Cajaput, Juniper or Lavender essential oils

1 drop of Turmeric essential oil.

Apply mixture and rub/scrub lightly

Wash with water.

Do not use soap on the skin.

**Acne Free essential oil blend can then be applied. Use either a dry skin blend that contains carrier oil, or use a blend specifically for oily skin.*

Essential oil blends can be made for Vata with equal amounts of :	*Essential oil blends can be made for Pitta & Kapha with equal amounts of :*
Sandalwood	Sandalwood
Jatamasi	Rose
50% sesame oil base	Lavender
	50% jojoba oil base

Be sure to follow your Ayurvedic diet and avoid foods that could aggravate the condition. Keep skin clean; wash often with a pH balanced soap (do not use regular soap). Avoid makeup and clogging of the skin pores while healing the acne.

Self Care

Flaxseed or Evening Primrose oil for hormonal balance.

Vitamin C with bioflavonoids : Pittas do best with Sago Palm or Ascorbate C - 3,000 mg.

Facial Sauna

General cautions : Do not squeeze or burst boils or acne spots as the infection may spread. Seek professional advice for recurrent boils.

AIDS

This is a disease of the immune system where the body is run down due to stress, poor diet, excessive sexual activities, drugs, alcohol, or through diseased blood transfusions. This is a Vata/Pitta condition with both doshas involved.

Feelings and Emotions : Guilt, shame, confusion about sexuality.

Cell Salts : Silica

Diet	*Vitamins & Minerals (Daily)*	*Essential Oils (Always dilute)*	*Herbs*	*Alternative Therapy*	*Avoid*
Ayurvedic	A: 50,000 IU	Sandalwood : PV-Ko	Isatis : PKV+	Chakra balance	Masturbation
diet for	E: 600 IU	Tea Tree: VPK=	Suma: PK-V+	Energy work	Spices
body type	C: 10,000 mg	Saffron: VPK=	Saw Palmetto: V-PK+	Acupuncture	Smoking
		Jatamasi: VK-P+	Ginko biloba: VPK=	Massage	Alcohol

Yellow vegetables	B-Complex: 200 mg.	Geranium: PK-V+	Shilajit: PKV+	Counseling	Sodas
		Egg Lecithin: 20 gms	Myrtle: PKV+		Red meat
	3 x per day	Cumin: VPK-	Guggul: KV-P+		Sugar
Shitaki mushrooms	Digestive Enzyme	Rose: VPK=	Sandalwood: PV-Ko		Reduce sexual activities
	Zinc: 50 mg		Red Clover: PK-V+		
	Acidophilus: 3 times/day		Brahmi PKV=		
Meat broth	Copper: 3 mg		Sarsaparilla: PV-KLo		
	RNA-DNA : 1500 mg.		Coriander: PVK-		
Immune soup	Sustain (Metagenics)		Ashwagandha: VK-P+		
	Q 10: 100 mg		Marshmallow: PV-K+		
			Diamond Ash: VPK=		
Sesame oil	Germanium : 200 mg.		Aloe Vera Gel: VPK=		
			Triphalla: VPK-		
			Immune support+ (Banyan herbs)		

Chayanprash	Medicated Oil :	
	Amla: VPKo	Trikatu: VK-P+
Lotus seeds		
Almonds		
Ghee		
Medicated Jelly (Chyavanprash)		

Vatas: Need to increase digestion. Take Trikatu (2 tablets) before each meal during lunchtime with yogurt and fennel.

• **Pitta** : Use ginger, coriander, cardamon, acidophilus.

Herbal Brew

Vata		*Pitta*		*Kapha*	
Astralagus	2 oz.	Saffron	1 oz.	Burdock	2 oz.
Ashwagandha	1 oz.	Rheumania	2 oz.	Plantain	3 oz.
Saw Palmetto	1 oz.	Astralagus	3 oz.	Solomon's Seal	1 oz.
Liquorice	2 oz.	Brahmi	2 oz.	Gokshura	1 oz.
Ligustrum	1 oz.	Sarsaparilla	2 oz.	Saffron	1 oz
Shatavari	3 oz.	Gokshura	1 oz.	Saw Palmetto	2 oz.
Bala	1 oz	Plantain	2 oz.		
Ginseng	1 oz.	Sandalwood	3 oz		
		Solomon's Seal	2 oz.		

Drink

Turmeric	1 Tbs.
Aloe vera	1 Tbs.

Mix all ingredients together. Use 1 teaspoon per cup of water, and drink 3 times a day.

Self-Massage (Abyangha)

Self-massage is very important. The following recipes are for preparing your own massage oil.

Vata	Brahmi	30 drops
	Sandalwood	20 drops

	Cumin	10 drops
	Jatamasi	15 drops
	Himalayan Cedarwood	20 drops
	Sesame oil	4 oz.
Pitta	Brahmi	30 drops
	Sandalwood	20 drops
	Cumin	10 drops
	Rose	20 drops
	Lavender	15 drops
	Sunflower oil or Ghee	4 oz.

Self-Care

Breathwork, Meditation, Mantra

ALCOHOLISM

Alcoholism can be associated with repressed feelings and emotions consistent with "holding on" or hiding. A poor diet and a deficiency of nutrients can also result in addiction. Alcohol raises Pitta, blocking the functions of the liver and pancreas.

Feelings and Emotions : Suspicion of self. Lack of self-love.

Diet	Vitamins & Minerals (Daily)	Essential Oils (Always dilute)	Herbs	Alternative Therapy	Avoid
Pitta	A: 2,000 IU	Geranium: PK-V	Aloe Vera: VPK=	Counseling	Sugar
Ayurvedic	B-Complex: 300 mg.	Sandalwood: PV-Ko	Gentian: PK-V+	Emotional release	Drugs
diet	B-12:30 mcg.	Rose: VPK=	Turmeric: KV-Po	Tarpana massage	Coffee
	E: 150 IU	Jatamasi: KV-P+	Barberry: PK-V+	Therapeutic touch	Fried foods
Wheat germ	C: 2,500 mg.	Bergamot: VK-P+	Brahmi: PKV=	Energy work	
	Selenium: 1,000 mg.		Skullcap: PV-Vo	Pancha Karma	
	Magnesium: 500 mg.		Hops: PK-V+		
	Zinc: 50 mg.	For withdrawal	Burdock: PK-V+		
	Nicotinic Acid: 500 mg.	symptoms:	Milk Thistle: PK-V+		
	B2 - Riboflavin: 200 mg.	Melissa: PKV-	Passion Flower: PK-V+		
	Amino Acid : 100 mg.	- Marjoram: KV-P+	Dandelion: PK-V+		
		-Ylang Ylang: PV-K+	Amla: PV-Ko		
	Catechin: 100 mg.	-Lavender: PK-Vo			
	L-Glutathione: 300 mg		Ayurvedic Formulas:		
	L-Glutathione: 300 mg		-Bhanta Rasayana: VPK-		
	Pantethine: 300 mg.-		- Saraswati: VPK-		
	2-3 × per day		- Chjyavanprash: VP-K+		
	B6 - Pyrodoxine: 100 mg.		-Amla: PV-Ko		

B1 - Thiamine: 100 mg.
Folic Acid: 50 mcg.
A good Multi-Vitamin
Evening primrose: ½ gram
3 × per day

Herbal Brew

Vata		Pitta		Kapha	
Brahmi	1 oz.	Dandelion Root	2 oz.	Ginger	2 oz.
Ginger	2 oz.	Burdock Root	2 oz.	Burdock Root	2 oz.
Coriander	2 oz.	Brahmi	1 oz.	Peppermint	1 oz.
Skullcap	2 oz.	Milk Thistle	2 oz.	Cardamon	1 oz.
Saraswat	1 tsp.	Mint	2 oz. (or add 1)	Passion Flower	2 oz.
		Lobelia	1 oz.	Ginger	1 oz.
Drink 4 to 6 cups per day		Gentian tablets	2 tablets	Turmeric	1 tablet

ALLERGIES

Caused by low immunity and/or long term use of allopathic drugs particularly antibiotics. The body is not able to produce antihistamines because of stress, poor diet, overwork, nervousness, environmental pollution, or food allergies. More common in Vata body types because of their weak digestive system and sensitivity. Pitta types often suffer more with skin rash or sweating type allergies. Kaphas usually experience sinus congestion, hay fever, or water retention.

Feelings and Emotions : Something, someone is irritating them. Life is too much. Feeling overwhelmed.

Diet	Vitamins & Minerals (Daily)	Essential Oils (Always dilute)	Herbs	Alternative Therapy	Avoid
Ayurvedic	A: 25,000 IU	Myrtle: KP-V+	Bayberry: KV-P+	Tarpana	Foods which are
diet for	E: 200 IU	Saffron: VPK=	Calamus: VK-P+	Nasya	common allergens:
body type	C: Ascorbate 2000-3000 mg.	Eucalyptus : KV-P+	Mullein : PK-V+	Pancha	-Wheat
Yellow	B-12: 100 mcg. (4 weeks)	Lavender: PK-Vo	Elecampane: VK-P+	Karma	-Dairy
vegetables	B-Complex: 100 mg.	Patchouli: VP-K+	Basil: VK-P+		-Beef
Shitaki	Bioflavonoids: 1000 mg.	Peppermint: PK-Vo			-Corn
mushrooms	Pantothenic Acid: 2500 mg.	Camphor: VK-P+			-Citrus
Rotation diet	Molybdenum: 50 mg.	Cubeb: VK-P+	Nutmeg: VK-P+		-MSG
Raw foods	Quercetin: 100 mg.	Spruce: VK-P+	Cardamon: VK-P+		-Soy
& juices	Linoleic Acid: 200 mg.	All Chamomiles: VPK-	Fennel: VPK=		-Sugar
Elimination	Lactobacillus: ¼ tsp. 3 × day	Rosemary: KV-P+	Coltsfoot: PK-Vo		
diet	Acidophilus: 3 × a day	Angelica: VPK=	Cloves: VK-P+		

Immune building diet	Bifido bacteria: 3 × a day	Lemon Balm: KP-Vo	Eucalyptus: KV-P+
	Catechine : 100 mg.	Basil : VK-P+	Aloe Vera: VPK=
		Echinacea: PK-V+	Immune support (Banyan Herbs)
		Rose: VPK=	Lobelia: K-PV+
			Ephedra: K-VP+
			Angelica: VPK = P+ (in excess)
			Vasa: PK-V+
			Kola: VPK-
			Trikatu: VK-P+
			Triphalla: VPK-
			Guduchi: VPK+
			Brahmi: PKV=

Herbal Brew

Vata		Pitta		Kapha	
Eucalyptus	1 oz.	Elecampane	2 oz.	Ephedra	2 oz.
Elecampane	1 oz.	Coriander	1 oz.	Elecampane	1 oz.
Ginger	2 oz.	Vasa	2 oz.	Peppermint	1 oz.
Cardamon	1 oz.	Peppermint	1 oz.	Horehound	1 oz.
Cloves	1 oz.	Mullein	2 oz.	Mullein	2 oz.
Liquorice	2 oz.	Brahmi	1 oz.		

Drink 4 cups in-between meals. Add warm milk at night. Avoid milk if there are dairy allergies; substitute rice or soymilk.

Vata & Kapha

Warm compress over the chest with equal amounts of :

Encalyptus 5 drops
Camphor 5 drops
Rosemary 5 drops
Myrtle 5 drops

Mix with 2 Tbs. of mustard or canola oil

Warm the oil and apply to chest. Cover the chest with wool cloth for 15 minutes.

Repeat 2-3 times per week.

Pitta

Compress should be at room temperature.

Cilantro juice - 3 times per day

Drink - VKP

Mix :	Lemon Balm	5 drops	Take essential oil blend and use
	Rose	3 drops	2 drops in 8 oz. of water once per day.
	Chamomile	3 drops	

More on Herbs

Vata & Kapha : Take 2 tablets of Trikatu before every meal. 1 tsp. coriander before each meal.

Vata-Pitta-Kapha : Take 500 mg. of Triphalla at bedtime.

Eyewash to Reduce Redness in Eyes

Make infusion of 1 oz. Chrysanthemum herb in 2-oz. water - or use Eyebright.

Strain well. It is best to use cotton cloth on strainer.

Keep formula refrigerated. Wash eye 3 times per day.

Self Care

Essential oil inhalation every 2 hours

Colon cleanse

Compresses over the area

Vaporizer at night in the bedroom with essential oils

ALOPECIA (Hair Loss)

At first, the hair begins to thin slowly in patches eventually being followed by baldness. It can result from old age, radiation, endocrine disorders, hormone imbalance, sudden weight loss, stress, overwork, pregnancy, or heredity factors. When the condition is due to heredity, one needs to begin to work on it at an early age. Vitamin and mineral deficiency can also be consistent with alopecia.

Feelings and Emotions : Anger, irritability. Thinking too much. Having to do the right thing. Compulsiveness

Diet	Vitamins & Minerals (Daily)	Essential Oils (Always dilute)	Herbs	Alternative Therapy	Avoid
Ayurvedic	B-Complex: 200 mg.	Ginger: VK-P+	Bhringaraj: VPK=	Shirodhara	White sugars
diet for	F: 100 mg.	Brahmi: VPK-	Alfalfa: PK-V+	Head massage	Over eating fruit
body type	Inositol: 100 mg.	Coriander: VPK-	Brahmi: VPK=		Fried foods
Protein foods	Folic Acid: 150 mcg.	Gold Chamomile: KP-V+	Ginger: VK-P+		Coffee
	C: 3000 mg.	Birch: PK-V+			Tobacco
Foods high	E: 150 IU	Sandalwood: VP-Ko	Rose Petals: VPK=		Hot spicy foods
in sulfur	Lecithin: 2 tablets	Aloe Vera: VKP-	Sage: KV-P+		Stress
Eggs	before meals		Rosemary: KV-P+		Hormone therapy
	Choline: 100 mg.	Medicated oils:	Aloe Vera: VPK-		
Legumes	Zinc: 50 mg.	- Bhringaraj: VPK=	Nettles: PK-V+		
	Multi-Vitamin	- Amla : PV-Ko	Burdock: PK-V+		
Cabbage	Multi-mineral	- Brahmi: VPK=	Yarrow: PK-V+		
Sunflower	Flax oil: 2 tsp.		Yucca: VPK-		
seeds					
Juice therapy	Amino Acids Complex	Vegetable oils:			

Copper: 100 mg. - Coconut: P-K+Vo
Iodine : 100 mg. - Sesame: V-PK+

Hair Oil Formulas

Vata		Pitta		Kapha	
Sesame Oil	1 oz.	Coconut or Jojoba oil	1 oz.	Almond oil	1 oz.
Rosemary	10 drops	Brahmi	10 drops	Sage	10 drops
Brahmi	5 drops	Sandalwood	5 drops	Rosemary	10 drops
Sandalwood	5 drops	Coriander	10 drops	Coriander	10 drops
Coriander	5 drops	Birch	5 drops	Brahmi (gotu kola)	10 drops
Chamomile	5 drops	Chamomile	5 drops		

Mix all ingredients. Apply on scalp for 20 minutes before shampooing.

Herbal Brew

Vata		Pitta		Kapha	
Brahmi	2 oz.	Brahmi	2 oz.	Yarrow	1 oz.
Rosemary	1 oz.	Rose Petals	1 oz.	Brahmi	2 oz.
Sage	1/2 oz.	Coriander	1 oz.	Coriander	2 oz.

Ginger	2 oz.	Chrysanthemum	2 oz.	Ginger	2 oz.
Coriander	1 oz.	Mint	1 oz.		
Bhringaraj	1 oz.	Chamomile	½ oz.		

Self-Care

Yoga : headstand (inversion therapy) — Stress reduction tapes — Oil treatments for the hair

Head massage/scalp massage — Add herbs and essential oils to shampoo and conditioner

ALZHEIMERS

Another name for Pre-senile Dementia, which begins with personality changes, difficult communication, and mood swings. Vata types can become "spacey" and leave out words when speaking. Pitta types can become irritable and on edge about life. Kapha types shut down communication and become disoriented. Causes are hereditary, with some controversy about other possible causes, namely; excess amounts of aluminium, silicon, sulfur, and calcium. Hair analysis can be used as a diagnostic tool for monitoring any heavy metals within the body. Chelation can remove them and increase arterial blood flow.

Feelings and Emotions : Life is becoming too much. Life is overwhelming, not worth dealing with.

Cell Salts : Silica; Kalphos; Potassium phosphate

Diet	Vitamins & Minerals (Daily)	Essential Oils (Always dilute)	Herbs	Alternative Therapy	Avoid
Ayurvedic	B-Complex: 200 mg.	Brahmi: VPK-	Brahmi: VPK=	Head massage	Aspirin
diet for	B-12: 200 mcg.	Ginger: VK-P+	Ginko biloba: VPK-	Chelation	Antacids
body type	A: 100,000 IU	Ashwagandha: VK-P+	Basil : VK-P+	Shirodhara	All products with

Foods high	Beta-Carotene: 1500 IU	Amla: VPK	Rosemary: KV-P+	Nasya	aluminium:
in minerals	C: 2500-3000 gm.	Cyperus: PKV-	Dandelion: PK-V+	Hair analysis	- Makeup
Fiber	E: 150 IU	Basil: VK-P+	Myrrh: KV-P+	Pancha Karma in	-Baking Powder
(oat bran)	Selenium: 200 mcg.	Cardamon: VK-P+	St. John's Wort: PK-V+	the early stages	- Shampoo
Foods rich	Boron: 100 IU	Hyssop: VK-P+	Calamus: VK-P+		- Cookware
in sulfur	Zinc : 50 mg.	Mint: PK-Vo	Irish Moss: V-PK+		- Deodorant
(legumes)	Co Q-10: (2) 50 mg.:	Lemongrass: PK-Vo	Lotus Seeds: PV-K+		- Beer cans
Oats	2 × day	Camphor: KV-P+	Jasmine Flowers : PK-V+		Fried foods
		Angelica : VPK =	Mental clarity (Banyan Herbs)		
Lots of	Lecithin: 200 mg.		Burdock: PK-V+		
yellow &	L-lysine: 4 tables daily	Bergamot: VK-P +	White Musal: VPK-		Fast foods
orange	L-phenylalamine: 100 mg.		Cardamom: KV-P+		
vegetables	Amino Acid Complex:		Chryanthemum : PK-V+	**Ayurvedic Herbal Formulas:**	
Kidney beans	700-900 mg. 2 x day		Ghee: PV-K+		-Triphalla: VPK
Lots of	Germanium: 75 mg.		Chicory Root: PK-V+		-Trifolia: VK-P+
seaweed	DHEA: 150 mg.				
Potassium broth					
Juice fasting					
Ghee					
Salmon / Sardines					

Herbal Brew

Vata		Pitta		Kapha	
Basil	1 oz.	Brahmi	2 oz.	Chicory Root	2 oz.
Brahmi	2 oz.	Ginko biloba	1 oz.	Cardamon	1 oz.
Rosemary	1 oz.	Dandelion	1 oz.	Spearmint	1 oz.
Cardamon	1 oz.	Chrysanthemum	2 oz.	Irish Moss	1 oz.
Calamus	1 oz.	Burdock	1 oz.	Burdock	1 oz.
Ginko biloba	2 oz.	Jasmine	1 oz.	Ginko biloba	2 oz.
		Peppermint	1 oz.		

Potassium Broth

Cut all ingredients. Add to two quarts of water and bring to a boil. Cover. Simmer for two hours.

Vata		Pitta		Kapha	
Potatoes & peelings	5	Peelings of sweet potatoes	5	Potatoes & peelings	5
Carrots	4	Parsley	½ bunch	Parsley	1 bunch
Ginger, fresh	2"	Cilantro	1 bunch	Ginger	3"
Celery	½ stalk	Mint	½ bunch	Juniper berries	1 handful
Cilantro	1 bunch	Yellow squash	2	Cilantro	1 bunch

Spinach	½ bunch	Coriander seeds	½ oz.	Spinach	½ bunch
Watercress	½ bunch	Borage	½ oz.	Borage	1/8 oz.
Tomatoes	2	Water	2 quarts	Carrots	4
Water	2 quarts			Water	2 quarts

Prevention Massage

Basil	5 drops	Lemongrass	3 drops
Camphor	3 drops	Angelica	2 drops
Bergamot	3 drops	Base Oil	4 oz.

Self-Care

Use essential oils in an aromatherapy lamp when studying or during activities that require concentration and memory.

Inhalations: Three times per day- especially with essential oils of Rosemary, Basil, Mint, and/or Lemon.

Early prevention: Alzheimer's can be prevented when symptoms begin to appear.

Abyangha (self massage)

AMENORRHIA

It is the absence of menstruation, which can be due to low caloric intake or excessive exercise that lowers the body weight and body fat. It is also consistent with low protein or low mineral levels. Long term incidence may cause bone loss.

Feelings and Emotions : Fear of the unknown.

Cell Salts : Nat Sulph; Calci-Phos

Diet	Vitamins & Minerals (Daily)	Essential Oils (Always dilute)	Herbs	Alternative Therapy	Avoid
Ayurvedic	B-6: 200 mg.	Cyperus: VPK-	Saffron: VPK=	Acupuncture	Exercise
diet for	Folic Acid: 50 mcg.	Valerian: VK-P+	Ignatia: PK-V+	Rolfing	Weight loss
body type	E: 150 IU	Angelica: VPK-,	Nettle Leaf: PK-V+	Ayurvedic	Excess protein
	Calcium: 1200 mg.	P + (in excess)	Dong Quai: VK-Po	consultation	Stress
Spices	Magnesium: 100 mg.	Basil: VK-P+	Rose: VPK=	Therapeutic	Birth control pills -
	Evening Primrose:	Sage: VK-P+	Ginger: VK-P+	touch	"post pill
Sesame seeds	200 mg.	Clary Sage: VPK-	Cyperus: VPK	Woman's support	syndrome"
	Flax Seed Oil: 200 mg.	Geranium : PK-Vo	Squaw Vine: PK-V+	group	
Saffron rice			Angelica: VP-P+ (in excess)		
			Aloe Vera: VPK=		
			Fennel: VPK=		
			Black Cohosh: PK-V+		
			Vitex: VPK-		
			Yarrow: PK-V+		
			Cotton Root: V-KP+		
			Cinnamon: VK-P+		

Herbal Brew

Vata		Pitta		Kapha	
Ginger	2 oz.	Nettles	2 oz.	Vitex	2 oz
Catnip	2 oz.	Shatavari	1 oz.	Ginger	1 oz.
Angelica	2 oz.	Mint	1 oz.	Angelica	2 oz.
Rose Petals	2 oz.	Fennel	1 oz.	St. John's Wort	1 oz.
Vitex	1 oz.	Black Cohosh	1 oz.	Yarrow	2 oz.
Shatavari	1 oz.	Chamomile	1 oz.	Cyperus	1 oz.
		Rose Petals	1 oz.		

Drink 4 times per day

Vata		Pitta		Kapha	
Vitex	1 oz.	Chamomile	2 oz.	Angelica	1 oz.
Rose Petals	2 oz.	Yarrow	2 oz.	Motherwort	1 oz.
Angelica	2 oz.	Blessed Thistle	1 oz.	Ginger	2 oz.
Cinnamon	1 oz.	Motherwort	1 oz.	Cinnamon	1 oz.
Ginger	1 oz.	Rose Petals	1 oz.	Yarrow	2 oz.
Cotton Root	1 oz.	Hibiscus	1 oz.	Hibiscus	1 oz.

Drink 4 times per day

All Doshas :

Two weeks before periods, drink 1 cup daily.

Vata : Aloe Vera Gel with Basil or Ginger added.

Pitta : Aloe Vera Gel with ½ tsp. Fennel or Mint added.

Kapha : Aloe Vera Gel with Turmeric added.

Self-Care

Supportive counseling	Aromatherapy (especially in the morning)
Abdominal massage	Dance movement

ANAEMIA

A blood disorder caused by a deficiency of iron and minerals, where the blood becomes thin and weak. There are many kinds of anaemia: Micro Cystic - VK; Sickle Cell - VK; Side Roblastic - VK; Metablastic - PK. Vatas may experience copper skin, insomnia, dizziness, constipation, or dehydration. Pittas have fevers, inflammation, thirst, and yellow on the eyes and skin. Kaphas often have water retention, fatigue, tiredness or pale, almost white skin.

Feelings and Emotions : Feeling tired of life.

Diet	Vitamins & Minerals (Daily)	Essential Oils (Always dilute)	Herbs	Alternative Therapy	Avoid
Ayurvedic diet for body type	B-Complex: 200 mg. A-E: 450 IU (easier) Folic Acid : 200 mcg.	Chamomile: VPK Lemon Thyme: PK-Vo	Aloe Vera: VPK= Bibhitaki: PK-Vo Amalaki: PV-Ko	Naturopath & Ayurvedic consultation	Blood cleansers Excessive exercise Iron Ferrus Sulfate

	B2 - Riboflavonoids:	Saffron: VPK=
Bone soup	25-30 mg.	Shatavari: PV-K+
	B1 - Thiamin: 100 mg.	Manjishta: PK-V+
Sesame seed	Folate: 300 mcg. -especially during pregnancy (for anaemia)	Punarnava: PK-V+
		Agrimony: PK-V+
Pomegranate juice	Copper: 50 mg.	Yellow Dock: PK-V+
	Iron : 100 mg.	Shata Root: best taken in tablet form
	Zinc: 40 mg.	
Spinach	Hydrochloric Acid: 2 before protein meals	Fo Ti : PV-K+
Carrots		
Molasses	Iron (Ferrus Fumerate): 80 mg.	**Ayurvedic Formulas:**
Beets	-(helps in constipation)	-Chyavanprash: VP-K+
Organic whole milk		-Triphalla: VPK-
		-Iron Ash: VPK
Red organic meats		

Herbal Brew

Vata		Pitta & Kapha	
Amalaki	1 oz.	Yellow Dock	2 oz.

Shatavari	2 oz.	Bibhitaki	1 oz.
Ashwagandha	1 oz.	Peppermint	1 oz.
Lotus	1 oz.	Nettles	1 oz.
Fo Ti	1 oz.	Barberry	1 oz.
Ginger	1 oz.	Agrimony	1 oz.
Raspberry Leaves	½ oz.	Dandelion Root	2 oz.
Comfrey	1 oz.		

Recipies

Saffron	½ gram
Milk or Yogurt	1 cup
Molasses	1 tsp.

Take 3 times per day with 1 teaspoon of ghee.

General caution : Seek professional advice to determine the type of anaemia you have before home treatment

ANOREXIA - BULIMIA

Anorexia and bulimia involve suppression of the digestive fire due to eating and vomiting or skipping meals. People with this condition usually have the tendency to make poor food choices. Vatas tend to fast and feast. Pittas often have burning in the stomach. Kaphas force themselves to throw up.

Feelings and Emotions : Low self esteem. Fear of gaining weight. Distorted view of self. Sees self as overweight, even when emaciated.

Diet	Vitamins & Minerals (Daily)	Essential Oils (Always dilute)	Herbs	Alternative Therapy	Avoid
Ayurvedic diet for body type	B-Complex: 200 mg.	Ginger: VK-P+	Comfrey: PV-K+	Counseling	All sugars - until the condition is under control
Lots of digestive spices (especially carminative)	Good Multi-Vitamin	Cardamon: VK-P+	Ashwagandha: VK-P+	Massage	Depressing situations
Lots of green leafy vegetables	Zinc: 50 mg. with every meal	Bergamot: VK-P+	Slippery Elm: PV-K+	Breathwork	
	Pancreatic Enzymes: 2 with each meal	Orange: VK-P+	Cardamon: VK-P+	Therapeutic touch	
	Comfrey: 2 with each meal	All Citrus: VK-P+	Ginger: VK-P+	Polarity therapy	
	Pectin: 2 with each meal	Rose Geranium: PK-V+	Fennel: VPK=		
	Papaya Enzymes: 2 tablets before meals	Clary Sage: VPK	HIng: VK-P+		
	Trikatu: 2-3 before meals	Sandalwood: PV-Ko	Valerian: VK-P+		
		Lemongrass: PK-Vo	Nutmeg: VK-P+		
		Bay: VPK+	Lemongrass: PK-Vo		
		Angelica: VPK= P + (in excess)	Angelica: VK-P+		
			Chitrack: VPK		
			Shatavari: PV-K+		
Lots of yellow (Vata) vegetables			Hingatash: VK-P+		
Hing with all beans			Chyavanprash: VP-K+		
Kicharee			Ashwagandha Compound: VK-P+		

Herbal Brew

Kapha		Vata		Pitta	
Ginger	2 oz.	Ashwagandha	2 oz.	Fennel	1 oz.
Orange Peel	1 oz.	Angelic	2 oz.	Mint	2 oz.
Cardamon	2 oz.	Slippery Elm	2 oz.	Coriander	2 oz.
Basil	1 oz.	Comfrey	1 oz.	Comfrey	1 oz.
Lemongrass	2 oz.	Liquorice	2 oz.	Liquorice	1 oz.
Cinnamon	1 oz.	Ginger	2 oz.	Slippery Elm	1 oz.
Fennel	1 oz.	Coriander	1 oz.		
Mint	1 oz.	Shatavari	1 oz.		

MORNING BREAKFAST

Oats or any other grain	
Slippery Elm powder	2 Tbs.
Ginger	½ tsp.
Cardamon	½ tsp.
Coriander	¼ tsp.
Cinnamon	½ tsp.
Kicharee	equal amount of rice, mung dahl, and spices

Cook oatmeal. Add slippery elm, all spices, and kicharee

TAKE

Vata & Kapha: Trikatu - 3 tablets before each meal for 2 weeks, then 2 tablets before meals for 1 month, then 1 tablet before meals for 3 months.

ANXIETY

Anxiety can be associated with excitement, panic, apprehension, or feeling unsure. It is often elevated by too much coffee, drug usage, excess sugar in the diet, feeling troubled, or not trusting the process of life. Vata types may experience anxiety more often than the other body types.

Feelings and Emotions : No trust of self. Mistrust in general.

Diet	Vitamins & Minerals (Daily)	Essential Oils (Always dilute)	Herbs	Alternative Therapy	Avoid
Ayurvedic	B-Complex: 200 mg.	Jatamasi: KV-P+	Chamomile: PK-Vo	Massage	Sugar
diet for	B6 Pyridoxine: 100 mg.	Sandalwood: VP-Ko	Chrysanthemum : PK-V+	Therapeutic touch	Coffee
body type	B1 Thiamine: 100 mg.	Lavender: PK-Vo	Skullcap: PK-Vo	Tarpana	Cigarettes
	B3 Niacinamide: 500 mg.	Vetiver: V-KP+	Valerian: VK-P+	Reiki	Processed
Lots of yellow	2 x day	Ylang Ylang: PV-K+	Kava Kava: PV-K+	Counseling	foods
vegetables	Calcium: 300-750 mg.	Chamomile: VPK-	Passion Flower: PK-V+	Shirodhara	Alcohol
	(in extreme cases)		Bala: PV-Ko		
Lots of roots	L-tryptophan: 100 mg.		Bhringaraj: VPK=		
vegetables			Jasmine Flower: PK-V+		
			Alum Root: PK-V+		

Catechu: KP-V+
Myrrh: KV-P+
Katuka: PK-V+

Herbal Brew

Vata Tea		Pitta & Kapha Tea	
Kava Kava	2 oz.	Chamomile	2 oz.
Valerian	1 oz.	Brahmi	1 oz.
Liquorice	1 oz.	Skullcap	2 oz.
Fennel	2 oz.	Passion Flower	2 oz.
		Jasmine Flower	1 oz.

At night, drink tea with warm milk.

Self-Care

Abyangha massage: every morning with relaxing formula.

Massage head at night with essential oil formula.

Inhalation : every 2 hours with essential oil of your choice.

Put drops of essential oil on your disk, work area, or pillow; can also use a diffuser.

Meditation : add drop or two of essential oil on your third eye area (on forehead, in between the eyes).

ARTERIOSCLEROSIS

This is the degenerative condition of the arteries caused by the accumulation of lipids or plaque on the arterial wall. It begins at an early age. Often, one-year-old babies show lesions in the aorta. This buildup of mineral deposits and fats on the arterial walls causes blockages, which result in thickening or solidifying of blood, high cholesterol, and circulatory problems. The presence of a diagonal crease on the earlobe correlates very well with the degree of arteriosclerosis. The earlobe is richly vascularized, and a decrease in blood flow over time is believed to indicate a collapse of the vascular bed, which is indicated by a specific crease on the earlobe.

Feelings and Emotions : Feeling constricted and trapped in the body.

Diet	Vitamins & Minerals (Daily)	Essential Oils (Always dilute)	Herbs	Alternative Therapy	Avoid
Ayurvedic	B-6: 300 mg.	Sandalwood : PV-Ko	Cayenne: KV-P+	Massage	Carbon monoxide
diet for	Omega 3oils:	Lemon: PV-Ko	Comfrey: PV-K+	Hypnosis	Barium
body type	Multi-vitamin	Juniper: KV-P+	Goldenseal: PK-V+	Chelation	Organophosphates
Raw carrots		(in excess)	Rosehips: V-KP+	Shirodhara	Glues in solvents
		Cardamon: VK-P+	Burdock: PK-V+	Pancha Karma	Heat
		Myrrh: VK-P+	Arjuna: PK-V+	Biofeedback	Cold
	Multi-mineral	Rose: VPK=	1-3 gms day		Carbon disulfide
	E: 200 IU	Orange: VK-P+	Guggal: KV-P+		Cigarettes
	C: 1,500 mg.		Saffron: VPK=		The pill; estrogen
Lots of fiber	B3- Niacin: 200 mg.		Salvia danshen: KV-P+		Second-hand smoke

Psyllium seed	Magnesium/Calcium:	Hawthorn Berries: V-KoP+	Sedentary lifestyle
Guar gum	500 mg.	Ginger : VK-P+	Red meat
Pectin	Pantethine: 900 mg.	Cardamon: VK-P+	Saturated fats
Oat bran	Mesoglycan: 100 mg.	Cinnamon: VK-P+	Sugar
(not wheat	Evening primrose: VPK	Brahmi: VPK=	Milk
bran)	200 mg. 2 x per day	Garlic: VK-P+	Coffee
		Ashwagandha: VK-P+	Alcohol
		Aloe Vera: VPK=	Stress
		Horsetail: PK-V+	Suppressing emotions
			Salt

Herbal Brew						**Recipe**	
Vata		**Pitta**		**Kapha**		**Kapha & Vata :**	
Comfrey Root	2 oz.	Brahmi	2 oz.	Guggul	2 oz.	Arjuna powder	1 Tbs.
Ginger	1 oz.	Burdock	2 oz.	Ginger	2 oz.	Guggul powder	1 Tbs.
Rosehips	2 oz.	Red Clover	1 oz.	Cinnamon	1 oz.	Take 2 tsp. twice a day with lunch .	
Ashwagandha	2 oz.	Mint	1 oz.	Cardamon	1 oz.	and dinner	
Cinnamon	1 oz.	Cinnamon	½ oz.	Burdock	1 oz.	**Pitta :**	
Cardamon	1 oz.	Cardamon	½ oz.			Arjuna powder	1 Tbs

Brahmi powder	1 Tbs.
Take 2 tsp. (or 1,000 mg) with lunch & dinner.	

Self-Care

Imagery	Stress management
Lifestyle modification	Yoga
Exercise	Meditation

ARTHRITIS

A degenerative disease that is very common. An autoimmune disorder often consistent with extreme pain and swelling of the joints, degeneration of the cartilage, and/or weakening of the bones. Pittas often suffer with inflammation (heat makes it worse). Vatas generally have aching and dryness (cold increases pain). Kaphas usually experience swelling. It can be caused by poor diet, poor digestion, and/or a low immune system. Rheumatism is a more advance condition often affecting all joints; it is more easily diagnosed with blood work.

Feelings and Emotions : Holding on to anger and resentment. Something is eating you. Stuck, not moving forward.

Diet	Vitamins & Minerals (Daily)	Essential Oils (Always dilute)	Herbs	Alternative Therapy	Avoid
Elimination diet	B-Complex: 100 mg. -(esp. B-15)	Brahmi: VPK-	Guggul: VK-P+	Light massage	Sugar
		Oregano: VK+P+			Dairy
Ayurvedic	C: Ascorbate:	Cyperus: PKV-	Sandalwood: PV-Ko	Sauna	

diet for	2000-3000 mg.	Sandalwood: PV-Ko	Dashmool: VK-P+	Steam	Meat
body type	E: 400 IU	Peppermint: PK-Vo	Galangal: VK-P+		
Food	F: 200 mg.	Chamomile: VPK+	Guduchi: PK-V+		
combining	D: 500 IU	Cypress: VKP+	Aloe Vera: VPK=		
Potassium	K: 200 IU	Eucalyptus: KV-P+	Neem: PK-V+		
broth	B3 - NIacin: 100 mg.	Sweet Marjoram:	Ginger: VK-P+		Acid foods
Nuts	B5 - Pantothenic Acid:	KV-P+	Cyperus: PKV-		White flour
(soaked)	1000-1500 mg.	Rosemary: KV-P+	Chaparral: PK-V+		Cayenne
	Magnesium: 200 mg.	Lavender: PK-Vo	Turmeric: KV-Po		
	Glucosamine Sulfate:	Juniper: KV-P+	Angelica: VK-P+		
	200 mg.	Medicated Oils:	(do not use if tumor or fibroid)		
	A good Multi-Mineral		Kaishore Guggulu (Banyon herbs)		
			Purnana Vadi Guggulu		
			Gentian: PK-V+		
		- Maharayan: VPK	Buckhorn: PK-V+		
	Calcium: 1500 mg.	- Narayan: VPK	Black Cohosh: PK-V+		
		- Saharshardi: VP-K+	Myrrh: KV-P+		
		- Brahmi oil (or			
		mustard oil): VPK	**Ayurvedic Formulas:**		
		- Yogaraj Guggul	- Trikatu, 2 tablets before meals.		
			-Triphalla, 4-6 tablets at bedtime.		

Herbal Recipes

Herbal Paste

Mix all ingredients together, apply them on joint, let dry.

Vata

Juice of ½ lemon
1 tsp. Bentonite clay
½ tsp. Ginger powder
1 tsp. Sandalwood
¼ tsp. Mustard oil

Pitta

2 Tbs. Sandalwood powder
10 drops Cyperus essential oil
5 drops Peppermint oil
¼ tsp. Coconut oil or Brahmi oil
1 tsp. Bentonite clay

Kapha

1 tsp. Calamus powder

Herbal Brews

Vata

Ashwagandha	2 oz.
Valerian	1 oz.
Ginger	1 oz.
Angelica	1 oz.
Dashmoola	2 oz.
Chamomile	1 oz.
Rosemary	½ oz.

Pitta

Burdock	2 oz.
Skullcap	1 oz.
Guduchi	2 oz.
Chamomile	2 oz.
Liquorice	1 oz.

Aloe Vera gel 3 x day (best fresh)

Kapha

Cinnamon	2 oz.

1 tsp. Bentonite clay
½ tsp. Ginger powder
1 tbs. rubbing alcohol
¼ tsp. Cayenne
¼ tsp. Mustard oil

Ginger	2 oz.
Cyperus	2 oz.
Yucca	2 oz.
Lingusticun	2 oz.
Turmeric powder ½ tsp.	

Take

Kapha: Triphalla at night; Guggul in the morning (2 tsp. or 200 mg)

Pitta : Castor oil - 1 Tablespoon at night

Kapha: 1 tsp. Ginger & 1 cup water 2 times per day before meals.

Massage Formula

Cypress	10 drops	Juniper	10 drops
Eucalyptus	5 drops	Rosemary	5 drops
Peppermint	5 drops	Vegetable oil	2 oz.

Self Care	Ice packs for Pitta	Exercise	Hot Baths	1 to 3 day fast
	Basti oil enemas	Colon Cleanse	Castor oil compresses	

General cautions : For severe arthritis, consult a professional practitioner. Do not take devil's claw, black cohosh or celery during pregnancy.

ATHLETE'S FOOT

Athlete's foot involves susceptibility to infection by mold-like bacteria, yeast, fungi, parasites, and viruses. Fungus results from "creatures of darkness", moisture, and heat. It is necessary to strengthen the immune system. Athlete's foot can be exacerbated by poor food combining, too much starch, sugar, fried foods, and direct contact in public showers (wear sandals). Vatas may experience dryness, cracking, and itchiness. Pittas and Kaphas experience discomfort between the toes, foul odor, redness, defoliation of skin, cracking, and puss.

Feelings and Emotions : Stagnation. Afraid to move forward. Confusion.

Diet	Vitamins & Minerals (Daily)	Essential Oils (Always dilute)	Herbs	Alternative Therapy	Avoid
Ayurvedic	E: 250 IU	Tea Tree: VPK=	Echinacea: PK-V+	Acupuncture	Sugars
diet for	C: 1,500 mg.	Clove Oil: VK-P+	Liquorice: VP-K+		Wine
body type	Selenium: 100 mcg.	Anise: VK-P+	European Mistletoe: VK-P+		Sodas
Eat a well	Zinc: 100 mg.	Basil: VK-P+	Black Walnut: PKVO		Fried foods
balanced	Beta-Carotene: 2000 IU	Tarragon: VK-P+	Korean Ginseng: V-KPo		Alcohol
diet	(critical)	Marigold (Tagetes):	Siberian Ginseng: V-KPo		Grains
Lots of raw	A: 10,000 IU (until clear)	PK-V+	Barberry: PK-V+		Fruit
vegetables	B-6: 200 mg.	Lemongrass: PK-Vo	Aloe Vera: VPK=		Fermented food
Green juice	Thymus Extract: 2 tablets	Cajaput. KV-P +	Turmeric: VK-Po		
Food	Chlorophyll: 2 Tsp.,	Trifolia: VK-P+	Marigold: PK-V+		
combining	2 x per day.	Turmeric: VK-Po	Burdock: PK-V+		
Cave man	Q-10: 100 mg.	Yarrow: VPK-	Dandelion: PK-V+		
	Iron: 400 mg.	Thyme: VK-P+	Red Clover: PK-V+		
		Chamomiles: VKP-	Peppermint: PK-Vo		
		Niaouli: VPK-	Ginger: VK-P+		
diet: (no	Colloidal Silver		Goldenseal: PK-V+		
sugars, low			Pau d'Arco: PK-V+		

fruit, no grains, some starches,
lots of green proteins, oils)
Rotation diet
(for allergies)

Herbal Brew

Vata		Pitta		Kapha	
Ginger	2 oz.	Echinacea	2 oz.	Mint	1 oz.
Prickly Ash	1 oz.	Mint	1 oz.	Burdock	2 oz.
Coriander	2 oz.	Burdock	2 oz.	Echinacea	2 oz.
Lavender	1 oz.	Red Clover	1 oz.	Ginger	1 oz.
Astragalus	1 oz.	Dandelion	1 oz.	Dandelion	2 oz.

Anti-Fungal Powder

Arrowroot	4 Tbs.
Goldenseal powder	1 Tbs.
Marshmallow	2 Tbs.
Black Walnut powder	2 Tbs.
Turmeric powder	1 Tsp.

Mix all ingredients together. If the powder is grainy, put it in a coffee or nut grinder. Mix well. Store this powder in a sealed container. Apply to feet as needed. This same mixture can be used as a footbath. Steep herbs in water. Strain,. Soak feet.

Self-Care

Foot baths

Walk barefoot when possible (except public baths)

Spray essential oils in shoes

BACK PROBLEMS

It can result from old injuries, heredity, accidents, poor posture, organ weaknesses, malfunctioning vertebrae, birth defects, and/or long periods of sitting. Vatas are prone to extreme back pain. Pittas may experience inflammation or burning. Kaphas tend to experience swelling.

Feelings and Emotions : Not feeling supported.

Diet	Vitamins & Minerals (Daily)	Essential Oils (Always dilute)	Herbs	Alternative Therapy	Avoid
Ayurvedic	B-Complex: 2 tablets	Lavender: VK-Vo	Kava Kava: PV-Ko	Chiropractic	Unsupervised
diet for	B5 - Pantothenic Acid:	Ylang Ylang: PV-K+	Passion Flower: PK-V+	treatments	exercise
body type	2,500 mg.	Rosemary: VK-P+	Skullcap: PK-V+	Raindrop therapy	Over eating
	Magnesium: 800 mg.	Brahmi: VPK-	Valerian: VK-P+	Acupuncture	Over stretching.
Foods rich	Calcium: 800 mg.	Eucalyptus: KV-P+	Chamomile: PK-Vo	Physical therapy	Over bending
in calcium	C: 3000 mg.	Juniper: KV-P+	Guggul: KV-P+	Massage	Jumping

& Magnesium	Cypress: VKP+	Cyperus: VPK	When caused by digestive & assimilation problems:	Running
	Valerian: VK-P+	Jatamasi: KV-P+	- Colonics	
	Geranium: PK-V+	Nutmeg: VK-P+		
Green, leafy vegetables	Chamomile: VPK-	Oat Straw: VPK-K+		
	Blended oil cream	St. John's Wort: PK-V+		
	Mahanarayana tail	Jasmine Flower: PK-V+		
	*Moov	Lotus seeds: PV-K+		
		Dashmoola: VK-P+		

* *Product of* Paras Pharmaceuticals Ltd.

Herbal Brew

Vata		Pitta		Kapha	
Brahmi	2 oz.	Brahmi	2 oz.	Brahmi	1 oz.
Valerian	1 oz.	Chrysanthemum	2 oz.	Valerian	1 oz.
Ginger	1 oz:	Chamomile	1 oz.	Guggul	2 oz.
Oatstraw	1 oz.	Skullcap	1 oz.	Passion Flower	2 oz.
Lotus Seed	1 oz.	Jasmine Flowers	1 oz.	Skullcap	1 oz.
Jatamasi	2 oz.	St. John's Wort	1 oz.	Mint	1 oz.
		Mint	1 oz.		

Bedtime: Drink ½ cup tea with ½ cup warm milk. Add 1-Tbs ghee, Mix well.

Compresses with Essential Oils

Vata & Kapha

Ginger Powder	2 Tbs.
Water	4 Tbs.
Lavender essential oil	5 drops
Eucalyptus oil	5 drops (or any oils of your choice)

Paste will get hot. Take it off after 5-10 minutes, or when it begins to burn.

Self Help

Basti oil enema	Compresses
Magnetic Blend	Yoga

General cautions: Back problems need specialist care. For chronic or severe back pain, seek the advice of a professional practitioner to gain the most benefit from herbal medicine.

BAD BREATH

Bad breath can be caused by a number of reasons or conditions, including tooth decay, poor digestion, liver trouble, catarrh, poor food combining, lack of chlorophyll in the diet, or a congested colon. This often inflicts Pitta with the feeling of sourness in the mouth.

Feelings and Emotions : Unpleasant smell.

Diet	Vitamins & Minerals (Daily)	Essential Oils (Always dilute)	Herbs	Alternative Therapy	Avoid
Ayurvedic	Acidophilus: 2 caps	Peppermint: PK-Vo	Peppermint: PK-Vo	Ayurvedic	Poor food
diet for	3 x day	Thyme: VK-P+	Rosemary: KV-P+	consultation	combinations
body type	Chlorophyll: 2 tsp.	Bergamot: VK-P+	Myrrh: VK-P+	Colonics	Mucous forming
or anti-	2 x day	Fennel: VPK=	Goldenseal: PK-V+	Dental visits	foods
Pitta diet	B-Complex: 200 mg.	Eucalyptus: KV-P+	Ginger: VK-P+	Pancha Karma	Constipation
Pungent	Digestive enzymes	Clove: VK-P+	Fennel: VPk=	treatments	Negative emotions
herbs	C: 1,500 mg.	Tea Tree: VPK=	Mint: PK-V+		Tongue scraping
Fried foods	PABA: 100 mg.		Trikatu: VK-P+		
Fruits					
Proper food	Magnesium: 200 mg.				
combining	Zinc: 50 mg.				
Lots of	Triphala: 3-6 tablets				
greens	at night with tea				
Lots of					
vegetables					

Herbal Brew

Vata		Pitta		Kapha	
Ginger	2 oz.	Mint	1 oz.	Angelica	2 oz.
Cardamon	1 oz.	Coriander	2 oz.	Angelica	1 oz.
Coriander	2 oz.	Chamomile	2 oz.	Cardamon	2 oz.
Fennel	1 oz.	Fennel	2 oz.	Basil	1 oz.
Angelica	1 oz.			Rosemary	1 oz.

Self-Care

Fennel or Anise essential oil on the tongue	Flossing	Tongue Cleaning
Mouthwash	Fasting	

BI-POLAR - (MANIC-DEPRESSIVE)

This is a chemical imbalance in the brain where the person changes from low depressive states to very high energetic states. It can be caused by hereditary factors, severe birth trauma, stress, environmental pollutants, over-exposure to chemicals, or a B-vitamin deficiency. Vatas experience bouts of anxiety, fear, or nervousness, and their moods will swing both high and low. Pittas often struggle with anger and irritability. Kaphas become depressed, along with problems of phobia and paranoia.

Feelings and Emotions : Unsure of life. General insecurity.

Diet	Vitamins & Minerals (Daily)	Essential Oils (Always dilute)	Herbs	Alternative Therapy	Avoid
Ayurvedic diet for body type	B-Complex 2 tablets; 3 x day C: 3,500 mg. B-12: 500 mcg./or shots	Brahmi VPK- Basil: VK-P+	Basil: VK-P+ Brahmi: VPK- Rosemary: KV-P+ Skullcap: PK-Vo	Counseling Shirodhara Tarpana B-12 shots: (2-3 times per week)	Foods high in vanadium Herring Sardines White sugar Alcohol Hallucinogenic drugs
Lots of green, leafy vegetables	B6 - Pyridoxine: 100-200 mg. L-Phenylalanine: 300 mg. (for 2 months)	Rosemary: VK-P+ Myrtle: PK-V+ Lavender: PK-Vo Chamomile: VPK-	Passion Flower: PK-V+ Chrysanthemum: PK-V+ Peppeımitn: PK-Vo Calamus: VK-P+		
Carbo-hydrates	Blue-green algae: 2-tsp. 3-x day Primrose: 500-mg.	Myrrh: Kv-P+ Frankincense: KV-P+			
Seaweeds	1-3 x day Amino Acid Complex : 2-x day Natural Lithium : 300-400 mg. Spirulina: 2-tsp. 3-x day Folic Acid: 500-600 mcg.				

Herbal Brew

Vata		Pitta		Kapha	
Calamus	1 oz.	Chrysanthemum	2 oz.	Skullcap	1 oz.
Brahmi	2 oz.	Skullcap	1 oz.	Calamus	1 oz.
Ginger	1 oz.	Brahmi	2 oz.	Chrysanthemum	2 oz.
Basil	2 oz.	Mint	1 oz.	Basil	1 oz.

Self-Care

Breathing exercises Yoga
Meditation

BLACK EYE

This is an effusion of blood under the loose skin over and around the eyes. Can be caused by an injury or weak kidneys. With Vatas the eye becomes yellow, Pittas experience a black eye, and Kapha's eye may turn dark brown. Dark circles under the eyes.

Feelings and Emotions : Angry.

Cell Salts : Calcium Fluoride

Diet	Vitamins & Minerals (Daily)	Essential Oils (Always dilute)	Herbs	Alternative Therapy	Avoid
Ayurvedic	C: 25,000 mg.	*Hydrosols:	Arnica: KV-P+	Reiki	Fried foods

diet for	K: 200 mcg.	Lavender: PK-Vo	Comfrey: PV-K+	Therapeutic Touch	Congesting foods
body type	B-Complex: 100 mg.	Rose: VPK=	Aloe Vera: KPV	Homeopathics	Watching TV
Foods high in	P: 200 mg.		Chamomile: PK-Vo	Shirodhara	
bioflavonoids			Cinnamon: VK-P+		
Cooling foods			Ginger: VK-P+		

* *Hydrosols are composed of the water remaining after the distillation of essential oils. This water is suitable for eye washing.*

Herbal Brew			**Self-Care**
Vata	**Pitta**	**Kapha**	**Comfrey ointment**
Comfrey-equal amounts	Mint-equal amounts	Ginger-equal amounts	Cool compresses with rose or
Ginger	Chamomile	Mint	neroli essential oil
Cinnamon			Ice compresses
			Inhalations

Mix in equal parts and drink until eye has cleared.

BLEEDING

It can be caused from a injury or an accident. Nosebleeds are common for Vatas; Pittas and Kaphas experience more head injuries. Women, especially Pitta types, have excessive bleeding during menstruation or menopause. Haemorrhoids are common with constipation and straining which cause Frank "Red" blood with stool. Bleeding ulcers are a Pitta condition and cause a black tarry stool.

Feelings and Emotions : Not feeling harmonious. Scattered.

Cell Salts : Ferr phos, Iron phosphate.

Diet	Vitamins & Minerals (Daily)	Essential Oils (Always dilute)	Herbs	Alternative Therapy	Avoid
Anti-Pitta	A: 5,000 IU	Cajaput: KV-P+	Comfrey: VP-K+	Therapeutic touch	Dairy
Diet	K: 500 mcg.	Tea Tree: VPK=	Plantain: PK-V+	Reiki	Hot spices
Astringent	B17:2 grams with meals	Cypress: VPK+	Yarrow: PK-V+		Meat
foods	Calcium: 800 mg.	Lavender: PK-Vo	Horsetail: PK-V+		Excess salt
Green	Magnesium: 500 mg.	Chamomile: VPK-	Calendula: PK-V+		
vegetables		Tagetes: VK-P+	Shepherd's Purse: PK-V+		
Wheatgrass		Sandalwood: PV-Ko	Cayenne: VK-P+		
juice			Aloe Vera Gel: VPK=		
Liquid			Witch Hazel: PK-V+		
chlorophyll			Alum Root: PK-V+		

Herbal Brew

Drink for two weeks :

Horsetail	1 oz.
Plantain	2 oz.
Calendula	1 oz.
Shepherd's Purse	1 oz.
Witch Hazel	2 oz.
Fennel	2 oz.

Self-Care

Direct pressure can be applied onto the cut to stop the blood flow.

When in the wild, Plantain can be used as a natural Band-Aid.

Nosebleeds : Put head back. Place a copper penny on forehead. Hold the head back for 15 minutes.

Salves

Cold baths

Cold compresses

Ice

BRUISES

Bruises are more or less extensive injuries of the deeper part of the skin and underlying tissues, accompanied by an outpouring of blood from damaged vessels. The simplest type of bruise is one in which the deeper layers of the skin are damaged, causing a slight bluish discoloration. When a sever blow occurs, the muscles may be bruised and torn without an opening in the skin. The resulting effusion of blood may cause a large swelling which sometimes results in the formation of an abscess. If the bruise is close to a bone, it can become calcified.

Feelings and Emotions : Guilty, Self-punishment.

Cell Salts : Calcium Fluoride

Diet	Vitamins & Minerals (Daily)	Essential Oils (Always dilute)	Herbs	Alternative Therapy	Avoid
Ayurvedic	C: 2,000 mg.	Pine: KV-P+	Arnica: KV-P+	Reiki	Dairy
diet for	3 x day	Amber: VPK-	Triphala: VPK-	Therapeutic touch	Clogging

body type	D: 200 IU	Orange: VK-P+	Guggal: KV-P+	Aura balancing	foods
Berries	Bioflavonoids: 500 mg.	Bergamot: VK-P+	Camphor: KV-P+	Chakra balancing	
Cherries	B-Complex: twice a day	Lavender: PK-Vo	Salvia: KV-P+		
Proteins	Folic Acid: 300 mcg.	Cardamon: VK-P+	Turmeric: VK-Po		
Green	Iron: 40 mg.	Lemon: PV-Ko	Comfrey: PV-K+		
vegetables	F: 200 IU	Lime: PK-V+	St. John's Wort: PK-V+		
Cooling	P: 200 mg.	Yarrow: VPK+	Red Clover: PK-V+		
foods	K: 200 mg.		Burdock: PK-V+		

Bruise Herbal Brew

Vata		Pitta		Kapha	
Skullcap	1 oz.	Marshmallow	1 oz	Ginger	2 oz.
Ginger	1 oz.	Mints	2 oz.	Mint	1 oz.
Rosehips	2 oz.	Comfrey	2 oz.	Lemongrass	2 oz.
Comfrey	1 oz.				

Self-Care

Castor Oil Pack

Ice Compresses

Cold Water Baths

General caution: Seek immediate medical attention for serious bruising or grazes, especially if the pain has not considerably lessened after 24 hours.

BURNS

Burns are injuries caused by dry heat or scalds caused by moist heat. Burn injuries can also occur through contact with electric wires or with acids or other chemicals. Simple sunburn produces redness and disappears quickly. More severe burns produce blisters, tissue damage (scars), severe deformations, and sometimes-even death.

Feelings and Emotions : Feeling aggravated with life. Tired of life. Burnout.

Cell Salts : Calcium Fluoride

Diet	Vitamins & Minerals (Daily)	Essential Oils (Always dilute)	Herbs	Alternative Therapy	Avoid
Pitta	C: 1,000 mg.,	Sandalwood: PV-Ko	Aloe Vera Gel: VPK-	Chakra Balance	Heat
reducing diet	every hour	Vetiver: V-KP+	Chickweed: PK-V+	Energy Work	Warm water
High caloric	B-Complex: 200 mg.	Lemongrass: PK-Vo	Comfrey: PV-K+	Cranial Sacral	Ointment
diet	Potassium: 200 mg.	Lavender: PK-Vo	Coriander: VPK+	Colour Therapy	Butter
High protein	A: 75,000 IU	Blue Chamomile: PV-K+			
diet	E: 200 IU after	Coriander: VPK-	Plantain: PK-V+		
Lots of fluids	each meal	Tea Tree: VPK=	Slippery Elm: VP-K+		
Fresh fruits	PABA: 200 mcg.		Shepherd's Purse: PK-V+		
Fresh	D: 600 IU		Turmeric: VK-Po		
vegetables	F: 300 mg.				
Rosehips	Zinc: 40 mg.				
Cherries					

Green peppers

Citrus

Cooling foods

Self-Care

Immediately immerse the burned area in cool or ice water for 5-10 minutes (within a 20-minute period)

Cold compresses	Liquid honey
Comfrey poultice	Apple cider vinegar
Saline water	Ghee or coconut oil with lavender, apply to the affected area.

Salve - with cooling oils of coconut or sunflower.

CANCER

Cancer is a process of the cells reproducing out of control and attacking other tissues of the body. Rebelling against the central authority of the body/mind. It can be caused by chronic constipation, poor digestion, food sensitivity, poor diet, suppressed emotions, lack of spiritual connection, exposure to chemicals, and environmental hazards. Vatas are more prone to colon, bone, stomach cancers and dry tumors; Pittas are more prone to liver, stomach, pancreas, skin, brain, and lymph cancer. Kaphas are more prone to melanoma,. tumors, lung, and breast cancer.

Feelings and Emotions : Self hate, criticism, judgements, and belief in suffering and separation.

Diet	Vitamins & Minerals (Daily)	Essential Oils (Always dilute)	Herbs	Alternative Therapy	Avoid
Ayurvedic	A: 100,000 IU	Ginger: VK-P+	Chaparral : PK-V+	Ayurvedic	Canned foods

diet for	C: 10,000 mg.	Rose : VPK=	Essiac Blend: PR-V+	consultation	Processed foods
body type	E: 75,000 IU	Lavender: PK-Vo	Burdock: PK-V+	Biofeedback	Sugars
Cleansing	F: 200 mg.	Yarrow: PK-V+	Astralagus: VP-K+	Sound therapy	High protein
Short period	Calcium: 800 mg.	Rose Geranium: PK-V+	Pippali: VK-P+	Pancha Karma	Refined grains
of fasting	Potassium: 800 mg.	Sandalwood: PV-Ko	Ashwagandha: VK-P+	Tarpana	Junk foods
Foods which	Chromium: 100 mcg.	Saffron: VPK=	Guduchi: PK-V+	Wholistic	Sour foods
support the	B-complex: 200 mg.		Solomon's Seal: PV-K+	medical doctor	Diary
immune			Yarrow: PK-V+		Meat
system	B17 (laetrile): 200 mg.		Goldenseal: PK-V+		Fried foods
Shitaki	B12: 400 mcg.		Turmeric: VK-Po		Iron supplements
mushrooms	Niacin: 160 mg.		Manjishta: PK-V+		All chemicals
Yellow &	Soybean extract: 1 bottle		Ginger: VK-P+		Household
orange	once day for 2 months then		Saffron: VPK=		cleansers
vegetables	½ bottle once day until remission		Haritaki: VK-Po		
Raw foods	Q-10: 100 mg.		Guggul: KV-P+		
Wheatgrass			Myrrh: KV-P+		
Alfalfas			Brahmi: VPK-		
Barleygrass			Calamus: VK-P+		
Green juices					
Dandelion greens					

Herbal Brew

Vata		Pitta & Kapha
Astralagus	1 oz.	Essiac Blend
Ginger	1 oz.	10 drops Chaparral
Burdock Root	1 oz.	
Slipper Elm	1 oz.	

Vata : Need tonics, colon cleansers, and digestive aids.

Pitta: Need blood purifiers.

Kapha : Need strong expectorants.

General cautions : Patients are advised to consult the doctor.

CANDIDIASIS

This is a yeast type fungus infection which is able to live in many parts of the body where there is moisture and wetness, such as: intestines, mouth, sinuses, lungs, urinary tract, and the vagina. Candida easily multiply with poor diet (sugar and yeast), weakening the immune system and digestive tract causing many problems in them. This condition can be triggered by antibiotics and birth control pills. In Vata body types it creates allergies, dryness, constipation, muscle pain, and adrenal insufficiency. In Pitta types, there can be rashes, athelete's foot, jock itch, and heartburn. In Kapha body types, it may cause water retention, congestion, depression, diabetes, and kidney problems.

Feelings and Emotions : Not trusting the flow of life.

Diet	Vitamins & Minerals (Daily)	Essential Oils (Always dilute)	Herbs	Alternative Therapy	Avoid
Ayurvedic	A: 25,000 IU (unitl clear)	Trifolia: VK-P+	Prickly Ash: VK-P+	Chiropractic	Antibiotics
diet for	B-Complex: 200 mg.	Tea Tree: VPK=	Hing: VK-P+	treatments	Fermented foods
body type	Biotin: 300 mcg.	Cloves: VK-P+	Aloe Vera: VPK=	Naturopathic	Nut butters
Cleansing diet	B12 Shots 1 x week	Rosewood: VK-P+	Asafoetida: VKP+	consultation	Pickles
Proteins	Megadolophilus: ¼ tsp.	Rosemary: VK-P+	Katuka: PK-P+	Ayurveda	All yeast foods
Colloidal	3 x day	Peppermint: PK-Vo	Barberry: PKV+	consultation	& breads
silver	Caprylic Acid:	Tarragon : VK-P+	Goldenseal: PKV+	Pancha Karma	Chemical cleansers
Raw foods,	2 caps 3 x day	Palmarosa: VPK-	Pau d' Arco: PKV+		Acid foods
(kapha,	Selenium: 200 mcg.	Myrrh: KV-P+	Cardamon: PK-V+		
pitta)	*Niastatin	Bergamot: KV-P+	Bay: VKP+		
Rotation diet	(powder/oral form)	Bay: VKP+	Ginger: VK-P+		

* *Doctor's prescription required. This is the only antibiotic that does not kill friendly bacteria within the body.*

Herbal Brew

Vata		Pitta		Kapha	
Prickly Ash	2 oz.	Pau d'Arco	2 oz.	Pau d'Arco	2 oz.
Ginger	1 oz.	Barberry	1 oz.	Katuka	1 oz.
		Mint	1 oz.	Cardamon	1 oz.

Morning : Drink 2 Tbs. Aloe Vera juice in 8-oz water.

Salve

Beeswax	1 part
Vegetable oil	3-5 parts
Essential oils of your choice	40 drops

Melt wax. Add vegetables oil. Test consistency with cold spoon.

Add more wax for hardness; oil for softness.

Let cool.

Add essential oils.

Self-Care

Use Hing with cooking of all beans and soups.

CANKER SORES

Canker sores appear as a swelling in the mouth and progresses into an ulcerated lesion, with much pain and burning. They are caused by stress, poor diet, too much sugar, and/or deficiencies of B-12 and iron. Pittas may experience inflammation with puss. Vatas may experience dryness and pain. Kaphas may experience large sores with swelling (puss).

Feelings and Emotions : Not good enough. Too much stress.

Cell Salts : Calcium Sulph

Diet	Vitamins & Minerals (Daily)	Essential Oils (Always dilute)	Herbs	Alternative Therapy	Avoid
Ayurvedic	A: 1000 IU	Tea Tree: VPK=	Burdock: PK-V+	Acupuncture	Wheat
diet for	B-Complex: 2 tablets	Bergamot: VK-P+	Golden Seal: PK-V+	Therapeutic Touch	Cheese
body type	2 x per day	Geranium: PK-V+	Pau d'Arco: PK-V+	Reiki	Tomato
	Folic Acid: 400 mcg.	Cajaput: KV-P+	Neem: PK-V+	Chakra Balancing	Lemon
	B-12: 300 mcg.	Frankincense: VK-P+	Red Clover: PK-V+	Shirodhara	Pineapple
Elimination	Iron: 100 mg.	Myrrh: VK-P+	Guduchi: PK-V+		Sugar
diet	Copper: 40 mg.	Neem: PK-V+	Comfrey: VP-K+		Mustard
	Zinc: 50 mg.	Lavender: OK-Vo	Red Raspberry: PK-V+		Vinegar
Chlorophyll	B-5: 150-200 mg.	Sandalwood: PV-Ko	Red Root: PK-V+		Most citrus
	L-lysine: 2500 mg.		Slippery Elm: VP-K+		
	Amino Acid Complex:				
	2 tablets 2 x day				

Herbal Brew

Vata Tea		Pitta-Kapha Tea	
Comfrey	1 oz.	Burdock	1 oz.
Chitrak	1 oz.	Red Clover	1 oz.
Cardamon	1 oz.	Pau d'Arco	1 oz.
		Mint	2 oz.
		Guduchi	2 oz.

Salve

Beeswax	1 part
Vegetable Oil	3-5 parts

Essential Oils - 30 drops per ounce of beeswax.

In a small pan, melt the wax and vegetable oil. Remove from stove.

Add essential oils. Let cool.

Apply to Canker Sore

Vata-Kapha : Mix 2 drops Aloe Vera Gel with ½ tsp. Turmeric and 1 drop essential oil.

Pitta : Mix 2 drops Aloe Vera Gel with 1/3 tsp. Sandalwood powder and 1 drop Sandalwood essential oil.

CHICKEN POX

It is highly contagious viral disease that is characterized by generalized skin eruptions, which commonly afflects children. One attack usually protects one against the disease for life. The rash first shows up across the trunk, arms, and face as red bumps that contain drops of clear fluid eventually breaking out to form a crust. This cycle continues for 3 or 4 days. The patient should be isolated for 10-14 days.

Feelings and Emotions : Sensitive to the opinions of others.

Cell Salts : Aconite, Belladonna and Pulsatila

Diet	Vitamins & Minerals (Daily)	Essential Oils (Always dilute)	Herbs	Alternative Therapy	Avoid
Ayurvedic	A: 25,000-100,000 IU	Peppermint: PK-Vo	Echinacea: PK-V+	Homeopathics	Scratching
diet for	(unitl clear)	Geranium: PK-V+	Cayenne: KV-P+		Heating foods
body type	E: 50 IU	Blue chamomile: PV-K+	Chickweed: PK-V+		Massage
	Multi-Mineral	Lavender: PK-Vo	Cleavers: PK V+		Hot baths
Protein	Potassium: 1000 mg.	Clary Sage: PVK-	Lobelia: K-VP+		
	Zinc: 10 mg.	Rose: VPK=	Red Clover: PK-V+		
Light diet	RNA & DNA 3 x day,	Sandalwood: PV-Ko	Burdock: PK-V+		
	until condition clears				
	C: 2,500 mg.				

Herbal Brew

Vata		Pitta		Kapha	
Chamomile	1 oz.	Chickweed	½ oz.	Mint	½ oz.
Rosehips	1 oz.	Burdock	1 oz.	Burdock	1 oz.
Mix with Berry juice	½ cup	Chamomile	1 oz.	Mix with Apple juice	8 oz
		Mix with Apple juice	8 oz.		

Mix ½-cup tea with ½-cup juice and drink every 2 hours.

Children

Echinacea 10 drops every 2 hours - until rash is gone.

Self-Care

Take a cotton ear swab. Apply Blue Chamomile essential oil, dab lightly on all sores.

Chickweed bath — Cool baths with Chamomile

Chickweed ointment — Basti oil enema

General cautions Always consult a professional practitioner if you have, or suspect you have, shingles. Take professional advice if you notice a sudden change to a wart.

CHRONIC FATIGUE

Caused by a virus related to Epstein Bar Herpes family, affecting with flue type symptoms, as well as low energy. Vata's experience extreme tiredness, loss of appetite, anxiety, intestinal problems, mood swings, and muscle pain. Pitta's experience fevers, liver problems, irritability, and swollen glands. Kapha's experience respiratory problems, depression, sleepiness, and spasms

Feelings and Emotions : Tired of not knowing what one's life purpose is all about.

Cell Salts : Silica oxide

Diet	Vitamins & Minerals (Daily)	Essential Oils (Always dilute)	Herbs	Alternative Therapy	Avoid
Ayurvedic	A: 50,000-100,000 IU	Angelica: VPK-	Astralagus: VK-P+	Colour therapy	Frequent flying
diet for	C: 5,000-8,000 mg.	Lavender: PK-Vo	Ashwagandha: VK-P+	Reiki	Radiation
body type	B-Complex: 100 mg.	Immortelle: VPK-	Shatavari: PV-K+	Tarpana	Chemical cleansers
	Megadolphilus : 3 x day	Saffron : VPK=	Brahmi: VPK-	Dance	Processed foods
Yogurt	E: 800 IU	Bergamot: VK-P+	Ginger: VK=P	Acupuncture	Fried foods
	Calcium: 1200 mg.	Myrtle: PK-V+	Fennel: VPK=	Life purpose	Poor food
Juices	Magnesium: 1,000 mg.		Saw Palmetto: V-PK+	counseling	combining
	Bioflavonoids: 300 mg.		Solomon's Seal: PV-K+		Yeast
Sesame seeds	Selenium: 200 mcg.				All chemicals
	Zinc: 50 mg.		Chrysanthemum: PK-V+		Preservatives
	Potassium: 100 mg.		Fo-Ti: PV-L+		Fluorescent lights
	DHEA: 50 mg. 2 x day				Overuse of
Nutmilk					computers

Herbal Brew

Vata		Pitta		Kapha	
Astralagus	equal amounts	Shatavari	equal amounts	Ashwagandha	2 oz.
Saw Palmetto		Brahmi		Ginger	2 oz.
Solomon's Seal;		Fo Ti		Guggul	2 oz.
Ashwagandha		Fennel			
Ginger		Chrysanthemum			
Shatavari					

Self-Care

Yoga

Meditation

Waling

Dancing

COLITIS

Irritation and inflammation of the colon, poorly formed stools, and pain due to toxins in colon. Vata's experience food sensitivities and irregular bowel movements; Pitta types may experience severe inflammation; Kapha types may lose weight and have loose stools with mucous.

Feelings and Emotions : Experiencing lack of support, fear, and insecurity.

Diet	Vitamins & Minerals (Daily)	Essential Oils (Always dilute)	Herbs	Alternative Therapy	Avoid
Ayurvedic	A: 25,000 IU	Helichrysum: PK-V+	Bayberry: PK-V+	Massage	Red meat
diet for	B-Complex: 200 mg.	Tea Tree: VPK=	Katuka: KP-V+	Biofeedback	Dairy
body type	C: 4,000 mg.	Geranium: PK-V+	Aloe Vera: VPK=	Reiki	Sulpha drugs
Oat bran	Multi-vitamin	Sandalwood: VP-Ko	Cyperus: VPK	Therapeutic	Fried foods
Steamed	Calcium: 800 mg.	Myrrh: VK-P+	Chamomile: PK-Vo	touch	Sugars
vegetables	Magnesium: 700 mg.	Cypress: VKP+	Dandelion: PK-V+	Gem Therapy	Alcohol
Cabbage	Zinc: 50 mg.	Chamomile: VPK-	Comfrey: VP-K+	Colour Therapy	Spicy foods
juice	Bioflavonoids: 1,000 mg.		Papaya: PK-Vo	Food allergy	Allergic foods
Carrot juice	Acidolophilus: 3 x day		Alum Root: PK-V+	testing	Yeast foods
Baked foods			Triphalla: VPK-		
Broiled foods			Marshmallow: PV-K+		
Stearned foods			Fennel: VPK=		
Rotation foods			Coriander: VPK=		
Allergy/			Nutmeg: VK-P+		
avoidance diet			Mint: PK-Vo		
Cave man diet					

Herbal Brew

Vata		Pitta		Kapha	
Katuka	1 oz.	Papaya Leaves	1 oz.	Fennel	1 oz.
Cyperus	1 oz.	Chamomile	1 oz.	Mint	1 oz.
Comfrey	1 oz.	Dandelion	1 oz.	Cyperus	1 oz.
Coriander	1 oz.	Alum Root	1 oz.	Katuka	1 oz.
Nutmeg	½ oz.	Fennel	1 oz.		

Self-Care

Relaxation techniques

Meditation

Yoga

COMMON COLD

Infection due to low immunity describes the common cold. Pittas get fevers and sometime diarrhea. Vatas may experience restlessness, pain in the joints, sneezing, and/or headaches. Kaphas suffer from congestion and excess mucus.

Feelings and Emotions : Not paying attention to one's needs. Confusion. Stressed.

Diet	Vitamins & Minerals (Daily)	Essential Oils (Always dilute)	Herbs	Alternative Therapy	Avoid
Kelp	A: 1500 IU	Eucalyptus: VK-P+	Slippery Elm: PV-K+	Homeopathy	All dairy
	Beta-Carotene: 15000 IU	Rosemary: KV-P+	Ginger: VK-P+	Saunas	Sugar
Garlic detox	B-Complex: 3 tablets	Myrtle: PK-\ +	Echinacea: PK-V+	Music therapy	
	C: 5000-10000 mg.	Lavender: KP-Vo	Goldenseal: PK-V+	Colour therapy	
Fast	Amino acids	Sandalwood: PV-Ko	Astralagus: PV-K+		
		PepperMint: PK-VO	Mint: PK-Vo		
Colloidal		Camphor: KV-P+	Clove: VK-P+		
Silver		Cinnamon: VK-P+	Basil: VK-P+		
			Yarrow: PK-V+		
Ayurvedic diet		Hyssop: KV-P+	Elderberry: KP-Vo		
for body type		Anise: VK-P+	Shatavari: PV-K+		
		Basil : VK-P+	Ajwan: VK-P+		
Plenty of fluids		Angelica: VPK=, P+	Triphalla: KVP =		
		Lemon Balm: PK-Vo	Liquorice: VP-K+		
			Lemongrass: PK-Vo		
			Burdock: KP-V+		

Herbal Brew

Vata		Pitta		Kapha	
Basil	1 oz.	Elder berries	1 oz.	Burdock	1 oz.
Astralagus	2 oz.	Echinacea	1 oz.	Lemongrass	1 oz.
Elder berries	1 oz.	Shatavari	1 oz.	Clove	½ oz.
Ginger	1 oz.	Mint	1 oz.	Cinnamon	½ oz.
Cinnamon	1 oz.	Burdock	2 oz.	Elder berries	2 oz.
Shatavari	1 oz.			Mint	½ oz.
				Ginger	½ oz.

Drink herbal blend 3 times a day.

Inhalation Therapy

Vata		Pitta		Kapha	
Lemon	3 drops	Mint	3 drops	Lemon	3 drops
Ginger, fresh	3 inch piece	Lime	2 drops	Ginger	2 inch piece
Eucalyptus	3 drops	Myrtle	2 drops	Camphor	2 drops

Self-Care

Aromatherapy inhalations	Steam
	Hot bath
	Rebounder
	Foot baths
Dry skin brushing	Colon cleanse
Necessary to increase the digestive fire - use spices for appropriate dosha (body type)	

Cough		Cold Remedy Massage Blend	
Myrtle	1 drop	Basil	3 drops
Hyssop	1 drop	Angelica	2 drops
Anise	1 drop	Eucalyptus	5 drops
Honey	2 Tbs. Take 2 x per day	Lemon Balm	3 drops
		Vegetable Oil	2 oz.

General caution Seek professional advice if fingers and toes frequently become cold and numb. Also remember that in the very young and very old, even a common cold can develop into pneumonia. Always seek professional advice if symptoms persist or suddenly get worse.

COMMON DISEASES OF INFANTS & CHILDREN

The following herbs are considered particularly suitable for children, easing symptoms and speeding recovery. Most of the remedies are best given as infusions, and can be given in a bottle. Infusions can be flavoured with honey or maple syrup if necessary, but they are better given unsweetened. The dosages given are for 1-6-year-olds, but they can be adjusted to suit other age groups.

Seek Immediate Professional advice for

Severe diarrhoea or vomitting; a temperature of 39°C (102°C); fever with convulsions; breathing difficulties; unusual drowsiness; high-pitched crying.

Cautions : Do not give babies under 6 months any medicine without professional advice. Give children under 1 year pasteurized honey. Unpasteurized honey in rare cases can cause food poisoning.

General Ailments

Infants and children are susceptible to a wide array of ailments.

Digestive upsets that result in diarrhoea and constipation can be the result of food intolerance or allergy in infants, especially when foods such as dairy produce are being introduced into the diet. Other minor digestive upsets due to infection or inflammation can cause loss of appetite.

Colic is a spasm of the gut causing cramping pain in the abdomen. It usually occurs during the first 3 months of life, particularly after feeding in the evening, when the digestion may not be working so well.

Nappy rash occurs when urine, moisture and irritants in the nappy cause the baby's skin to become red, sore and damp. It is essential to clean the baby thoroughly at each nappy change. Ensure that cloth nappies are thoroughly rinsed, avoid leaving a wet, chafing nappy on the baby and remove the nappy completely whenever possible.

Cradle cap is a thick yellow-brown encrustation on the baby's scalp, caused by over-activity of the sebum oil glands.

Headaches, colds, catarrh and chesty coughs are common problems in childhood and often respond well to herbal treatment.

Insomnia is a common childhood problem even though children require more sleep than adults and should sleep with ease. Over-excitement, teething, a wet nappy, or being too hot or cold may interfere with sleep patterns. Herbs such as lime will encourage a relaxed night's sleep.

Dosage

The dosages on this page are for 1-6-year-olds. For other ages, adapt the dose as follows:

6-12 months old - 1/3 dose

7-12 years old - 1½ dose

(a) Digestive upsets, wind & colic

The following infusions are suitable for infants over 6 months. For those under 6 months, the infusions can be taken by breast-feeding mothers.

Herb Ginger (*Zingiber officinale*)

Remedy : Give ¼ level tsp of powder with ½ cup of hot water 1-2 times a day.

Herb : German chamomile (*Chamomilla recutita*)

Remedy : Make an infusion with 1 level tsp to 1 cup of water. Give up to 3 cups a day.

Herbs : Anise (*Pimpinella anisum*), Fennel (*Foeniculum vulgare*)

Remedy : Make an infusion with 1 level tsp of either of the seeds to 1 cup of water. Give up to 2 cups a day.

Herb : Slippery elm (*Ulmus rubra*)

Remedy : Mix 1 tsp of powder with hot water to make a paste, then blend with cold or warm water as required and flavour with honey, chinnamon or maple syrup. Give up to 50 g powder in doses during the day.

(b) Constipation

Herbs: Linseed (*Linum usitatissimum*), Slippery elm (*Ulmus rubra*)

Remedy : Give 1 tsp of linseed of slippery elm with a large glass of water each day.

(c) Diarrhoea

Herbs : Agrimony (*Agrimonia eupatoria*), Common plantain (*Plantago major*)

Remedy : Make an infusion using 15 g of either herb to ½ litre of water and given up to 2 cups each day.

(d) Headaches

Herbs : Lime (*Tilia* spp.), Lemon Balm (*Melissa officinalis*)

Remedy : Make an infusion using either herb and give 1-2 cups a day.

(e) Nappy rash & inflamed skin rashes

Herb Chickweed (*Stellaria media*)

Remedy : Apply ointment 1-2 times a day.

Herb Marigold (*Calendula officinalis*)

Remedy : Apply ointment or cream to clean, dry skin at each nappy change.

Note : for nappy rash, the ointment is best.

Herbs Marigold (*Calendula officinalis*), Nettle (*Urtica dioica*).

Remedy : Make an infusion with 1 level tsp of each herb to 1 cup of water. Give 1-2 cups a day.

(f) Cradle cap

Herb Olive (*Olea europaea*)

Remedy : Apply olive oil to the affected area 1-2 times a day.

(g) Colds, Catarrh & Chesty coughs

Herb Thyme (*Thymus vulgaris*)

Remedy : Make an infusion with 1 level tsp herb to 1 cup of water. Give 1-2 cups a day.

(h) Earache

Herb Garlic (*Allium sativum*)

Remedy : Break open a garlic oil capsule, put 1 drop on to cotton wool and plug into the ear.

(i) Teething

Herbs German chamomile (*Chamomilla recutita*), Slippery elm (*Ulmus rubra*)

Remedy : Give German chamomile infusion (see Digestive Upsets) or make a paste from slippery elm powder and the infusion, and rub on the gums.

(j) Difficulty in Sleeping

Herbs German chamomile (*Chamomilla recutita*), Lime (*Tilia* spp.)

Remedy : Make an infusion using either herb and give 1-2 cups before bedtime.

CONSTIPATION

Constipation is the retention of waste materials in the body. Some indications of accumulation of toxins in the colon include a coating at the back of the tongue, bloating, gas, and abdomianl pain. Cultures consuming high fiber diets (100-170 grams daily) have a transit time of 30 hours and a fecal weight of 500 grams, whereas the typical low fibre diets (+20 grams daily) have a transit time of 48+ hours and a fecal weight of 100 grams. This condition is more common to a Vata body type. It affects other doshas under extreme circumstances, such as when traveling.

Feelings and Emotions : Holding on. It's hard to let go.

Cell Salts : Magnesium Phosphate

Diet	Vitamins & Minerals (Daily)	Essential Oils (Always dilute)	Herbs	Alternative Therapy	Avoid
Ayurvedic	Folic Acid: 200 mcg.	Rose: VPK=	Plantago PV-K+	Massage	Anti-depressants
diet for	A: 25,000 IU	Trifolia: VK-P+	Haritaki: VK-Po	Acupuncture	Anticholinergics
body type	B-Complex: 100 mg.	Ginger: VK-P+	Flaxseed: V-KoP+	Pancha Karma	Antacids
Drink plenty	B1: 100 mg.	Anise: VK-P+	Cumin: PKV=		Tobacco
of water	Choline: 500 mg.	Fennel: VPK=	Garlic: KV-P+		Cocaine
Ground	Inositol: 500 mg.	Cumin: VK-P+	Rose: VPK=		Amphetamines
seeds	B3 - Niacin: 300 mg.	Rosemary: VK-P+	Aloe Vera: VPK=		Mineral Oil
Lightly	C: 1000 mg.	Calamus: VK-P+	Senna: PK-V+		Laxatives (addictive)
cooked	Calcium: 200 mg.	Cyperus: VPK-	Barberry: PK-V+		Bad food combinations
whole bran	Potassium: 300 mg.	Cypress: VKP+	Yellow Dock: PK-V+		Fried foods
Soaked nuts	E: 150 IU	Lemon: PV-Ko	Cascara sagrada: PK-V+		Anti-Psychotics
	F: 200 IU	Lavender: PK-Vo	Cayenne : VK-P+		Sugar

	Black Pepper: VK-P+	Beta-Blockers
	Triphalla: VK-Po	
	Lemon Peel: PV-Ko	Cheese
Vata:	Ginger : VK-P÷	Muscle Relaxants
- Light cooked apple	Pippali : VK-P+	Yogurt
with cinnamon & ginger	Punarnava: PK-V+	Bread
	Bibhitaki: KP-Vo	Pastries
	Triphala: VPK; 4-6 tablets;	Fried foods
Pitta & Kapha:	at night with tea or milk	Pork/Meats
-Raw Grated Vegetables	Slippery Elm : PV-K+	Dry foods
	Oregon Grape: PK-V+	Inactivity
	Rhubarb: PK-V+	

Herbal Brew

Vata		Pitta		Kapha	
Ginger	2 oz.	Mint	1 oz.	Rose Petals	2 oz.
Slippery Elm	2 oz.	Bibhitaki	2 oz.	Pippali	1 oz.
Plantain	2 oz.	Haritaki	1 oz.	Ginger	2 oz.
Rose Petals	1 oz.	Cascara sagrada	1 oz.	Haritaki	1 oz.
Bibhitaki	1 oz.	Rose Petals	1 oz.		
Tamarind	1 oz.				

Self-Care

Exercise daily

Yoga: sun salutation

Meditation

Relaxation

Fasting/Light Diet

Self-massage, especially the abdomen

Basti (oil enema)

Castor Oil Pack

General caution : Seek professional advice for persistent constipation.

COUGHS AND BRONCHITIS

Coughing is usually a reaction to irritant particles in the bronchial tubes. It is worthwhile considering the type of cough you have and where it is centred. Herbal remedies can then be chosen to work effectively to clear or ease the cough.

Productive, Chesty coughs may produce white, yellow or green phlegm.

Unproductive coughs are dry and irritant and often take a long time to clear.

Bronchitis occurs when the lining of the lungs' airways becomes inflamed, resulting in a chesty cough, possible breathlessness and a raised temperature, Use both an external and an internal remedy.

Herbs : Thyme is an effective antiseptic for the whole system. Liquorice acts as a soothing expectorant for persistent coughs and makes any remedy more palatable. Take plenty of garlic to fight bronchitis.

General caution : Seek professional advice if a cough lasts for more than I week without a cold or infection.

General Remedy

Herb : Thyme (*Thymus vulgaris*)

Remedy : Take 5 cups of infusion a day.

Dry Coughs in the Throat and Chest

Herbs : Balm of Gilead (*Populus candicans*), Thyme (*Thymus vulgaris*), Lliquorice (*Glycyrrhiza glabra*).

Remedy : Make an infusion using equal parts of thyme, balm of Gilead buds and liquorice powder. Take $^1/_2$ cup 6 times a day, or mixequal parts of each tincture and take 1 tsp up to 5 times a day with water. Reduce the dosage as the cough eases.

Cautions : Seek professional advice if no improvement occurs after 1 week. Do not take liquorice if pregnant.

Chesty Coughs & Bronchitis

Herbs : Elecampane (*Inula helenium*), Eucalyptus (*Eucalyptus globulus*), Liquorice (*Glycyrrhiza glabra*).

Remedy (Internal) : Make a decoction of elecampane and take 2-3 cups a day. Add 5 g of liquorice powder to the decoction to improve the flavour if desired.

Note : For acute bronchitis and coughs, add 5 g of eucalyptus leaf to the decoction.

Caution : Do not take elecampane during pregnancy.

Herbs : Echinacea (*Echinacea* spp.), garlic (*Allium sativum*)

Remedy : (Internal) : Take $^1/_2$ tsp of echinacea tincture with water 2-3 times a day, or take tablets. In addition, eat 2 garlic cloves daily.

Herbs : Thyme (*Thymus vulgaris*), Cajuput (*Melaleuca leucadendron*), Eucalyptus (*Eucalyptus globulus*).

Remedy : (External) : Mix 5 drops each of eucalyptus and thyme essential oils with 2 tsp of olive or sunflower oil. Massage over the chest and back, up to twice a day, Alternatively, burn 5-10 drops of one of the oils in a burner for 30 minutes.

Caution : Do not apply thyme oil during pregnancy.

CYSTITIS

It is the inflammation or infection of the bladder. Urination for Vata will be scanty and painful; Pitta may experience some puss: and Kaphas may experiences puss and swelling.

Feelings and Emotions : Not wanting to connect. Wanting to be alone. Feeling irritation.

Diet	Vitamins & Minerals (Daily)	Essential Oils (Always dilute)	Herbs	Alternative Therapy	Avoid
Ayurveda	A: 50000 IU (until clear)	Juniper VK-P+	Barberry: PK-V+	Therapeutic	Sugar
diet for	B-Complex: 50 mg.	Sandalwood: PV-Ko	Garlic: VK-P+	touch	Refined carbohydrates
body type	Beta-carotene: 20000 IU	Cajeput: VK-P+	Goldenseal: PK-V+	Chakra	Full strength
Acidophilus	C: 500 mg. every 2 hours	Bergamot: VK-P+	Uva-Ursi: PK V+	balancing	fruit juice
after meals	D: 600 IU	Eucalyptus: KV-P+	Black Pepper: VK-P+	Reiki	Coffee: decaf
Cranberry	E:600 IU	Lavender: PK-Vo	Fennel: VPK=	Counseling	and regular
juice	Choline: 100 mg.	Pine Needle: KV-P+	Buchu Leaves: PK-V+		Caffeine in all forms
Watermelon	Calcium: 300 mg.	Benzoin: VPK-	Brahmi: VPK-		Cigarettes
Propolis	Magnesium: 200 mg.	Cedarwood: PK-V+	Mint: PK-Vo		Alcohol
Cranberries	Potassium: 200 mg.	Frankincense: VK-P+	Coriander: VPK-		Dehydration
16 oz. of	Biofavonoids: 1 gm.	Niaouli: PK-V+	Cilantro: PK-Vo		Stress
Juice daily	Zinc: 30 mg.	Tea Tree: VPK=	Dandelion: PK-V+		Poor hygiene
Restrict		Trifolia: VK-P+	Ginger: KV-P+		Red pepper
calories			Gokshura: KVP+		Hot spices
			Chandraprabha: K-VP+		Garlic
					Onions

Herbal Brew

Vata		Pitta & Kapha	
Fennel	1 oz.	Uva Ursi	1 oz.
Coriander	1 oz.	Buchu Leaves	1 oz.
Ginger	2 oz.	Dandelion	2 oz.
Black Pepper	2 oz.	Fennel	2 oz.
		Coriander	2 oz.
		Ginger	2 oz. (Kapha only)

Self-Care

Douche

8 oz. of water

3 drops of Tea Tree essential oil

2 drops of Dhavana essential oil

General cautions : Seek immediate professional help if cystitis is severe or recurrent, there is blood in the urine, or pain around the kidneys or small of the back.

DIABETES

Diabetes appears in two forms: Diabetes Mellitus and Diabetes Insipidus. Diabetes Mellitus involves the inability to assimilate food, and it primarily affects the function of the liver and the pancreas. Diabetes Insipidus is characterized by constant thirst and an excessive flow of urine. This condition can be caused by excess consumption of sugar and Kapha-producing food due to a low pancreatic function. It can also be inherited. Vata urine tends to be like butter or sesame oil in advanced stages with a noticeable loss of bladder control and weak muscles. Pitta urine can be very alkaline, combined with bladder and kidney inflammation. It can also be acidic and bluish or red due to toxicity in the kidneys. Moreover, vision can rapidly weaken. Kaphas may experience very poor digestion, sweet smelling urine containing mucous, excessive urination, or cold hands and feet.

Feelings and Emotions : Not enjoying the sweetness of life. Not being on purpose.

Diet	Vitamins & Minerals (Daily)	Essential Oils (Always dilute)	Herbs	Alternative Therapy	Avoid
Ayurvedic	Zinc: 30 mg.	Lavender: PK-Vo	Blueberry Leaf : PK-V+	Sound therapy	Alcohol
diet for	Iron: 50 mg.	Myrtle: PK-V+	Turmeric: KV-Po	Massage	All sugars
body type	Magnesium: 500 mg.	Eucalyptus: VK-P+	Myrrh: VK-P+	Acupuncture	Restrict starches
Bitter melons	Amino Acids	Camphor: KV-P+	Aloe vera: VPK=P-	Pancha Karma	(carbohydrates)
Complex	Calcium: 400 mg.	Juniper Berry: KV-P+	Gentian: PK-V+	treatments	White potatoes
carbo-	C: 1000-3000 mg.	Hyssop: K-P+	Katuka: VPK	Therapeutic	Rice
hydrates		Geranium: PK-V	Neem: PK-V+	vomiting	Processed foods
	Manganese: 500 mg.		Barberry: PK-V+		Dairy
	B Complex: 200 mg.		Goldenseal: PK-V+		Fat
	B1: 100 mg.		Black Pepper: VK-P+		Stress
Ghee:	B2: 10 mg.		Cayenne: VK-P+		
1-2 Tbs.	B6: 100 mg.		Ginger: VK-P+		
2-3-x day	B12: 400 mcg.		Ginseng: V-KPo		

Lots of water	B3 - Niacin: 100 mg.	Comfrey: PV-K+	**Ayurvedic Herbs:**
Lots of	Potassium: 300 mg.	Wintergreen: PK-Vo	Chandraprabha: VPK-
greens	Pangamic Acid: 200 mg.	Dandelion Root: VK-P+	Shilajit: VPK-
Liquorice ghee	Co Q-10: 80 mg.	Buchu leaves : PK-V +	Trikatu: VK-P+
Milk-	D: 400 IU	Raspberry Leaves: PK-V+	Triphalla: VPK
(10 gm)	E: 400-1200 IU	Eucalyptus: VPK+	Guggul: PKV+
Nuts	F: 2 Tbs. cold pressed	Yarrow: PK-V+	Gurmar: PK-V+
Protein	vegetable oil or 6 capsules	Bitter Root: PK-V+	
Stevia	Chromium: 200-400 mcg.	Vanadium: 100 mcg.	
		Red Root: PK-V+	
		Marshmallow: PV-K+	

Herbal Brew

Vata		Pitta		Kapha	
Eucalyptus	1 oz.	Mint	1 oz.	Eucalyptus	1 oz.
Rosemary	½ oz.	Lavender	1 oz.	Red Clover	2 oz.
Yellow Jasmine	1 oz.	Burdock	1 oz.	Ginger	1 oz.
Dashmoola	2 oz.	Red Clover	1 oz.	Yarrow	1 oz.
Ginger	2 oz.	Raspberry Leaves	1 oz.	Dandelion	1 oz.
		Dandelion	1 oz.		

Drink tea all day between meals.

Trifala : 2.000 mg. at night (all doshas) **Gurmar or Shardunikha:** Take 3 tablets 3 x a day before meals with tea.

Self-Care

Exercise (walking, swimming, etc.)
Inhalation of essential oils: 3-4 times per day
Turmeric Rice: Cook rice with 1 Tbs. Turmeric
Meditation
Mantra
Yoga

DYSMENORRHIA (PAINFUL MENSTRUATION)

Sometimes accompanied by incapacitating cramps and often nausea and diarrhoea. It has been determined that an excess of a certain type of prostaglandin is found in the uterus. Prostaglandins are chemicals found in the body, one of which causes contractions of the uterine and intestinal muscles. With too much prostaglandin, the rhythmic contractions of the uterus during menstruation become longer and tighter, keeping oxygen from the muscles. It is this lack of oxygen that we perceive as pain. Vata experiences light menstruation, along with severe pain. Pitta may have the opposite effect with heavy bleeding and painful diarrhea. Kapha suffers from clots, water retention, and fatigue.

Feelings and Emotions : Not having good feelings about their feminine energy. Sexual guilty.

Cell Salts : Magnesium Phosphate

Diet	Vitamins & Minerals (Daily)	Essential Oils (Always dilute)	Herbs	Alternative Therapy	Avoid
Ayurvedic	E:400 IU, 2 x day	Clary Sage: VPK-	Dong Quai: VK-P+	Massage	Caffeine
diet for		Geranium: PK-V+	Uva-Ursi: PK-V+	Bio-feedback	Sodas
body type	Evening Primrose Oil	Lavender: PK-Vo	Crampbark: KV-P+	Acumpuncture	Salt

	1000 mg.	Yarrow: PK-V+	Blue Cohosh: KV-P+	Tarpana	Sugar
Seaweeds		Fennel: VPK=	Fennel: VPK=	Therapeutic touch	Alcohol
or kelp	Calcium: 1,000 mg.	Cypress: VKP+	Ginger Root: VK-P+	Reiki	IUD
	Magnesium: 600 mg	Chamomile: VPK-	Valerian. VK-P+		Fasting
Whole grains	Iron : 30 mg.	Jasmine: PK-V+	Cinnamon: VK-P+		Light diet
	Iodine: 200 mcg.	Peppermint: PK-Vo	Raspberry Leaf: PK-V+		when
Legumes	B Complex: 200 mg.	Sage: VK-P+	Vitex: VPK-		Vata
	C: 2000 mg.	Tarragon: VK-P+	Yarrow: PK-V+		
Vegetables	Pantothenic acid: 200 mg.	Thyme: VK-P+	Hops: PK-V+		
& fruits			Nettles: PK-V+		
			Alfalfa: PK-V+		
Brewer's yeast			Liquorice: PV-K+		
			Lemongrass: PK-Vo		
Add turmeric to rice			Motherwort: PK-V+		
and vegetables			Dandelion: PK-V+		
			Shepeherd's Purse : PK-V+		
			Black Currant : KP-V+		
			Turmeric: VK-Po		
			Cardamon: VK-P + (in excess)		

Herbal Brew

Vata		Pitta		Kapha	
Cramp Bark	2 oz.	Yarrow	2 oz.	Raspberry Leaf	2 oz.
Shatavari	2 oz.	Shatavari	2 oz.	Ginger	1 oz.
Ginger	1 oz.	Motherwort	1 oz.	Vitex	1 oz.
Cinnamon	1 oz.	Fennel	1 oz.	Lemongrass	1 oz.
Liquorice	1 oz.	Vitex	1 oz.	Uva Ursi	1 oz.
Vitex	2 oz.	Nettles	1 oz.	Nettles	1 oz.

Drink 2-3 cups daily, beginning two weeks before menstruation.

Self Care

Exercise	Regular sleep schedule
Compresses	Warm bath with essential oils of clary sage, lavender, and geranium.
Compress over the abdomen	Vaginal massage (by GYN, midwife, mate, or self)
Breathwork	

EARACHE

Earaches are due to inflammation in the middle ear. This may be due to chronic or acute infections, eczema, wax, neuralgia or infected teeth. Other causes may be colds, tonsillitis, allergies, or measles. Vatas may experience dryness, scalyness, or severe pain and inflammation. Pittas may experience burning pain. Kaphas may experience congestion, pain and drainage.

Feelings and Emotions : Not wanting to hear which is being spoken about. For children, when there is too much fighting going on in the home, they may get an earache.

Cell Salts : Kalimur (Potassium Chloride)

Diet	Vitamins & Minerals (Daily)	Essential Oils (Always dilute)	Herbs	Alternative Therapy	Avoid
Ayurvedic diet	A: 100,000 IU	Camphor: KV-P+	Astralagus: VP-K+	Chiropractic	All dairy
for body type	C: 2500 mg.	Lavender: PK-Vo	Mullein: PK-V+	Cranial sacral	Bread
	Thymus gland extract:	Cajeput: KV-P+	Echinacea: PK-V+	Reiki	containing
Elimination	50 drops per day	Niaouli: PK-V+	Hops: PK-V+	Therapeutic touch	milk
diet for	Zinc: 100 mg.	Savory: KV-P+	Oregano: VKP+	Ear candling	Simple
2 weeks	Biofavonoids: 200 mg.	Clove: VK-P+	Boneset: PK-V+	Sound therapy	carbohydrates
	Evening Primrose: 200 mg.	Eucalyptus: VK-P+	Lobelia: K-PV+		Eggs
Rotation diet	Flax Seed Oil : 200 mg.	Pine: KV-P+	Manjishta: PK-V+		Wheat
		Geranium: PK-V+	Dashmoola: VK-P+		Corn
Lemon juice		Juniper: KV-P+	Castor Root: V-PK+		Oranges
		Immortele: PKV-	Vatsanabha: VPK+		Peanut butter
			Vitex: VPK-		
		Medicated Oil:	Bhringaraj: VPK=		
		Garlic with olive oil	Ginger: VK-P+		
		Mullein oil	Hing: VK-P+		

Herbal Brew

Vata & Kapha		Pitta	
Lemon juice	1 oz.	Lemon juice	1 oz.
Ginger, fresh	2-inch piece	Fennel seed	1 Tbs.
Water	3 cups	Water	3 cups
In blender, mix ginger, water, and lemon juice; add honey or sucanat to taste. Blend well. Strain. Drink 3 times per day.		*In blender, mix fennel water, and lemon juice; add maple syrup to taste. Blend well. Strain. Drink 3 times per day.*	

Recipes

1. 40 drops pure lemon juice with 2 Tbs. of water. Put 3 drops in ear 3 times per day.
2. On a cotton ball put 2 drops of lavender, lemon or niaouli. Fold corners of ball and place cotton in outer ear.
3. From "Back to Eden", by Jethro Kloss: Bake a large onion until soft. Tie it over the ear.
4. A hot foot bath with 1-Tablespoon mustard seed vegetable oil and essential oil of choice.
5. Mullein flower oil - 4 drops.
6. Use 1 pinch Hing (asafoetida) with one drop of essential oil and mix well. Place in the center of cotton ball and fold corners. Then place in ear and make sure the mixture on the cotton does not touch the ear.

Choose one of the above recipes. Then, using your thumbs, massage around the outside of the ear with a cooling essential oil of your choice. Massage with downward movements. Be sensitive.

Self-Care

Warm compresses around the ear.

ECZEMA (ATOPIC DERMATITIS)

A disease of the skin which is not contagious but can be inflammatory. It can be due to disturbances of the digestive organs, blood conditions or external irritants such as heat, cold or irritants from plants. Eczema appears in three different varieties. Eczema rubrum, Eczema erythermatosum, or Eczema pustulosum. It is a skin condition with characteristic symptoms of itchiness, inflammation, thick or day skin or skin lesions such as scratches, papules, patches of redness, weeping, scaling or blistering. It is most commonly found on the face, wrists and insides of the elbows and knees.

Feelings and Emotions : Anger, guilt, blame.

Cell Salts : Calc Sulph (calcium sulfate)

Diet	Vitamins & Minerals (Daily)	Essential Oils (Always dilute)	Herbs	Alternative Therapy	Avoid
Ayurvedic diet	B Complex: 200 mg.	Bergamot: VK-P+	Marshmallow: PV-K+	Therapeutic touch	Stress
for body type	C: 3,000 mg. (ascorbate)	Chamomile: VPK	Bupleurum: PKV+	Reiki	Dairy
	D: 500 IU	Eucalyptus: VK-P+	Isatis: PKV+	Acupuncture	Wheat
Legumes	PABA: 200 mg.	Helichrysum: PKV+	Blackthorn: PKV+	Colour therapy	Sugar
	Biotin: 300 mcg.	Juniper: KV-P+	Hawthorn Berry: V-KPo	Counseling	Caffeine
Wheatgrass	Choline: 200 mg.	Lavender: PK-Vo	Liquorice Root: VP-K+		Fatigue
	Inositol: 100 mcg.	Melissa: PK-Vo	Burdock Root: KP-V+		Sour foods
Green	E: 500 IU	Patchouli: VPK	German Chamomile: VPKo		Pungent foods

vegetables	Niacin: 100 mg.	Rosewood: K-VP+	Neem: PK-V+	Salt
Ghee	Flaxseed Oil: 1 teaspoon	Geranium: PKV+	Pau d'arco: PK-V+	
	3 x day (300 mg.)	Sage VK-P+		
		Hyssop : PKV+	Red Clover: PK-V+	
		Rosemary: P-VP	Yellow Dock: PK-V+	
	Evening Primrose Oil:	Myrrh: KV-P+		
	400 mg.		Calendula: PK-V+	
	A: 50,000-75,000 IU	Rose: VPK=	Aloe vera: VPK=	
	for 3 months	Neem: PK-V+	Chickweed: PK-V+	
	Zinc: 50 mg.		Dandelion: KP-V+	
	Zinc Skin Ointment		Plantain: KP-V+	
	Bioflavonoids: 200 mg.		Yarrow: PK-V+	
	Magnesium: 600 mg.		Turmeric: VK-Po	
	Sulfur Skin Ointment		Barberry: PK-V+	
	Silica: 25 mg.		Guggul: KV-P+	
			Milk Thistle : PV-K+	
			Shatavari: PV-K+	
			Aloe Vera Gel: VPK=	
			Saffron: VPK=	
			Goldenseal : PK-V+	
			Nettles: PK-V+	
			Gokshura: PK-Vo	

Herbal Brew

Vata		Pitta		Kapha	
Chamomile	2 oz.	Pau d'arco	1 oz.	Red Clover	1 oz.
Licorice	1 oz.	Dandelion	2 oz.	Milk Thistle	1 oz.
Shatavari	2 oz.	Yarrow	2 oz.	Dandelion	2 oz.
Hawthorn	2 oz.	Plantain	1 oz.	Plantain	2 oz.
Marshmallow	½ oz.	Calendula	2 oz.	Burdock	2 oz.
Chickweed	1 oz.				

Drink throughout the day - as many as 6 cups.

Poultice

Mix Aloe vera Gel or Ghee and Turmeric (equal amounts)

Make a paste

Apply to the area

In the Morning

In blender mix Aloe vera Gel and Turmeric (equal amounts)

Drink before breakfast

Neem - Lavender Salve

1 part beeswax

3 parts oil

Melt beeswax in a pan over low temperature. Remove from stove. Add vegetable oil or jojoba oil. Add 50 drops essential oils. Put in refrigerator for 15 minutes to cool. Take out. Apply to areas needed.

Self-Care

Drink fresh cilantro juice

Colon cleanse

Turmeric creme

Neem-Lavender salve

To avoid scratching, cover the affected area with an absorbent, non-irritating material such as cotton.

General caution : If there is no improvement or if the condition deteriorates, consult a professional practitioner.

EDEMA

Water retention caused by weakening of the kidneys. Most common during old age. A Kapha condition affecting all doshas. Vatas experience dry skin, and tissues become spongy; Pitta may experience swelling, inflammation, and the skin holding the imprint of the finger when pressed; Kapha's have moist skin and feels damp when pressed with fingers. Can be caused by poor diet, poor food combining, pregnancy, PMS, and food allergies. Caution: Edema could be an indication of kidney or heart failure.

Feelings and Emotions : Fear of letting go.

Cell Salt : Silica Natrium Phosphate

Diet	Vitamins & Minerals (Daily)	Essential Oils (Always dilute)	Herbs	Alternative Therapy	Avoid
Kapha diet	A: 25,000 IU	Sandalwood: VP-Ko	Ashwagandha: VP K+	Sauna	Dry foods (Vata)
best for Pitta	C: 2,500 mg.	Lavender: PK-Vo	Sarsaparilla: VPK+	Massage	Corn
	B-Complex: 200 mg.	Juniper: VK-P+	Marshmallow: VPK+	(Lymph Drainage)	Salt
Rotation diet	B6: 100 mg.	Coriander: VPK	Dandelion: PKV+	Acupuncture	Sodas
		Parsley: KVP+	Nettles: PK-V+	Therapeutic touch	Foods high-sodium
Diet must be			Coriander: VKP-		White sugar
modified			Chickweed: PK-V+		Chips
			Uva Ursi: PKV+		Pretzels
			Burdock: PKV+		Birth control pills
			Cleavers: PK-V+		
Cilantro			Goshkura: PKVo		
			Lemongrass: VK-P+		
			Purnarnava: PKV+		
			Chandraprabha: VK-VP+		
			Fennel: VPK=		
			Chicory: PK-V+		
			Lavender: PK-Vo		
			Juniper: KV-P+		
			Kudzy: PVK+		
			Brahmi: PKV		
			Red Clover: PK-V+		

Herbal Brew

Vata		Pitta		Kapha	
Sarsaparilla	1 oz.	Dandelion	1 oz.	Buchu Leaves	1 oz.
Coriander	½ oz.	Nettles	½ oz.	Juniper	½ oz.
Lemongrass	½ oz.	Fennel	½ oz.	Uva Ursi	½ oz.
Ashwagandha	½ oz.	Coriander	½ oz.	Nettles	½ oz.
		Burdock	½ oz.	Lemongrass	½ oz.

Self-Care

Compress over kidneys

Kidney Flush

Exercise

Dry skin brushing

FERTILITY PROBLEMS IN WOMEN

Although much more research is needed, herbal medicine does appear to increase fertility in women who are trying to conceive, especially if the problem is related to hormonal imbalances, age or the amount of mucus produced by the cervix. Where there appears to be no physical problem preventing conception, for example a blocked fallopian tube. ovarian cysts or internal scarring, herbal medicines are well worth trying. Diet, exercise and lifestyel may also play a significant role in improving fertility.

Aiding Conception

Herb : Agnus castus (*Vitex agnus-castus*)

Remedy : Take tablets or take 20-40 drops of tincture with water each morning for a maximum of 3 months at a time.

Herb : Chinese angelica (*Angelica sinensis*)

Remedy : Take tablets or make a decoction using 12 g of root to 750 ml of water and drink each day for up to 3 months.

Caution : Discontinue if you become pregnant.

Low sex drive

Herb Schisandra (*Schisandra chinensis*).

Remedy : Soak 5 g (a small handful) of berries in water overnight. Strain the berries and make a decoction with 250 ml of water. Brew for 15 minutes and take the dose each day.

Note : Traditionally, this remedy is taken for 100 days to raise sexual energy and vitality. (It is safe to take it for this period).

FERTILITY PROBLEMS IN MEN

Impotence in men is a common problem and herbal medicine has been used throughout history to help restore healthy sexual function. A low sperm count, which is a common cause of infertility, is often related to lifestyle and general states of health.

Saw palmetto is a tonic herb that increases stamina. It benefits the male sexual organs and is reputed to increase potency.

Withania is an all-round tonic that is not as stimulating as ginseng, but is nonetheless helpful in restoring normal vitality after a long-term illness or stress.

General Vitality

Herb : Withania (*Withania somnifera*)

Remedy : Take 2 g of the dried root a day, either by chewing it, or taking it is powder form mixed with honey and, if required, water. Take for up to 6 weeks.

Impotence and Premature Ejaculation

Herb : Ginseng (*Panax ginseng*)

Remedy : Take 0.5-1 g up to 3 times a day for 6 weeks at a time, either by chewing the root, cooking it in a soup or stew, or taking it in tablet form.

Note : Ginseng is the best-known remedy for this condition. However, schisandra (*Schisandra chinensis*) berries also benefit male sexuality. Take as listed above in Fertility Problems in Women under Low Sex Drive for up to 6 weeks.

Caution : Do not take caffeine while taking ginseng.

Herb : Saw palmetto (*Sabal serrulata*)

Remedy : Take ½ tsp of tincture with water up to 3 times a day for up to 6 weeks.

FEVER

A fever occurs when the body temperature becomes elevated due to a high Pitta state or due to an infection in the body. Fevers are good for the body during illness because they help burn out toxins in the body. Many natural physicians encourage a low fever (under 105° F) and do not recommend suppression of the fever.

Feelings and Emotions : Burning up inside.

Diet	Vitamins & Minerals (Daily)	Essential Oils (Always dilute)	Herbs	Alternative Therapy	Avoid
Pitta Diet	C: 2,000 every 2 hours	Lavender: PK-Vo	Yarrow: PK-V+		Iron
	A: 50,000 mg.	Rose: VPK=	Echinacea: PK-V+		Zinc

Many fluids	Chamomile: PK-Vo	Feverfew: PKV+	Aspirin
	Fennel: VPK=	Pokeroot: PK-V+	No minerals
Lots of vegetable juices	Coriander: PKV=	Hyssop: K-P+	
	Hyssop: KV-P+	Lobelia Extract : K-PV+	
	Basil: VK-P+	Lemongrass: PK-Vo	
Green juices	Sandalwood: PV-Ko	Coriander: VPK-	
	Geranium: PK-V+	Fennel: VPK=	
	Rose: VPK=	Tulsi: VK-P+	
	Cyperus: PKV-	Catnip: PK-Vo	
	Juniper: VK-P+	Blackthron: PK-V+	
		Fenugreek: VK-P+	
		Rose petals: PKV=	
		Ginger: VK-P+	

Herbal Brew

Vata		Pitta		Kapha	
Fenugreek	2 oz.	Yarrow	2 oz.	Ginger	2 oz.
Basil	2 oz.	Rose Petals	1 oz.	Yarrow	2 oz.
Ginger	2 oz.	Fennel	1 oz.	Fenugreek	1 oz.
Catnip	2 oz.	Feverfew	1 oz.	Basil	1 oz.
		Coriander	1 oz.		
		Erand	1 oz.		

Self care

Foot Bath

In a basin of very warm water, add 10 drops of essential oils.

Sit in chair with feet in basin of water.

Cover person with blankets

Cold sheet treatment

Prepare a hot bath.

Add essential oils: 10 drops yarrow, 10 drops cypress, and 10 drops juniper.

Put a sheet in the freezer or in ice water.

Put the person in the bath with a cool compress on the head - add more hot bath water to tolerance.

Drink a cup of the herbal blend for specific body type. This will cause sweating.

When the sweat breaks, remove them from bath.

Wrap in cold sheet from freezer.

Around the cold sheet, wrap with wool blanket(s).

Crush 2 cloves garlic; mix with petroleum jelly; apply to bottoms of feet/ cover with wool socks.

Fever should spike in 10-15 minutes with profuse sweating; then fever drops to normal.

When you remove the sheet, it is often tinged brown with impurities from the skin.

FIBROCYSTIC BREAST

Fibrocystic breast consists of lumps of a soft, moveable nature found in the breast tissue. They can increase in size and cause pain during menstruation. The main cause is hormonal imbalance and it can be aggravated by poor diet and stress.

Feelings and Emotions : Old hurt and pain relating to male energy.

Diet	Vitamins & Minerals (Daily)	Essential Oils (Always dilute)	Herbs	Alternative Therapy	Avoid
Ayurvedic diet	A: 15,000 IU (until clear)	Dhavana: VPK-	Shatavari: PV-K+	Ayurvedic	Alcohol
for body type	Beta-carotene: 20,000 IU	Clary sage: VKP-	Squaw vine : PKV+	consultation	Animal fat
Whole grains	B-1: 150 mg.	Geranium: PK-V	Pokeroot: PK-V+	Therapeutic Touch	Rancid foods
Kelp	B-6: 150 mg.	Sage: VK-P+	Mullein: PK-V+	Colon cleansing	Meat
Spirulina	C: 4,000 mg.	Cypress: VKP+	Red Clover: VK-P+	Acupuncture	Coffee
Bee pollen	E: 500 IU	Borage Oil: PK-V+	Dandelion: PK-V+		Black tea
Wheatgrass	Evening Primrose: 400 mg.	Castor Oil: V-KP+	Jatamasi: VK-P+		Soda
Mushroom	Q10: 100 mg.		Black Pepper: VK-P+		
Kelp	Selenium: 200 mcg.		Cayenne: VK-P+		
Seed nuts	Germanium: 100 mcg.		Saffron: VKP=		
			Ginger: VK-P+		

Herbal brew

Vata		Pitta		Kapha	
Shatavari	2 oz.	Shatavari	2 oz.	Shatavari	2 oz.
Jatamasi	1 oz.	Dandelion	1 oz.	Red Clover	1 oz.
Guggul	2 oz.	Red Clover	1 oz.	Poke Root	1 oz.
Black Pepper	1 oz.	Mullein	1 oz.	Guggul	1 oz.
		Squavine	1 oz.		

Drink

Saffron with rice milk, soymilk or low fat milk - 3 times per day.

Self-Care

Warm compresses with castor oil.

FIBROIDS

Fibroids are benign tumors that can occur throughout the body. They usually occur in the smooth muscle such as Uterine and Breast areas. Vata may experience pain and fear; Kaphas' fibroids may swell and become damp; Pitta suffers from inflammation and excessive bleeding.

Feelings and Emotions : Wanting to give birth to something.

Cell Salt : Silica

Diet	Vitamins & Minerals (Daily)	Essential Oils (Always dilute)	Herbs	Alternative Therapy	Avoid
Ayurvedic diet	B-Complex: 200 mg.	Lavender: PK-Vo	Chaparral: PK-V+	Acupuncture	Hormone
for body type	Niacin: 200 mg.	Frankincense: KV-P+	Pau d' Arco: PK-V+	Reiki	replacement
	Pantothenic Acid:	Bergamot: VK-P+	Yellow Dock Root: PK-V+	Homeopathics	drugs
Dark green	1000 mg.	Clary Sage: VPK-	Wild Yam: VP-Ko	Therapeutic	Dairy
leafy vegetables	C: 2000 mg.	Dhavana: PVK-	Dandelion: PK-V+	touch	Eggs
Spirulina	F: 200 mg.	Tea Tree: VPK=-	Burdock: PK-V+		Red meat
Whole grains		Cyperus: PKV-	Yarrow: PK-V+		Fat
Green drinks		Frankincense: VK-P+	Ginger: VK-P+		Dong Quai
Fresh fruit			Shatavari: PV-K+		
			Cotton Root Bark: V-KP+		
			Triphalla: VPKo		
			Cyperus: PKV-		
			Vitex: PKV-		

Herbal Brew

Vata		Pitta		Kapha	
Ginger	equal parts	Dandelion	equal parts	Pippali	equal parts
Wild Yam Root		Cyperus		Ginger	
Myrtle		Vitex		Barberry	

FLATULENCE

Flatulence is a collection of gas in the stomach or bowels. Gas may produce unpleasant rumblings in the bowels, farting, or burping. The cause is usually fermentation set up by yeast overgrowth, poor food combining, junk food diet, stress, or hurried eating. Vata people are very susceptible to gas. Vegetarians can become low in hydrochloric acid. Older people lose their digestive powers.

Feelings and Emotions : Gripping fear.

Cell Salts : Magnesium Phosphate

Diet	Vitamins & Minerals (Daily)	Essential Oils (Always dilute)	Herbs	Alternative Therapy	Avoid
Ayurvedic diet	B1 : 100 mg.	Lavender: PK-Vo	Liquorice: VPK+	Homeopathics	Improper food
for body type	B5: 2500 mg.	Bergamot: VK-P+	Rhubarb: PK-V+	Ayurvedic consultation	combining
	B-Complex: 200 mg.	Chamomile: PK-Vo	Coriander: VKP-	Pancha Karma	Unsoaked legumes
Acidophilus	Multi-vitamin	Coriander: VPK-	Cumin: PK-V+		Repressed emotions
	Multi-mineral	Eucalyptus: KV-P+	Garlic: KV-P+		Too much vitamin C
Primadophilus		Fennel: VPK=	Mustard: KV-P+		Constipation
		Ginger: VK-P+	Nutmeg: VK-P+		
Food combining		Juniper: VK-P+	Turmeric: KV-Po		
		Myrrh: VK-P+	Tarragon: KV-P+		
Cave man diet		Nutmeg: VK-P+	Fennel: VPK=		
		Peppermint: PK-Vo	Valerian: VK-P+		

More fibre	Rosemary: KV-P+	Asafoetida: VK-P+
	Spearmint: KP-Vo	Pippali: VK-P+
	Tarragon: KV-P+	Cardamon: VK-P+
	Jatamasi: KV-P+	Clove: VK-P+
	Fennel: VPK-	Cinnamon: VK-P+
	Anise: VK-P	Catnip: PK-Vo
	Caraway: VK-P+	Ginger: VK-P+
		Horseradish: VK-P+
		Haritaki: VK-Po
		Amalaki: VP-Ko
		Bibhitaki: KP-Vo
		Hingwastika: VK-P+

Herbal Brew

Vata		Pitta		Kapha	
Cardamon	equal amount	Fennel	equal amounts	Cardamon	equal amounts
Ginger	equal amounts	Mint	equal amounts	Ginger	equal amounts
Anise	equal amounts	Coriander	equal amounts	Anise	equal amounts
Hing	1 pinch	Hing	1 pinch	Hing	1 pinch

Drink 1 cup before meals.

Massage formula for abdomen

Fennel	10 drops	Anise	5 drops	Vegetable oil	4 cz.
Coriander	10 drops	Caraway	5 drops		

Self-Care

Take bitters before each meal	Take sea salt	Food combining
Pinch of baking soda in warm water	Compress of ginger	Compresses
Castor oil	Basti oil enema	Colon cleansing

GALL BLADDER

The gall bladder is a companion to the liver and found underneath it, storing the bile produced by the liver, which releases the necessary bile for digestion of oils and fats. When the organ becomes weakened due to improper diet, it can produce gallstones, which are often crystallized forms of cholesterol combined with fat. Vata types experience gallstones with severe pain, nausea and dry stones; Pitta experiences yellow and green inflammation, and kapha experiences weight gain with a lot of phlegm, especially around the abdominal area, with stones that are round and whitish in colour.

Feelings and Emotions : Too controlling; not flowing with inner self. Indecisiveness. Not knowing when to be in control or when to let flow with life.

Cell Salts : Natrium Phosphate

Diet	Vitamins & Minerals (Daily)	Essential Oils (Always dilute)	Herbs	Alternative Therapy	Avoid
Ayurvedic	A: 25,000 IU (until clear)	Lemon: PV-Ko	Barberry Bark: PK-V+	Pancha Karma	Sweets
diet for	(beta-carotene best)	Coriander: PVK-	Dandelion: PK-V+	Acupuncture	Fats
body type	B-Complex: 150 mg.	Turmeric: VK-P+	Fennel: VPK=	Reiki	Fried foods
	12: 1,500 mcg.	Peppermint: PK-Vo	Coriander: VPK-	Colonics	Hydrogenated oils
Liquid	Choline: 500 mg.	Ginger: VK-P+	Peppermint: PK-Vo	Chiropractic	Meat
diet for	Inositol: 500 mg.	Lime: PK-V+	Gokshura: PK-Vo	treatments	Sugars
10 days	C: 25,000 mg.	Grapefruit: KV-P+	Katuka: PKV+	Acupressure	
	D: 400 IU		Corn Silk: PK-V+		
	E: 700 IU		Guduchi: PKV+		
			Ginger: VK=P+		
			Catnip: PK-Vo		
			Gravel Root : PK-V+		
			Triphalla Guggulu: VK-P+		

Herbal Brew

Vata		Pitta		Kapha	
Ginger	1 oz.	Dandelion	1 oz.	Guduchi	1 oz.
Fennel	1 oz.	Mint	½ oz.	Ginger	1 oz.
Coriander	1 oz.	Catnip	1 oz.	Mint	½ oz.
		Gravel Rot	1 oz.	Corn Silk	1 oz.

Gall Bladder Cleanse

Day 1 : Cut out all meat-flesh or fowl.

Day 2 : Cut out all diary products. Continue eating other foods.

Day 3 : Cut out all nuts and seeds.

Day 4 : Cut out all legumes, tofu and tofu products as well.

Day 5 : Cut out all grains.

Day 6 : Cut out all vegetables.

Day 7 : Cut out all fruits and drink nothing but apple juice; if allergic reaction to apple or oranges, use cranberry.

For 3 days : Drink 8 ounces of juice every 2 hours with the 2 capsules of Barberry Bark. This will soften the stones. Drink lots of water in between. Take an enema or colima every night.

On the evening of the 3rd Day : Take 4 ounces of olive oil and 4 ounces of lemon juice. Go to bed.

Next morning you should pass an oily bowel movement with green stones.

Go back to eating starting with vegetables as of day #6 above, reintroducing foods of day 6 through day 1 consecutively. You are back to normal eating. Be kind to yourself.

Self-Care

Compresses with essential oils	Castor oil pack
Colon cleanse	Basti oil enema
Fasting	Gall Bladder cleanse

GLAUCOMA

It is a condition of the eye in which increased pressure results in an imbalance between production and outflow of fluid. In acute glaucoma, obstruction to outflow is the main factor responsible for the imbalance. Since collagen is the most generous protein in the body, in the eye it gives strength to the tissues. Faulty collagen metabolism is often associated with this condition. Symptoms include eye discomfort or pain, blurred vision, poor night vision, poor peripheral vision and/or halos around lights. Vatas may experience extreme pain and nausea; Pittas may experience redness and blurred vision; and Kaphas may experience vomitting with whitish mucous.

Feelings and Emotions : Not wanting to see clearly.

Diet	Vitamins & Minerals (Daily)	Essential Oils (Always dilute)	Herbs	Alternative Therapy	Avoid
Ayurvedic diet	C & Bioflavonoids:	Sandalwood: PV-Ko	Bhringaraj: VPK=	Marijuana extract:	Belladonna
for body type	10,000-15,000 mg.		Triphala: VP-Ko	-need a doctor's	Dairy
	E: 400 IU	Hydrosol (essential	Bibhitaki: PK-Vo	prescription	Red meat
	Bioflavonoids: 1 gm.	oil water):	Chrysanthemum: PK-V+	Massage	Tobacco
	Corticosteroids	Lavender: PK-Vo	Eyebright: PK-V+	Netra Basti	Coffee
Oranges	B-Complex: 150 mg.	Rose: VPK=	Bilberry: VPK-	Acupuncture	Black tea
	A: 50,000 IU				Stress
	Thiamine: 100 mg.				
	Pantothenic Acid: 100 mg.				
	3 x day				
Grapefruit	Rutin: 50-mg. 3 x day				

	Trikatu: 2 tablets
All citrus	3 x day before meals
	Zinc (sulfate) : 50 mg.

Herbal Brew

Vata		Pitta & Kapha	
Chrysanthemum	1 oz.	Eyebright	1 oz.
Liquorice	2 oz.	Chrysanthemum	2 oz.
Lemon Peel	1 oz.		

NETRA BASTI

Make ghee, heat to body temperature 98.6°-100°F. Make thick bread dough (¼ pound of flour and water). Roll into a donut and place around the eye as a dam while lying on your back with one eye facing straight up. Pour warm ghee into eye dam. With eyes open, look in all directions and relax for 5-10 minutes. Drain by piercing dam with finger on outer side and draining ghee into small bowl or cup. Repeat on other eye.

Self-Care

Yoga (avoid inverted postures)

Topical application of Vitamin C

Eye Exercises

GOUT

This is type of arthritis caused by an increased concentration of uric acid in the body fluids. Inflammation is caused by uric and crystals in the joints, kidneys, tissues and tendons. It is considered to be the "Rich Man's Disease". Nearly one-half of all first gout attacks occur in the first joint of the big toe. Pitta will experience burning inflammation and pain; Vata will find dryness of the toes and nails; while Kapha retains water throughout the foot and ankle.

Feelings and Emotions : Impatience, the desire to control events.

Cell Salts : Sodium Sulfate

Diet	Vitamins & Minerals (Daily)	Essential Oils (Always dilute)	Herbs	Alternative Therapy	Avoid
Ayurveda diet	E: 800 IU	Basil: VK-P+	Devil's Claw: PK-V+	Colloidal nickel	Meat
for body type	Folic Acid : 100 mg.	Birch : PK-V+	Camphor: KV-P+	Energy work	Wine
	E: 200 mg.	Fennel: VPK=	Mugwort: VK-P+	Therapeutic touch	Alcohol
Plenty of fluids	Potassium: 3000 mg.	Hyssop: K-P+	Sarsaparilla: PV-Ko	Reflexology	Aspirin
	Phosphorus: 800 mg.	Lemon: PV-Ko	Amalaki: PV-Ko	Homeopathics	Excess of food
Cherries	Glutamic Acid: 200 mg.	Nutmeg: VK-P+	Gokshura: PK-Vo+		Trauma
	Magnesium: 1000 mg.	Thyme: VK-P+	Guggul: VK-P+		Purines
Blueberries	C: 2500 mg.	Cyperus: PKV-	Pippali: VK-P+		Organ meats
	Niacin: 200 mg.	Juniper: VK-P+	Skullcap: PK-Vo		Yeast
	Iron: 40 mg.		Valerian: VK-P+		Poultry
Vegetarian diet	Pantothenic Acid: 8000 mg.		Blue Violet: VK-P+		Lentils

Calcium: 1500 mg.	Burdock: VKP+	Anchovies
2-week vitamin therapy	Gentian Root: VKP+	Fats
Germanium: 200 mg.	Yarrow: VKP+	Overweight
	Plantain: VKP+	Protein
		Ginger
	Wood Betony: VKP+	Refined carbohydrates
	Broom: VKP+ Buckthorn Bark: VKP+	Protein supplements

Herbal Brew

Vata		Pitta		Kapha	
Sarsaparilla	2 oz.	Burdock	2 oz.	Plantain	1 oz.
Amalaki	2 oz.	Gokshura	2 oz.	Ginger	2 oz.
Ginger	2 oz.	Yarrow	1 oz.	Burdock	1 oz.
Valerian	1 oz.	Skullcap	1 oz.	Guggul	1 oz.
		Plantain	1 oz.	Gokshura	2 oz.

Self-Care

Foot baths

Colon Cleanse

HAEMORRHOIDS (PILES)

Consists of a varicose and inflamed condition of the veins at the lower end of the bowel. This can be divided into three types: external, internal and mixed. External piles, found outside the bowel, are covered by skin that is brown or purple in colour. Internal piles are within the opening covered by a mucous membrane and are red or cherry coloured. Mixed piles are situated on the margin and covered half by skin, half by mucous membrane. Pittas can experience much redness, inflammation, swelling, and the margin and covered half by skin, half by mucous membrane. Pittas can experience much redness, inflammation, swelling, and bleeding with burning and diarrhoea. Pain involves the bladder and all around the thigh area, with dry skin around the rectum and constipation. Kaphas may experience large, white swollen hemorrhoids, with mucus on the stool. Vatas experience dryness and cracking with sharp pain.

Feelings and Emotions : Anal-retentive. Holding on.

Cell Salts : Calcium Fluoride

Diet	Vitamins & Minerals (Daily)	Essential Oils (Always dilute)	Herbs	Alternative Therapy	Avoid
Ayurvedic diet	A: 25,000 IU	Cypress: VPK+	Bayberry: KV-P+	Acupuncture	Constipation
for body type	B-Complex: 200 mg.	Cajeput: KV-P+	Aloe Vera Gel: VPK=	Reiki	carbohydrates
	C: 2,000 mg.	Lavender: PK-Vo	Calamus: VK-P+	Therapeutic touch	Sedentary
Plenty of	E: 600 IU	Myrrh: VK-P+	Black Pepper: KV-P+		lifestyle
fluids	Bioflavinoids: 200 mg.	Tea Tree: VPK=	Yellow Dock: PK-V+		Sitting in
	Calcium: 800 mg.	Chamomile: VPK-	Haritaki: VK-Po		upright chair
Low cellulose		Basil: VK-P+	Alum Root: PK-V+		
		Clary Sage: VPK-	Pomegranate: PK-Vo		

Salads	Frankincense: KV-P+	Red Raspberry: PK-V+
	Helichrysum: PKV+	Marshmallow: PV-K+
	Juniper: KV-P+	Mullein: PK-V+
Green	Patchouli: VP-K+	Ginseng: V-KPo
vegetables	Peppermint: PK-Vo	Astralagus: PVK+
	Yarrow: PK-V+	Black Cohosh: PK-V+
Fresh fruits	Tagetes: VK-P+	Basil: VK-P+
		Dry Ginger: KV-P+
Radish juice		Turmeric: KV-Po
		Amalaki: PV-Ko
		Trikatu: VK-Po
		Triphala: PVK
		Guggul: KV-P+

Herbal Brew

Vata		Pitta		Kapha	
Astralagus	2 oz.	Chamomile	2 oz.	Pomegranate	2 oz.
Basil	1 oz.	Mullein	1 oz.	Basil	1 oz.
Pippali	1 oz.	Yarrow	1 oz.	Pippali	1 oz.
Ginger	1 oz.				

Pitta & Kapha Suppository recipe

½ oz. Witch Hazel Leaf or Bark

½ oz. Oak Bark (powdered)

1 oz. Cocoa Butter

Melt cocoa butter in frying pan.

Add herbs Castor oil

Remove from fire

Add essential oils: 5 drops of cypress

Form into bullet shaped suppositories ½" in diameter, 1" long

Lay on plate. Cover. Place in refrigerator to harden

Vata Suppository recipe

Tumeric Powder	½ oz.
Aloe Vera gel	½ tsp.
Slippery Elm	½ tsp.

Grind herbs in blender, mix 2 Tablespoons aloe vera gel with:

Ghee	2 tsp.

2 tsp.

Apply in rectal area

Refrigerate leftover

Use each night until well

Vata & Kapha Recipe

1 oz. vegetable oil

Add 5 drops Cypress essential oil (or any suggested essential oil)

Rub into anus and inject small amount with rectal syringe (or baby ear syringe)

Self-Care

Warm sitz bath

Witch hazel compresses

Wear pearls

Place 4-5 pears in water overnight and drink the water.

Ice packs

Crush black sesame seeds (3-4 gms.) in hot water and take a sitz bath.

When sitting for long periods, use a pillow

Vitamin E on rectum

HEADACHE

This is symptom rather than a disease. The possible causes of headaches include eyestrain, stress, tension, musculoskeletal problems, misaligned spine, sinus or ear infections, high blood pressure, allergies, caffeine withdrawal or coffee toxicity, P.M.S., chocolate, hormonal fluctuations, an imbalance in arteries in the head, TMJ problems, changes in barometric pressure, overdoses of vitamin A, low blood sugar, and hangovers. To treat headaches, you must become a detective. Vata headaches are severe and pounding and are often caused by constipation. Pitta headaches usually occur in the middle of the day and may be burning and throbbing relative to impure blood, anger, irritability, judgements, or too much heat in the body. Kaphas usually wake up with a headache; the pain is dull and could be related to sinus congestion.

Feelings and Emotions : Not being flexible. Stressed. What is it you don't want to do or look at?

Cell Salts : Kali-Phos; Mag-Phos; Natmure; Silica

Diet	Vitamins & Minerals (Daily)	Essential Oils (Always dilute)	Herbs	Alternative Therapy	Avoid
Ayurvedic diet for body type	Quercetin: 500 mg.	Eucalyptus: KV-P+	Feverfew: PK-V+	Acupuncture	Caffeine
	Magnesium: 500 mg.	Menthol: PK-V+	Yellow Jasmine: PK-V+	Massage	Cigarettes
	Evening Primrose: 1000 mg.	Camphor: VK-P+	Everlasting: VPK-	Colonics	Bad food

Rotation diet	A: 150 IU	Juniper: KV-P+	Valerian: VK-P+	Biofeedback	combinations
		(in excess)			
	B-Complex: 100 mg.	Bergamot: VK-P+	Sweet Woodruff: VPK+	Chiropractic	Wine
Plenty of	B1: 100 mg.	Hyssop: K-P+Vo	Cayenne Pepper: KV-P+	treatments	Steroids
water	B2: 10 mg. per meal	Lavender: PK-Vo	Eucalyptus: VK-P+	Dance	Dairy
Food diary	Pangamic Acid: 100 mg.	Tea Tree: VPK=	Goldenseal: PK-V+	therapy	Wheat
	Pantothenic Acid: 100 mg.	Cajeput: KV-P+	Willow Bark: PK-V+	Shiatsu	Beef
	C: 1000 mg.	Lemon: PV-Ko	Peppermint: KP-Vo	Trager work	
	E: 1200 IU	Peppermint: PK-Vo	Ginger: VK-P+	Cranial sacral	
	Calcium: 1,500 mg.	Geranium: PK-V+		Electrical	
	Iron: 80 mg.	Ginger: VK-P+		stimulation	
	Potassium: 3,000 mg.	Chamomile: PK-V+			
	Natural Lithium: 300 mg.				
	Megadophilus:				
	3 x day				

Herbal Brew

Vata		Pitta		Kapha	
Ginger	2 oz.	Feverfew	2 oz	Jasmine Flowers	2 oz
Valerian	1 oz	Sweet Woodruff	1 oz.	Mint	1 oz.
Eucalyptus	1 oz.	Willow Bark	1 oz.	Guduchi	1 oz.

Shatavari	1 oz.	Mint	1 oz.	Willow Bark	1 oz.
		Guduchi	1 oz.		

Cinnamon - Ginger Paste

Cinnamon	½ tsp.
Ginger	½ tsp.
Water	2 Tbs

Mix well. Apply to the head. Let dry for 5 minutes. Wash off. Add a cool cloth over the area.

Headache-Free

Essential oil blend as Navratna taila or Ghrit Kumari Oil can be directly applied to the area of pain. Massage. Keep away from the eyes. At night, massage the neck.

Self-Care

Meditation	Tai Chi	Food diary
Visualization	Yoga	Compresses at night with essential oils of your choice
Relaxation techniques	Dance	Diffusing essentials oils at night
Hot baths	Basti oil enemas	Inhalation of relaxing oil blends

General caution : For migraine or recurrent headaches, consult a professional practitioner to diagnose and treat the underlying cause.

HEART ATTACK

When an adequate blood supply can no longer reach the heart, part of the heart muscle dies from lack of oxygen and other nutrients. This is classified as a heart attack or myocardial infraction. Individuals who have experienced heart attacks best describe the symptoms as an extreme tightening across the chest region or a feeling of heaviness in the chest/heart area. There may be radiating pain down left arm. Vata may experience tremors, extreme pain, contractions in the chest area, constipation, and dry cough; prone to myocarditis and pericarditis. Pitta may experience sweating, burning pain in chest, fever, and poor sleep patterns; prone to congestive heart failure. Kapha may experience a feeling of heaviness around the heart, difficulty with walking, congestion, phlegm, and tiredness; prone to cardiac arrest.

Feelings and Emotions: "Life pressing on my chest". Stressed, angry, always doing something. Attached. Holding on.

Cell Salts : Calcium Fluoride

Diet	Vitamins & Minerals (Daily)	Essential Oils (Always dilute)	Herbs	Alternative Therapy	Avoid
Ayurvedic diet	Linseed Oil - 200 mg.	Cypress: VPK+	Thyme: VK-P+	Bio-feedback	Stress
for body type	E: 500 Iu	Geranium: PK-V+	Hyssop: K-P+	Massage	Smoking
	D: 600 IU	Ginger: VK-P+	Cinnamon Bark: VK-P+	Acupuncture	Alcohol
	A: 15,000 IU	Lavender: PK-Vo	Skullcap: PK-Vo	Colour therapy	Cadmium
When high Vata,	B-Complex: 100 mg.	Rosemary: KV-P+	Arjuna: PK-V+	Chiropractic	Oral
do Kapha-Pitta	C: 25,000 mg.	Ylang-Ylang: PV-K+	Ashwagandha: VK-P+	treatments	Contraceptives
diet with	F: 200 mg.	Melissa: KP-Vo	Guggul: KV-P+	Tarpana	Saturated fats
cooked foods		Orange: VK-P+	Vervain: PK-V+	Shirodhara	Gaining weight
		Peppermint: PK-Vo	Saffron: VPK=	Pancha Karma	Sugar

Drink colloidal water	Rose: VPK=	Tansy: PK-Vo	Chelation therapy	Suppressing emotions
	Myrrh: KV-P+	Hawthorn Berries: V-KoP+		Greasy foods
	Sandalwood: PV-Ko	Cardamon: VK-P+		Red meat
	Angelica: VPK=	Liquorice: VP-K+		Table salt
	Borage: PKV+	Comfrey: VP-K+		Dairy
	Cardamon: VK-P+ (in excess)	Solomon's Seal: PV-K+		
		Gotu Kola: VPK=		
		Motherwort: PK-V+		
		Blue Cohosh: KV-P+		
		Coriander: VPK-		
		Goldenseal: PK-V+		
		Sorrel: VKoP+		
		Valerian: VK-P+		

Herbal Brew

Vata Tea (*drink warm*)		**Pitta Tea (*drink at room temperature*)**		**Kapha Tea (*drink warm*)**	
Dashmoola	1 oz.	Solomon Seal	2 oz.	Cardamon	2 oz.
Ginger, fresh	1 oz.	Coriander	1 oz.	Hawthorn Berries	2 oz.
Ashwagandha	2 oz.	Gotu Kola	2 oz.	Motherwort	1 oz.
Liquorice	1 oz.	Licorice	1 oz.	Blue Cohosh	1 oz.
Guduchi	1 oz.	Colloidal silver	30 drops	Chitrak	1 oz.

Sorrel	1 oz.
Hawthorn Berries	2 oz.

Herbal Formula :1		Herbal Formula #2	
Arjuna Powder	½ Tbs.	Guduchi	½ tsp.
Dashmoola	½ tsp.	Arjuna	½ tsp.
Triphalla Powder	½ tsp.	Punarnava	1 tsp.
Guggul	¼ tsp.	Shatavari	1 tsp.
Mix all ingredients together with water as a tea; or put in a capsule. Take 3 times per day.		Mix with 1 cup milk, rice milk, or soymilk.	

Vata & Kapha : Take with 6 Triphalla tablets at bedtime.

Self-Care

Visualization	Yoga	Experiencing love
Relaxation techniques	Meditation	Parasite cleanse
Spend time in nature	Wearing gemstones: ruby, garnet, gold, silver, pearl, moonstone, emerald, jade, yellow sapphire, yellow topaz	

HEPATITIS

A virus or bacteria that has several types: A, B, non-A, and non-B being the most common. Hepatitis A is transmitted mostly through fecal contamination. Hepatitis B is transmitted through infected blood or blood products and, occasionally, through saliva or sexual fluids. Hepatitis non-A and non-B is contacted most often through blood transfusions. Hepatitis can also be caused by Type D virus, cytomegaloveries and Epstein-Barr virus. Pitta usually displays the yellow eyes and fever, while the distinguishing characteristic in Vata is pain, loss of appetite, anger, and resentment.

Feelings and Emotions : Anger. Lashing out and dumping emotions onto others.

Cell Salts : Sodium Phosphates.

Diet	Vitamins & Minerals (Daily)	Essential Oils (Always dilute)	Herbs	Alternative Therapy	Avoid
Ayurvedic diet	A: 1000 mg.	Chamomile: PK-Vo	Aloe Vera: VPK=	Lymphatic drainage	Saturated fats
for body type	C: 10-15 mg.	Cinnamon: VK-P+	Barberry: PK-V+	massage	Sugar
	B12: shots	Cypress: VPK+	Dandelion: PK-V+	Homeopathics	Flour
Low in	Folic Acid: 100 mg.	Eucalyptus: KV-P+	Gentian: PK-V+	Acupuncture	Fruit juice
saturated fats	Liver Extract:	Melaleuca: VKP	Rhubarb: PK-V+	Chiropractic	Honey
	500 mg. 3 x day	Peppermint: PK-Vo	Goldenseal: PK-V+	Ayurvedic	Animal fat
Anti-Pitta	Choline: 1 gm. 3 x day	Patchouli: VP-K+	Amalaki: PV-Ko	consultation	Meat
diet	Methionine: 1 gm. 3 x day	Rosemary: KV-P+	Bhringaraj: VPK=		Marijuana
	Free Form Amino Acid:	Ginger: VK-P+	Manjishta: PK-V+		Cigarettes
Raw green	2 gm. 3 x day	Rose: VPK=	Ginger: VK-P+		Amphetamines
vegetables &	Pangamic Acid: 100 mg.		Milk Thistle: OK-V+		Hot, spicy, sour
sprouts	F: 200 mg.		Rose: VPK=		& salty foods

Green juices	Liquorice: VP-K+	Anger
Kicharee	Horsetail: PK-V+	Resentment
	Turmeric: KV-Po	Depression
	Coriander: VPK-	Fish
	Guduchi: PK-V+	
	Sudan Shan : PKV	
	Chiretta: VPK-	
	Katuka: VKP+	

Herbal Brew

Vata		Pitta		Kapha	
Amla	1 oz.	Dandelion	1 oz.	Guduchi	1 oz.
Ginger	2 oz.	Barberry	2 oz.	Ginger	2 oz.
Liquorice	1 oz.	Katuka	2 oz.	Manjishta	2 oz.
Milk Thistle	2 oz.	Guduchi	1 oz.	Horsetail	1 oz.
Rose Petals	1 oz.	Liquorice	1 oz.	Coriander	1 oz.

Add 10 drops goldenseal extract to 1 cup tea.

Self-Care

Liver flush	Dry skin brushing
Compresses	Rebounder

HIGH BLOOD PRESSURE

Mild cases of high blood pressure and arteriosclerosis (hardening of the arteries) can benefit from herbs. Garlic thins the blood, reduces fatty deposits and lowers blood pressure; buckwheat and ginkgo aid circulation, reduce blood pressure and prevent arteriosclerosis; and ginger improves circulation, especially to the capillaries.

General caution : Seek professional advice, especially if already taking medication for a circulatory condition.

General Remedies

Herbs : Garlic (*Allium sativum*), Buckwheat (*Fagopyrum esculentum*)

Remedy : Take either herb in tablet form or eat 1-2 fresh garlic cloves each day.

Note : Garlic is most effective when used as a regular preventative, rather than a remedy.

Herb : Ginkgo (*Ginkgo biloba*)

Remedy : Take tablets or ½ tsp of fluid extract with water twice a day for 2-3 months at a time.

Herb : Ginger (*Zingiber officinale*)

Remedy : Take ¼ tsp of fresh ginger into your food each day.

HOT FLASHES

A condition that occurs with the onset of menopause and is accompanied by a decrease in estrogen levels. Hot flashes usually affect the head and upper body, but can cover the torso or entire body. The length and duration of hot flashes vary from a few seconds to more than ten minutes. After a hot flash, a woman can feel slightly damp or thoroughly drenched in perspiration: this occurs most commonly in Pitta types.

Feelings and Emotions : Stress, Lacking in trust.

Diet	Vitamins & Minerals (Daily)	Essential Oils (Always dilute)	Herbs	Alternative Therapy	Avoid
Pitta diet	B-Complex: 200 mg.	Basil: VK-P+	Valerian: VK-P+	Biofeedback	Hot rooms
	C: 1300 mg.	Thyme: VK-P+	Wild Yam: VP-Ko	Homeopathics	Heat
	Magnesium: 2000 mg.	Lavender: PK-Vo	Red Clover: PK-V+	Dance therapy	Stress
Eat small meals	Potassium: 200 mg.	Calamus: VK-P+	Oatstraw: PV-K+	Massage	Tension
Salads	E: 1200 IU	Sage: VK-P+	Chickweed: PK-V+		Caffeine
Wild yams	Selenium: 200 mg.	Rose: VPK=	Elder: PK-Vo		Hot drinks
Cooling food	Bioflavenoids: 200 mg.	Myrrh: VK-P+	Violet: PK-V+		Tobacco
Soybeans	Black Current Oil: 100 mg.	Bergamot: VK-P+	Dandelion: KP-V+		Marijuana
Greens	D: 500 mg.	Clary Sage: VKP-	Yellow Dock: PK-V+		Spicy foods
Protein		Fennel: VPK=	Black Cohosh: Vk-P+		Acid foods
		Peppermint: PK-Vo	Vitex: VKP-		Alcohol
	Iron: 30 mg.		Dong Quai: VK Po		Fatc
	B3: 100 mg.		Sage: VK-P+		
			Liquorice: PV-Ko		
			Black Haw: VKP+		
			Alfalfa: PK-V+		
			Raspberry: PK-ᐯ+		
			Black Currant : PK-V+		

Wormwood: PK-Vo
Fenugreek: VK-P+
Blessed Thistle: PK-V+
Elder Flower: PK-Vo
Chaparral: PK-V+
Damiana: K-Vo-P+
Saffron: VPK=
Manjishta: PK-V+
Ginseng: V-KPo
Shatavari: PV-K+

Herbal Brew

Vata		Pitta		Kapha	
Fenugreek	2 oz.	Red Clover	2 oz.	Blessed Thistle	2 oz.
Shatavari	2 oz.	Vitex	2 oz.	Elder Flowers	1 oz.
Valerian	1 oz.	Liquorice	1 oz.	Sage	1 oz.
Vitex	2 oz.	Red Raspberry	1 oz.	Red Clover	1 oz.
Liquorice	1 oz.	Alfalfa	1 oz.	Damiana	1 oz.

Self-Care

Cool footbaths	Cool full body baths	Wear silk
Exercise	Meditation	Positive mental attitude
Yoga : sun salutation	Essential oil patches	Meditation
Mantra	Breathing exercises	

HYPOGLYCEMIA

Hypoglycemia represents a sudden drop in blood sugar. The brain is highly dependent on glucose as an energy source. A drop in blood sugar results in the release of hormones that work to increase those blood sugar levels, with adrenaline being one of those hormones. Vatas may experience tremors, anxiety, nausea, headaches, and dizziness. Pittas experience sweating, extreme hunger and increase in heart rate; Kaphas experience clouded vision, confusion, and tiredness.

Feelings and Emotions : A powerless victim. Feeling "less than."

Diet	Vitamins & Minerals (Daily)	Essential Oils (Always dilute)	Herbs	Alternative Therapy	Avoid
Ayurvedic diet	B-Complex: 100 mg	Ginger: VK-P+	St. John's Wort: PK-V+	Massage	Alcohol
for body type	B-12: 1000 mcg.	Anise: VK-P+	Shatavari: PV-K+	Acupuncture	Skipping meals
	C: 3,000 mg.	Cardamon: VK-P+	Dong Quai: VK-Po	Reflexology	Candy bars
Low animal	Folic Acid : 800 mcg.	Basil: VK-P+	Barberry: PK-V+		Refined
protein	Magnesium: 340 mg.	Rosemary: VK-P+	Aloe vera: VPK=		carbohydrates
	for 6 weeks	Oregano: VKP+	Trikatu: VK-P+		Coffee
Shitaki	Amino Acid Liquids;	Thyme: VK-P+	Triphalla: VKPo		Marijuana

Mushrooms	1000 mg.	Geranium: PK-V+	Calumba: PK-V+	Chocolate
	Alpa: 400 mg.	Lemongrass: PK-Vo	Gentian: PK-V+	Milk
Blue-Green	Potassium: 200 mg.	Sandalwood: PV-Ko	Golden Thread: PK-V+	Goldenseal
Algae	Digestive Aid: Best to	Yarrow: PK-V+	Guduchi: PKV+	Black Tea
	take 2 before mealtime		White Poplar: PK-V+	Soft Drinks
	Comfrey/Pectin:		Peruvian Bark: PK-V+	
	before meals		Katuka: PVK	
Bitter greens	2 tables 2-x day		Neem: PK-V+	
	Chromium: 200 mg.		Shilajit: K-VP+	
Low	Manganese: 200 mg.		Chiarata: PVK-	
carbohydrates			Yellow Dock: PK-V+	
			Hawthorn Berries: V-KoP+	
Cinnamon	Aloe vera Gel: 1 Tbs. 3 x per		Cardamon: VK-P+	
	day with lemon & apple juice		Clove: VK-P+	
Peanut butter	L-Tryptophan: 6 gms.			
Spirulina	Bee Pollen: 1 tsp. per day			

Herbal Brew

Vata		Pitta		Kapha	
Angelica	2 oz.	Lemongrass	1 oz.	Cardamom	2 oz.
Astralagus	2 oz.	Lemongrass	1 oz.	Ginger	1 oz.
Oat Straw	2 oz.	Liquorice	1 oz.	Liquorice	1 oz.
Ginger	1 oz.	Astralagus	2 oz.	Peppermint	2 oz.
Ashwagandha	2 oz.	Peppermint	2 oz.	Lemongrass	2 oz.
Liquorice	1 oz.				

Pancreatic Soup

Vata		Pitta		Kapha	
Ginger	2 inches	Green beans (cut in small pieces)		Spinach	1 bunch
Sweet Potatoes	1	Brussel sprouts	¼ lb.	Ginger, fresh	2 inch
Carrots	4	Kale	1 bunch	Kale	1 bunch
Beet & Greens	1	Shitaki mushrooms	4 oz.	Brussel sprouts	¼ lb.
Celery stalks	4	Sweet potato	1	Celery	4 stalks
Shitaki mushrooms	4 oz.	Mint	¼ bunch	Parsley	½ bunch
Asparagus	½ lb.	Cilantor	½ bunch	Carrots	3
Turmeric	2 tsp.	Coriander	3 tsp.	Lemongrass	2 tsp.

Tomato	3	Water	1 quart	Onions	1
Onions	1			Garlic	2-3 cloves
Water	1 quart			Cumin	½ tsp.
				Water	1 quart

Chop all ingredients. Add potatoes, carrots and mushrooms to the water. Bring to a boil. Saute all herbs in ghee. Add sauteed herbs and greens to the pot of soup. Simmer for two hours.

Drink

In a blender, mix 2 tsp. Aloe vera Gel, the juice of 1 lemon. Add 4-oz, apple juice. Blend

Self-Care

Massage feet with oils.

Tai Chi	Yoga	Walking
Sunbathing	Meditation	Breathwork

INDIGESTION

Indigestion is when you experience burning and gas. This can be caused by too little hydrochloric acid as well as too much. It is more common for Pittas to experience hyperacidity with belching caused by sour food and too many sweets. Vatas can experience low hydrochloric acid and more gas fermentation due to weak digestion. Kaphas can experience excess mucous due to slow digestion. To determine if indigestion is excess acidity or lack of acidity, test your saliva with nitrosine paper. Average reading below 6.8 pH = hyperacidity. Average reading above 7.2 pH = lac of acidity.

Feelings and Emotions Unable to bring thoughts and desires into reality.

Cell Salts Potassium Phosphate

Diet	Vitamins & Minerals (Daily)	Essential Oils (Always dilute)	Herbs	Alternative Therapy	Avoid
Ayurvedic diet	B-Complex: 100 mg.	Coriander: VPK-	Asafoerida: VK-P+	Rotation diet	Coffee
for body type	B1: 100 mg.	Bay: VKP+	Dill: PK-Vo	Dairy diet	Tobacco
	B3: 100 mg.	Ginger: VK-P+	Aloe vera Gel: VPK=	Ayurvedic	Fats
Small, frequent	B12: 400 mcg.	Cinnamon: VK-P+	Liquorice: VP-K+	consultation	Beans
meals	Acidophilus: 2 tablets	Basil: VK-P+	Black Pepper: VK-P+		Antacids
	30 minutes	Clove: KV-P+	Pippali: VK-P+		
Take time to chew	before meal	Ajwan: VK-P+	Mint: PK-Vo		
	Lecithin: 800 mg.	Thyme: VK-P+	Coriander: VPK=		
Do not drink	Digestive Enzymes:	Mint: PK-Vo	Ajwan: VK-P+		
with meals	Papain - 2 before meals	Angelica: VPK=P+	Slippery Elm: VP-K+		
	Amino Acids: 2 with meals	Cardamon: VK-P+	Trikatu: VK-P+		
		Fennel: VPK=	Comfrey: PV-K+		
Bananas	Bromelain: 2 before meals	Peppermint: PK-Vo	Hingastash: VK-Po		
Cabbage juice	HCL: 2 tables with				
	protein meal				

Herbal Brew

Vata		Pitta		Kapha	
Comfrey	1 oz.	Coriander	1 oz.	Clove	1 oz.
Ginger	½ oz.	Fennel	½ oz.	Ginger	1 oz.
Cinnamon	½ oz.	Mint	½ oz.	Black Pepper	½ oz.
Liquorice	½ oz.	Liquorice	½ oz.	Coriander	½ oz.

Drink three cups per day before meals.

Drink first thing in the morning

Vata-Kapha

Lemon	1 oz.
Ginger, fresh	2 inch piece
Water	3 cups

Blend all together. Strain. Drink.

Pitta & Kapha

Lemon	1 oz.
Fennel or Coriander	1 tsp.

Blend all together. Strain. Drink.

Vata

Take hing (1/16 tsp. with ghee. Mix together. Follow with water -3 times per day)

Essential Oil Formula

Angelic	2 drops	Fennel	3 drops
Cardamon	2 drops	Peppermint	2 drops

Vegetable oil 2 oz.

Mix together. Place 2 drops in 8 oz. Drink daily. Only use good quality essential oils when taking orally.

Old Time Remedy

Baking soda	2 Tbs.
Water	8 oz. glass

Dill Infusion

Dill	4 tsp.
Water	8 oz. glass

Boil water. Place herbs in container. Then add water to dill in container. Steep 15 minutes. Take 4 times per day.

Self-Care

Cook all beans with hing.

Compress over the stomach area.

INFECTION

Caused by a foreign organism entering the body, which the body is unable to destroy due to a weakened immune system. It can spread into other body parts as well as the blood, and become systemic. Pitta experiences swollen glands, boils, and redness; Vata may get a sore throat, dry cough, dizziness, and headaches; Kapha is plagued by respiratory and sinus problems.

Feelings and Emotions : I am weak. I am a victim.

Diet	Vitamins & Minerals (Daily)	Essential Oils (Always dilute)	Herbs	Alternative Therapy	Avoid
Immune support	A: 75,000 IU (until clear)	Thyme: VK-P+	Astralagus: VK-P+	Color therapy	Allergic foods
	Zinc: 50 mg.	Eucalyptus: KV-P+	Burdock: PK-V+	Colonics	Dairy
Yellow foods	C: 10,000 mg.	Oregano: VK-P+	Goldenseal: PK-V+	Music therapy	Sugars
	Potassium: 1,000 mg.	Rosemary: KV-P+	Rosehips: V-PK+		Canned foods
Juice fasts	Bioflavinoids: 250 mg.	Saffron: VPK-	Manjishta: PK-V+		Meats
	Colloidal Silver: PK-V+		Katuka: PK-V+		
Vata immune soup			Echinacea: KP-V+		
			Bayberry: KV-P+		
			Isatis: VKP+		
Cleansing diet			Turmeric: KV-Po		
			Coriander: VKP=		
			Dandelion: KP-V+		
			Amla: PV-Ko		
			Juniper Berries: KV-P+ (drink a lot of water)		

Herbal Brew

Vata		Pitta & Kapha	
Amla	1 oz.	Barberry	1 oz.
Ginger	1 oz.	Fennel	2 oz.
Astralagus	2 oz.	Dandelion	2 oz.
Rosehips	2 oz.	Coriander	1 oz.
		Burdock	1 oz. (Kapha only)

Add goldenseal extract - 15 drops. Drink 6 cups per day, until symptoms are gone.

Self-Care

Warm & cold baths with essential oils

Colon cleanse

Steam

Rebounder

Dry skin brushing

INFLAMMATION

This is a heating condition in the body which is caused by injury, trauma, accident, toxic blood (Ama), stress, or infection. The internal organs can also become inflamed. This conditon is more common for Pitta types.

Feelings and Emotions : Not feeling centered in life.

Cell Salts : Ferr Phos; Iron Phosphate

Diet	Vitamins & Minerals (Daily)	Essential Oils (Always dilute)	Herbs	Alternative Therapy	Avoid
Ayurveda Diet	B-Complex: 200 mg.	Lavender: PK-Vo	Fenugreek: VK-P+	Colour healing	Hot, spicy
for body type	B5: 2,500 mg.	Chamomile (blue): PV-K+	Goldenseal: PK-V+	Reiki	food
	B12: 300 mg.	Cyperus: VPK-	Hops: PK-V+	Chiropractic	Alcohol
Raw foods for	E: 150 IU	Yarrow: PK-V+	Lobelia: K-PV+	treatments	Sugar
Pitta & Kapha	Flaxseed: 500 mg.	Sandalwood: PV-Ko	Marshmallow: PV-K+	Energy work	Junk food
		Juniper: KV-P+ (in excess)	Mugwort: VK-P+		
Food combining		Geranium: PK-V+	Sarsaparilla: PV-Ko		
		Rose: VPK=	Slippery Elm: VP-K+		
Lots of green		Trifolia: VK-P+	Solomon's Seal: PV-K+		
juice			Sorrel: V-PK+		
			Tansy: PK-Vo		
			White Pond Lily: PV-K+		
			Cyperus: PK-Vo		
			Witch Hazel: PK-V+		
			Smart Weed: PKV+		
			Hyssop : VK-P+		
			Chickweed: PK-V+		

Gum Arabic: PV-K+
Chamomile: PK-Vo
Yarrow: PK-V+

Herbal Brew

Vata		Pitta		Kapha	
Slippery Elm	1 oz.	Yarrow	2 oz.	Fenugreek	2 oz.
Sorrel	2 oz.	Chamomile	2 oz.	Witch Hazel	1 oz.
Fenugreek	2 oz.	Mint	2 oz.	Chickweed	1 oz.
Kava Kava	1 oz.	Hops	1 oz.		

Self-Care

Cold compresses

Ice therapy

Charcoal poultice

INSOMNIA

Insomnia is the inability to sleep soundly and undisturbed. Its most common causes are anxiety and pain, but it may also be a symptom of a serious disease. A major factor in sleeplessness is linked to the inability to cope with stress.

Feelings and Emotions : Anxious, stressful. Too many fearful thoughts.

Homeopathics: Kali Phos (potassium phosphate)

Diet	Vitamin & Minerals (Daily)	Essential Oils (Always dilute)	Herbs	Alternative Therapy	Avoid
Ayurvedic diet	B-Complex: 20 mg.	Lavender: PK-Vo	Hops: PK-V+	Therapeutic Touch	Late night TV
for body type	B6: 100 mg.	Chamomile: VPK-	Motherwort: PK-V+	Reiki	Caffeine
	B12: 100 mcg.	Camphor: VK-P+	Mullein: PK-V+	Counseling	Stimulants
Protein	Niacin: 100 mg.	Thyme: VK-P+	Vervain: PK-V+	Massage	Chocolate
	Pantothenic Acid:	Marjoram: VK-P+	Skullcap: PK-Vo	Shirodhara	Soda
Baked potatoes	2,000 mg.	Neroli: VP K+	Catnip: PK-Vo		Sugar
	C: 3,000 mg.	Rose: VPK=	Kava Kava: PVK		Stress
Sweetened milk	D: 500 IU	Sandalwood: PV-Ko	Passion Flower: PK-V+		
	Calcium: 1000 mg.	Ylang-Ylang: PV-K+	Valerian: VK-P+		
Bananas	before bedtime	Orange: VK-P+	Chamomile: PK-Vo		
	Magnesium: 1000 mg.	Coriander: VKP-	Jatamasi: KV-P+		
Herbal teas	before bedtime	Melissa: KP-Vo	Nutmeg: VK-P+		
	Phosphorous: 2000 mg.	Mandarin: PK-V+			
Rice & hot	Potassium: 2500 mg.	Rosemary: VK-P+			
sweetened milk	Melatonin: 100 mg.	Basil: VK-P+			
Wheat	Co Q-10: 100 mg.				
Oatmeal	DHEA: 50 mg.				
Almonds					

Walnuts

Oranges, Mandarins

Raisins

Foods containing

Tryptophan

Herbal Brew

Vata		Pitta		Kapha	
Valerian	1 oz.	Hops	1 oz.	Skullcap	1 oz.
Catnip	2 oz.	Skullcap	1 oz.	Valerian	1 oz.
Nutmeg	2 oz.	Chamomile	2 oz.	Hops	2 oz.
Jatamasi	1 oz.	Passion Flower	2 oz.	Passion Flower	2 oz.
		Brahmi	1 oz.		

Drink one cup after dinner. At bedtime, add milk.

Self-Care

Enemas	Leisurely walk before bedtime	Swimming
Warm baths	Hot bath before bed	Hot milk
Soft music	Meditation	Stress reduction techniques

Daily aerobic exercise	Yoga asana: "crocodile pose" (Makarasan)	Mantra repetitions
Massage head and shoulders	Abyangha at night (self massage)	Self-Reiki

Aromatherapy: Diffuse essential oils near bed or put a few drops of essential oil on your pillow.

General Cautions : Only take ginseng during the day and do not take with caffeine. Do not take continuously for more than 6 weeks. Do not take during pregnancy. Do not give to children under 12.

KIDNEY STONES

They are abnormal accumulations of mineral salts which form in the kidneys and are sometimes passed into the urinary tract. The formation of these stones may be due to overactivity of the parathyroid gland which causes elevated calcium levels in the blood. Stones area caused by poor diet, a weakening of the pancreas, and the reduction of enzymes. Pitta manifests acute infections, with wet yellow stones; Vata experiences colon pain with brown to black stones; while Kapha may find puss in their urine, along with stones composed of calcium.

Diet	Vitamin & Minerals (Daily)	Essential Oils (Always dilu	Herbs	Alternative Therapy	Avoid
Ayurvedic diet	A: 10,000 IU (until clear)	Juniper: KV-P+	Parsley: VK-P+	Massage	Dehydration
for body type	B2: 200 mg.	Cyperus: PKV-	Thyme: VPK+	Energy work	Infections
	B5: 1000 mg.	Orange: VK-P+	Corn Silk: PK-V+	Acupuncture	Prolonged bed rest
Apple juice	B6: 200 mg.	Lemongrass: PK-Vo	Dandelion: PK-V+		Vitamin B6 deficiency
Cilantro	C: 2500 mg.	Myrtle: KP-V+	Juniper: VK-P+		Magnesium deficiency
Lemon juice	E: 400 IU	Uva Ursi: PK-V+			Vitamin A deficiency
Water melon	F: 200 mg.	Marshmallow: PV-K+			Sugar
	Choline: 500 mg.	Horsetail: PK-V+			Food high in

Potassium: 1000 mg.	Gokshura: PK-Vo	oxalic acid
Magnesium: 500 mg.	Manjishta: PK-V+	Coffee
	Buchu Leaves: PK-V+	Black tea
	Plantain: PK-V+	Red meat
	Shilajti: VK-P+	Antacids
	Gravel Root : PK-V+	Dairy
	Cleavers: PK-V+	Alcohol
	Pashanbheda: VPK	Nightshade vegetables

Herbal Brew

Vata		Pitta		Kapha	
Lemongrass	1 oz.	Horsetail	1 oz.	Cornsilk	2 oz.
Coriander	2 oz.	Cilantro	2 oz.	Buchu Leaves	1 oz.
Goshkura	1 oz.	Plantain	1 oz.	Lemongrass	2 oz.
Marshmallow	2 oz.	Coriander	2 oz.	Horsetail	1 oz.

Take : 500 grams of Shilajit - 3 times per day with tea.

Self-Care

Compresses

Kidney flush

Purgatives

Basti oil enemas

LARYNGITIS

It is the inflmmation of the mucous membrane of the larynx, and may be either acute or chronic. It can come by exposure to cold increasing Vata, or through a congestion extending from the nose above, or from the bronchial tubes causing great redness for Pittas. Kaphas may experience swelling, and Vatas may experience dryness. Vatas may experience dry throat, loss of voice, or hoarseness. Pitta may experience yellow mucous and inflammation with fever. Kaphas may have swollen throat with much mucous.

Feelings and Emotions : Difficulty with speaking their truth.

Cell Salts : Kali Murr, Potassium Chloride

Diet	Vitamin & Minerals (Daily)	Essential Oils (Always dilute)	Herbs	Alternative Therapy	Avoid
Ayurvedic diet	A: 100,000 IU	Benzoin: VPK-	Amla: VP-K+	Breathing therapy	Dairy
for body type	B-Complex: 200 mg.	Sandalwood: VPKo	Goldenseal: PK-V+	Sound therapy	Overexposure to cold
	C: 3000-5000 mg.	Cajeput: VK-P+	Echinacea: PK-V+	Lymphatic drainage	Protein foods
Elimination	Zinc: 50 mg.	Fennel: VPK=-	Rosehips: V-PK+	Chakra annointment	
diet	Zinc lozenges every	Anise: VK-P+	Lemon Peel: PV-Ko	Neck massage	
	2-3 hours	Lemon: VP-Ko	Purnarnara: PK-V+		
		Thyme: VK-P+	Astragalus: PVK+		
		Oregano: VK-P+	Yarrow: KP-V+		

Cinnamon: VK-P+	Angelica: VK-Po
Clove : VK-P+	Ginger: VK-P+
Coriander: VPK-	Boneset: PK-V+
	Burdock: PK-V+
	Mint: PK-Vo
	Ephedra : K-VP+
	Sage: VK-P+
	Jasmine: PK-V+
	Elecampane: VK-P+
	Bibhitaki: KP-Vo
	Turmeric: VK-Po
	Licorice: VP-K+

Herbal Brew

Vata		Pitta		Kapha	
Rosehips	2 oz.	Yarrow	1 oz.	Sage	2 oz.
Lemon Peel or Orange Peel	1 oz.	Mint	1 oz.	Ginger	1 oz.
Astralagus	2 oz.	Burdock	2 oz.	Yarrow	1 oz.
Ginger	1 oz.	Jasmine	1 oz.	Elecampane	1 oz.
Cinnamon	½ oz.	Astralagus	1 oz.	Amalaki	2 oz.

Add 10 drops of goldenseal tincture per cup for all body types.

Gargle

4-5 times per day. Add to one cup of water:

Sandalwood	1 drop
Thyme	1 drop
Cajeput	1 drop

Inhalation

Repeat every three hours with one of the following oils:

Sandalwood	3 drops
Thyme	3 drops
Cajeput	3 drops

Self-Care

Steam bath

Inhalations

Fomentations

Vapour rub throat

LEUCORRHEA

A whitish, brown or yellow vaginal discharge with an abnormal odour and a stickiness. This condition creates irritation and discomfort. More common in Kapha women, yet all body types can be affected. Vata's get dryness with brown discharge and itchiness. Pitta's experience inflammation, external redness, burning, a cheese texture to the discharge, and a sour odour. Kapha's experience thick mucus, swelling and heaviness.

Feelings and Emotions : Feeling unsupported by male energies.

Diet	Vitamins & Minerals (Daily)	Essential Oils (Always dilute)	Herbs	Alternative	Avoid Therapy
Ayurvedic diet	A: 75,000 mg. (until clear)	Tea Tree: VPK=	Pau d'Arco: PK-V+	Vaginal massage	Refined sugar
for body type	B-Complex: 4 tablets	Dhavana: VPK-	Goldenseal: KP-V+	Rebirthing	Fructose
	(yeast free)	Trifolia: VK-P+	Raspberry Leaves: PK-V+	Tarpana	Fruit concentrates
Yeast free diet	Biotin: 100 mcg.		Myrrh: VK-P+		Mushrooms
	D: 100 IU		Echinacea: PK-V+		Yeasted breads
	Calcium: 800 mg.		Wild Yam: PV-Ko		Frozen foods
	Magnesium: 600 mg.		Prickly Ash: KV-P+		Canned foods
	F: 200 mg.		Alum Root: PK-Vo		Pickles
	Evening Primrose: 200 mg.		Turmeric: VK-Po		Smoked dried meat
	Caprylic Acid: 2 tablets		Aloe Vera: VPK=		Moldy foods
	B6: 200 mg.		Shatavari: PV-K+		
	Zinc : 40 mg.		Katuka: KP-V+		
	Iron: 100 mg.		Oak Bark: VP-K+		
	Megadophilus: 3 x day		Sarsaparilla: PV-Ko		

Herbal Brew

Vata		Pitta		Kapha	
Wild Yam	1 oz.	Katuka	1 oz.	Katuka	1 oz.
Sarsaparilla	1 oz.	Raspberry Leaves	1 oz.	Raspberry Leaves	1 oz.
Shatavari	½ oz.	Shatavari	½ oz.	Sage	2 oz.
Prickly Ash	1 oz.	Wild Yam	½ oz.	Alum Root	½ oz.

Drink until condition clears up. Take 10-15 drops of echinacea.

Pessary

An ancient herbal form of a vaginal suppository

Coconut oil	1/8 cup
Cocoa butter	1 oz.
Herb of your choice	3 oz.

(Preferably *goldenseal, pau d'Arco, shatavari, alum, myrrh and sage*)

Sift all herbs well with a colander. Melt cocoa butter. Add vegetable oil.

Add herbs until mixture thickens. Remove from stove. Add essential oils.

Make into small cylinders, approximately ½ the size of your "pinky" in diameter. Place in refrigerator to harden for 1 hour. Remove from refrigerator. Store in container in cool place

For use: insert into the vagina for 3 hours. Pitta's should wear a panty liner for protection. Remove. Douche to remove excess.

Douche with strong decoction

Yogurt	½ cup
Water	¼ cup
Apple cider vinegar	¼ cup
Tea tree essential oil	10 drops

When itching occurs, insert fresh aloe into the vagina.

Dryness

Essential oils	20 drops
Water	1 cup

Mix well. Soak a tampax. Squeeze excess water, then insert in vagina. Change when dry.

MENSTRUAL PROBLEMS

The menstrual cycle can be disturbed for many reasons, most of them relating to hormonal imbalances. Other causes include stress, too much or too little exercise, weight problems, food sensitivity of allergy, steroids, the contraceptive pill, chronic illness, vitamin and mineral deficiency and even excess caffeine, alcohol or smoking. To determine the underlying cause, it is important to consult a professional practitioner.

Taking remedies for menstrual problems : The remedies listed should all be taken at the appropriate point in the cycle for 2-3 cycles.

The normal menstrual cycle lasts about 28 days. IF this cycle varies greatly from one period to another without reason, it could be termed irregular.

Pre-menstrual tension (PMT) and period pain have many causes and are experienced at some stage by most women. Breast tenderness, sore nipples and fluid retention are common symptoms.

Heavy periods can result in anaemia. If your period lasts longer than 5 days or if you have to change your protection every 2 hours, your periods may be too heavy. Nettle (*Urtica dioica*) is an excellent tonic, especially for heavy bleeding, as it contains more iron than spinach and can be eaten as a nourishing vegetable.

Self-help

Combine herbal remedies with a diet high in fresh vegetables and fruit, and low in fatty foods, sugar and alcohol. Try not to smoke. Regular exercise, particularly of the waist and pelvis, is helpful, as is a relaxed attitude to life. All reproductive problems will benefit from this simple approach.

General caution : For any chronic menstrual problem, it is wise to seek professional attention, especially if your periods are very heavy or painful.

(a) Irregular cycle

Herb Agnus castus (*Vitex agnus-castus*)

Remedy : Take tablets, or take 1.5-2 ml of tincture with water each morning on waking for at least 2 months.

Herb Motherwort (*Leonurus cardiaca*)

Remedy : Make an infusino and take 1-2 cups a day for up to 3 monthly cycles.

Caution : Do not take if menstrual bleeding is heavy.

(b) Pre-Menstrual Tension

Herbs Vervain (*Verbena officinalis*), Lime (*Tilia* spp.)

***Remedy* (Internal) :** Make on infusion using either herb (or an equal mix of both) and drink up to 5 cups throughout the day.

Herb : Valerian (*Valeriana officinalis*)

***Remedy* (Internal) :** Take tablets containing valerian, or take 20-40 drops of tincture with water up to 5 times a day.

Herb : Rosemary (*Rosmarinus officinalis*)

***Remedy* (External) :** Make an infusion with 1 tbsp of dried or 2 tbsp of fresh leaves to 1 litre of water and strain into a warm bath each morning. Alternatively, add 5-10 drops of essentials oil to a bath.

Note : Also try the agnus castus remedy under Irregular Cycle above.

(c) Breast Tenderness & Sore nipples

Herb : German chamomile (*Chamomilla recutita*)

Remedy : Make a compress with an infusion of 50 g of herb and 250 ml of water. Place gently over the breasts. Repeat as often as required.

Herb : Marigold (*Calendula officinalis*)

Remedy : Apply ointment to the nipples. If breast-feeding, wipe off the ointment before feeding.

(d) Fluid Retention

Herb : Dandelion (*Taraxacum officinale*)

Remedy : Make an infusion with the leaves and drink up to 3 cups a day.

(e) Heavy menstrual bleeding

Herbs : Chuang xiong (*Ligusticum wallachii*), White peony (*Paeonia lactiflora*), Chinese angelica (*Angelica sinensis*), Rehmannia (*Rehmannia glutinosa*).

Remedy : Mix equal parts of each root and make a decoction using 15 gm of the mixture to 750 ml of water. Drink in 3 equal doses throughout the day.

Note : Any of these herbs will help, but they are best together, in which form they are known as Four Things Soup.

Herbs : Shepherd's purse (*Capsella bursapastoris*), Nettle (*Urtica dioica*).

Remedy : Make an infusion using 7.5 g of each herb (or 15 g shepherd's purse only) to 750 ml of water. Divide into 3-5 doses and drink throughout the day.

(f) Period Pain

Flavour the decoctions with 1 heaped tsp of caraway seeds (*Carum carvi*). Mix before decocting.

Herbs : Wild yam (*Dioscorea villosa*), cramp bark (Viburnum opulus), black haw (*Viburnum prunifolium*).

Remedy : Make a decoction using 15 gm of one root to 750 ml of water. Sip small amounts during the day; or take 2 tsp of tincture with water 3-4 times a day for up to 3 days, then reduce the dose to 1 tsp a day for 5 days, or take tablets.

Herb : White peony (*Paeonia lactiflora*)

Remedy : Make a decoction using 20 g of root to 750 ml of water. Sip throughout the day.

MONONUCLEOSIS

It is characterized by chronic fatigue. Indicative of a chronically depressed immune system. It is an infections disease believed to be caused by a virus, which affects the lymph nodes located in the neck, armpits and groin. Symptoms include sore throat, fever, chills, swollen glands, as well as fatigue.

Feelings and Emotions : Not wanting to deal with life; it's too much.

Diet	Vitamin & Minerals (Daily)	Essential Oils (Always dilute)	Herbs	Alternative Therapy	Avoid
Ayurvedic	A: 5,000 IU (until clear)	Eucalyptus: KV-P+	Saffron: VPK=	Counseling	Birth control pills
diet for	B1: 150 mg.	Lavender: PK-Vo	Echinacea: KP-V+	Massage	Stress
body type	B2: 100 mg.	Blue Chamomile: PV-Ko	Astralagus: VP-K+	Acupuncture	Cigarettes
Protein	B6: 200 mg.	Bergamot: VK-P+	Ashwagandha: KV-P+	Pancha karma	X-ray
Fruit	Biotin: 140 mcg.	Saffron: VPK=	Angelica: VK-Po	Lymphatic	Fat
Mineral	Chlorine: 150 mg.		Red Root: PK-V+	drainage	Alcohol
water	Pantothenic Acid: 200 mg.		Lemon Peel: VP-Ko	Chiropractic	
Brewer's	C (ascorbate): 6000 mg.		Ginger: VK-P+	treatments	
yeast	Potassium: 800 mg.		Red Clover: PK-V+	Chakra balancing	
Eggs	Raw Thymus Extract:		Burdock: PK-V+		
Brown Rice			Lemongrass: PK-Vo		
	30 drops 3x / day				
	Raw glandular complex:				
Basmati Rice	40 drops or 2 tablets daily				
Garlic, Onions					
Asparagus					

Herbal Brew

Vata		Pitta		Kapha	
Astralagus	1 oz.	Red Root	1 oz.	Burdock	1 oz.
Angelica	1 oz.	Astralagus	2 oz.	Echinacea	1 oz.
Ginger	1 oz.	Coriander	2 oz.	Ginger	2 oz.
Lemon Peel	2 oz.	Echinacea	1 oz.	Lemongrass	1 oz.
Ashwagandha	2 oz.				

Self-Care

Hot herbs

Rest

Yoga

Compresses

Inhalation of essential oils

Fasting

Abyangha - self massage

MORNING SICKNESS

This occurs due to the rapid hormonal changes. Very often this is caused by vitamin B deficiency or low enzyme function, particularly hydrochloric acid. Vata experiences dizziness, flatulence, stomach problems, fatigue, and bloatedness. Pitta's experience irritability, diarrhea, becomes upset easily, heartburn, fevers, cravings of sour foods, and heat waves. Kapha's experience sleepiness, tiredness, sweet and starch cravings, water retention, rapid weight gain, nausea, vomiting, and depression.

Feelings and Emotions : Uneasiness and uncertainty about the birth process.

Diet	Vitamin & Minerals (Daily)	Essential Oils (Always dilute)	Herbs	Alternative Therapy	Avoid
Ayurvedic	B-Complex:	Ginger: VK-P+	Wild Yam: VP-Ko	Acupuncture	Cigarettes
diet for	4 tablets daily	Fennel: VPK=	Fennel: VPK=	Ayurveda	White sugar
body type	(yeast free)	Chamomile: VP-K+	Ginger: VK-P+	consultation	Coffee
Oatmeal	Digestive Aids	Lavender: PK-Vo	Dandelion: PK-V+	Music therapy	Black Tea
	Multi-vitamin	Lemon: PV-Ko	Vitex: VPK-	Energy work	Refined
Soup with		Peppermint: PK-Vo	Peppermint: PK-Vo	Homeopathics	carbohydrates
digestive herbs			Red Raspberry: PK-V+		Avoid yeasts
			Rose Petals: VPK-		
Ginger snaps			Shatavari: PV-K+		
			Slippery Elm: VP-K+		
Peppermint snaps			Cardamon: VK-P+		
Whole grains			Papaya Leaves: PK-V+		

Herbal Brew

Herbal Tea (as Gurukul Chai or Pragya) for all doshas.

For all doshas

Ginger	equal amounts	Fennel	equal amounts
Mint	equal amounts	Vegetable oil	50%

Massage on stomach a few times per day.

Self-Care

Abyangha	Foot bath	Breathwork
Meditation	Mantra	Tai Chi

MUMPS

Mumps is an infectious disease which is most common in children and is characterized by inflammatory swelling of the parotid and other salivary glands. Mumps, most often, affects the young and can be infectious one week or longer after the swelling of the glands has subsided. Once contracted, most people have lifetime immunity.

Cell Salts : Aconite, Belladonna

Diet	Vitamin & Minerals (Daily)	Essential Oils (Always dilute)	Herbs	Alternative Therapy	Avoid
Ayurvedic	A: 800 IU	Lavender: PK-Vo	Mullein: PK-V+	Reiki	Contact
diet for	B-Complex: 300 mg.	Lemon: PV-Ko	Sage: VK-P+	Therapeutic Touch	Citrus
body type	Multi-Complex :	Camphor: VK-P+	Bayberry: KV-P+	Color Therapy	Dairy
Acidophilus	4 tablets/day	Geranium: PK-V+	Root Bark: VPK	Music Therapy	Sugar
Green Juice	(children: 2 tablets)	Cypress: VK-P+	Echinacea: PK-V+		Poor food

Green	C: 3000 - Adults	Tea Tree : VPK=	Ginger Root: KV-P+	combining
vegetables	1500 - Children	Juniper: KV-P+	Lobelia: K-PV+	
Apples	1000 - under 12 years	Fennel: VPK=	Witch Hazel: PK-V+	
			White Oak Bark: PK-V+	
			Peppermint: PK-Vo	

Herbal Brew

Vata		Pitta & Kapha	
Ginger	2 Tbs.	Mullein	2 tbs.
Chamomile		Witch Hazel	1 tsp.
	2 Tbs.	Peppermint	1 tsp.
Add honey & lemon to taste		Chamomile	1 tsp.
		Add equal amount of apple juice	

Self-Care

Poultice of flaxseed

Steam bath

Warm compresses

NEURALGIA (NERVE PAIN)

Neuralgia is the pain caused by an irritated, damaged or trapped nerve, which usually occurs in brief, severe bouts and can be felt shooting along the nerve. Although it is difficult to treat, the following remedies may bring relief to minor problems. St. John's' wort is analgesic and antiviral, helping to relieve sciatica (pain caused by a trapped spinal nerve) and head pain. Cloves have an anaesthetic effect and peppermint eases pain.

General caution : Seek professional advice if there is fever, or swelling of the gums with toothache.

General Remedies

Herbs : St. John's wort (*Hypericum perforatum*) lavender (*Lavandula officinalis*), clove (*Eugenia caryophyllata*).

Remedy : Apply neat St. John's wort infused oil to painful areas, or add 20 drops each of clove and lavender essential oil to 50 ml of St. John's worth infused oil and then apply every 2-3 hours as required.

Herb : Peppermint (*Mentha piperita*)

Remedy : Make an infusion with 25 g of herb to 750 ml of water and bathe the affected area. Alternatively, dilute 20 drops of essential oil in 50 ml of carrier oil and gently massage into the painful area.

Caution : Do not use on children under 5.

Head Pain

Herb : Clove (*Eugenia caryophyllata*)

Remedy : Mix ½ tsp of powder with water to make a thick paste and apply to the head.

Toothache

Herb : Clove (*Eugenia caryophyllata*)

Remedy : Chew a clove or rub 1-2 drops of neat essential oil on to the affected tooth 2-3 times a day for up to 3 days.

OLD AGE/THIRD AGE

Traditionally, as we age, the 'fire' within us glows less brightly and our vitality slowly weakens. Many herbal medicines are ideally suited to treating the health problems that begin when people reach their late fifties, such as circulatory problems, weak digestion and poor memory. The herbs recommended here can help to maintain good health, preventing or reducing the severity symptoms that are often accepted as an inevitable consequence of ageing. Self treatment for other problems often experienced later in life, such as arthritis, is suggested in earlier sections.

Important Note

- If taking conventional medication tell your doctor if you intend to take a herbal remedy. This is especially important for the elderly.
- All remedies on this page need to be taken continuously for up to 3 months.
- If you are aged over 70, take ¾ of the stated dose for remedies given on other pages in this book.

(1) Maintaining Vitality

There are many herbs that help to maintain vitality.

Thyme is a much underrated herb. Recent research has discovered that it has anti-ageing and tonic properties which maintain vitality, and reduce the chance of catching colds, flue and other respiratory infections.

Withania is an alternative to ginseng and is considered a tonic herb that prevents or slows ageing. It si particularly helpful for regaining strength after a long illness, and is reputed to prevent hair turning grey.

Ginseng is taken by the elderly to help cope with the harsh winters. It is an excellent tonic for old age, improving vitality and resistance to stress and infection. Take for long-term stress and convalescence.

General Remedy

Herb : Thyme (*Thymus vulgaris*)

Remedy : Make a standard infusion. Take 2-3 cups a day.

(a) Stress or convalescence

Herb : *Withania somnifera*

Remedy : Take 1 gm of the root 2-3 times a day, either by chewing it or chopping it and mixing with a little water.

Herb : Ginseng (*Panax ginseng*)

Remedy : Take 1 gm 1-2 times a day for up to 3 months. Chew the fresh or dried root, cook it in a soup, or take in tablet form. Wait 3-4 weeks before taking it again.

Caution : Do not take caffeine while taking ginseng.

Option : If ginseng is too stimulating, take 3 gm of codonopsis (*Codonopsis pilosula*) a day in the same way as ginseng. This has a milder, but nonetheless tonic and strengthening, effect.

(b) Nervous exhaustion & stress

Herb : Oats (*Avena sativa*)

Remedy : Eat 25 gm of oats each day. Alternatively, take ½ tsp. of the tincture twice a day.

(2) General Conditions

Conditions that arise through ageing need patient, long-term treatment.

Ginkgo is the oldest tree, and its leaves maintain good circulation to the head and brain, improving memory, concentration and energy levels. Evidence suggests it may reduce the risk of a stroke.

Garlic, has great value as a long-term dietary supplement, helping to maintain healthy circulation, balance blood sugar levels, reduce high blood pressure and fat levels in the blood, and improve resistance to infection, especially bronchitis.

Rehmannia, a Chinese tonic herb with strengthening and mildly stimulant properties, appears to lower blood pressure and blood fat levels. It is suitable for people who have a weak liver and metabolism.

Gentian, a bitter herb, helps the absorption of food by maintaining digestive secretions, which diminish with age. Aperitifs, usually flavoured with bitter herbs, such as gentian, are a traditional way of preparing a weak digestion for a heavy or rich meal.

(a) Failing memory & concentration

Herb : Ginkgo (*Ginkgo biloba*)

Remedy : Take ginkgo tablets. These need to be taken regularly for at least 3 months before there is a noticeable improvement.

(b) Poor circulation & high blood pressure

Herb : Garlic (*Allium sativum*)

Remedy : Take 1-2 raw cloves a day with food, or take garlic tablets or capsules on a regular basis.

Herb : Buckwheat (*Fagopyrum esculentum*)

Remedy : Make a standard infusion and drink up to 2 cups a day.

(c) Chronic Infections

Herbs : Garlic (*Allium sativum*), Echinacea (*Echinacea* spp.)

Remedy : Take 1-2 raw cloves of garlic each day with food, or take either herb in tablet or capsule form on a regular basis.

(d) Weakened liver & metabolism

Herb : Rehmannia (*Rehmannia glutinosa*)

Remedy : Chew 5 gm of root 1-3 times a day, or make a decoction with 5 gm of root to 250 ml of water and take 1-3 times a day.

(e) Weakened Digestion

Herb : Gentian (*Gentiana lutea*)

Remedy : Take 5-10 drops of tincture with water 30 minutes before eating, 3 times a day.

Caution : Do not take gentian if you suffer from acid indigestion or a peptic ulcer.

PARASITES

There are several different types of worms which can live in our intestines. Most commonly found are hookworms, tapeworms roundworms, and pinworms. Because infestation of these parasites irritate the lining of the intestines, nutrient absorption from food is severely limited. Symptoms of parasites manifest itself in the form of weight loss, hunger pains, anemia, loss of appetite, and diarrhea.

Feelings and Emotions : Not caring for self.

Cell Salts : Natrium Phosphate, Sodium Phosphate

Diet	Vitamin & Minerals (Daily)	Essential Oils (Always dilute)	Herbs	Alternative Therapy	Avoid
Ayurvedic diet for	A: 10,000 IU B1: 200 mg.	Ginger: VK-P+ Lemon: VP-Ko	Mugwort: KV-P+ Black Walnut: V-PK+	Colonics Colloidal silver	Drinking ground water

body type	B2: 100 mg.	Tea Tree: VPK=	Bibhitaki: KP-Vo	Colour therapy,	Some raw ocean fish
Elimination	B6: 100 mg.	Clove: VK-P+	Tansy: PK-Vo	especially red	Sugar
diet	B12: 30 mcg.	Fennel: VPK=	Neem: PK-V+		Improper food
Horseradish	K: 200 mcg.	Neroli: VP-K+	Wormwood: PK-Vo		combining
Mustard	F: 200 mg.	Tangerine: VP-Ko	Prickly Ash: KV-P+		Insufficiently
Onions	D: 500 IU	Bergamot: VK-P+	Garlic: VK-P+		cooked
Acidophilus		Chamomile: VPK-	Basil: VK-P+		meats, especially
Protein	Potassium: 800 mg.	Lavender: PK-Vo	Rhubarb: PK-V+		beef, pork, & fish
Spices in	Calcium: 2000 mg.	Melissa: VP-Vo	Pysillium Husk: VP-K+		Walking barefoot
cooking		Angelica: VPK-	Hyssop: VK-P+		Bad personal
	Magnesium: 600 mg.	Camphor: VK-P+	Mountain Savory: VK-P+		hygiene
Small amount		Sage: VK-P+	Oregano: VK-P+		
of fruit		Trifolia: VK-P+	Tarragon: VK-P+		
		Hyssop: KV-P+	Thyme: VK-P+		
			Nutmeg: VK-P+		
			Marjoram: VK-P+		
			Bayberry: VK-P+		
			Black Pepper : VK-P+		
			Bay Leaves: KV-P+		
			Cardamon: KV-P+		
			Cayenne: VK-P+		
			Horseradish: VK-P+		
			Mustard: VK-P+		

Rosemary: VK-P+
Aloe vera Gel: VPK=
Pomegranate : PK-Vo
Asafoetida: VK-P+

Herbal Brew

Vata & Kapha

Black walnut tincture :

Day 1 -	Take 2 drops 4 times a day with milk or juice.
	1 wormwood capsule, 200-300 mg before supper
	3 capsules of cloves 3 times a day before meals
Day 2 -	Take 3 drops of black walnut tincture four times a day
	1 wormwood capsule before supper
	3 capsules of cloves before supper
Day 3 -	Take 3 drops of black walnut tincture
Days 4 to 10 -	Take 3 capsules of wormwood per day with 2 capsules cloves and 2 drops walnut tincture
After 10 Days -	Take 3 capsules of wormwood per week with 1 clove tablet and 1 drop walnut tincture.

Pitta

Follow same procedure as above, except use barberry capsules instead of cloves.

Caution

Do not use during pregnancy.

Self-Care

Parasite cleanse

Zapper electrical device

Neem basti

Basti oil enema

PREGNANCY

Although in many cultures herbs have traditionally been taken throughout pregnancy, it is wise to take herbs medicinally only when essential. Some herbs such as German chamomile (*Chamomilla recutita*), lime (*Tilia* spp.,) and cornsilk (*Zea mays*) are very useful and can be taken safely for 2-3 weeks at a time during pregnancy. Other herbs should be avoided altogether, as they have constituents that stimulate the muscles of the uterus and, in large doses, could cause a miscarriage. It is safe to continue using herbs in cooking throughout pregnancy.

General Ailments

Pregnancy is a time of great change for the body. Many minor ailments can be relieved by homemade herbal remedies.

Morning sickness (sensations of nausea) need not be restricted to the morning. Generally starting in the 4th-6th week and lasting until the 14th-16th week, morning sickness has many causes, including hormone fluctuations, low blood pressure, low sugar levels, food allergies, poor diet and stress.

Oedema (fluid retention and bloating) is extremely common during pregnancy. Water seeps from the blood vessels into the surrounding tissue, causing puffiness. The ankles and calves are mostly affected.

Constipation often occurs as pregnancy develops. Pressure increases on the lower bowel, impeding circulation.

Heartburn (pain in the centre of the chest) may also be caused by increased pressure within the body.

Stretch marks sometimes appear as the body swells. They can be minimized by rubbing aloe vera gel or olive oil into the skin to maintain its elasticity.

Childbirth can be helped by drinking raspberry leaf tea, a traditional remedy that prepares the uterine muscles for labour and giving birth.

Seek immediate professional advice for

- Prolonged nausea causing an inability to eat properly and frequent vomitting leading to dehydration.
- Frequent urination lasting for more than 3 days (or with pain after 2 days)
- Breast pain with swollen glands under the arms or fever
- Fluid retention that has not reduced after 3 days.

Herbs during pregnancy

- For the first 3 months avoid all herbal remedies, including essential oils, unless professionally prescribed.
- The following herbs are particularly dangerous and should on no account be taken during pregnancy: Blue Cohosh (*Caulophyllum thalictroides*), Goldenseal (*Hydrastis canadensis*), Juniper (*Juniperus communis*), juniper (*Juniperus communis*), Pennyroyal (*Mentha pulegium*), Yarrow (*Achillea millefolium*) and therapeutic doses of Sage (*Salvia officinalis*).

(a) Morning sickness & nausea

The following remedies are an exception and can be taken during the first 3 months of pregnancy.

Herb : German chamomile (*Chamomilla recutita*)

Remedy : Make an infusion in a covered container. Sip small quantities during the day. Do not drink more than 5 cups a day.

Herb : Ginger (*Zingiber officinale*)

Remedy : Make an infusino with ½-1tsp of grated fresh ginger per cup of water. Sip small amounts frequently throughout the day, rather than drinking a whole cup at a time. Take a maximum of 3 cups a day.

Herb : Fennel (*Foeniculum vulgare*)

Remedy : Make an infusion with ½ tsp of seeds per cup of water and drink up to 3 cups a day.

(b) Oedema

Herb : Cornsilk (*Zea mays*)

Remedy : Make an infusion and drink up to 5 cups a day.

(c) Constipation

Herbs : Psyllium (*Plantago* spp.), linseed (*Linum usitatissimum*)

Remedy : Take 1-2 tsp of either of the seeds with a large glass of water each day or soak them in cold water overnight before taking.

Note : Eat more dried fruit, especially figs.

(d) Heartburn

Herb : Meadowsweet (*Filipendula ulmaria*)

Remedy : Make an infusion and drink 1-2 cups a day.

(e) Headache & Nervous Tension

Herb : Lime (*Tilia* spp.)

Remedy : Make an infusion and drink 3-4 cups a day.

(f) Preparing for Childbirth

Herb : Raspberry (*Rubus idaeus*)

Remedy : Make an infusion using 1 tsp of the chopped fresh or dried leaf per cup of water. Brew for 5-6 minutes and drink 1-2 cups a day during the last 10 weeks of pregnancy.

Cautions : Do not leave the infusion to brew for more than 5-6 minutes. Do not take until the last 10 weeks of pregnancy.

(g) Strength marks

Herbs : Aloe (*Aloe vera*), Olive (*Olea europaea*)

Remedy : Rub aloe vera gel over the affected areas or massage olive oil firmly into the skin 1-2 times a day.

(h) Anaemia & High Blood Pressure

See Anaemia.

(i) Haemorrhoids

See Varicose Veins & Hemorrhoids.

(j) Backache

See Back Problems.

(k) Varicose Veins

See Varicose Veins.

(l) Vaginal Thrush

See Fungal Infections.

(m) Bladder & Kidney Infections

See Gall Bladder and Kidney stones etc.

(n) Healing after childbirth

See Cleansing Wounds & Healing Wounds.

PRE-MENSTRUAL SYNDROME (P.M.S.)

PMS consists of a reoccurrence of symptoms around the menstrual cycle. These symptoms include depression, feelings of being bloated, moodiness, anxiety, tension, tiredness, cramps, backache, tender breasts, forgetfulness, irritability, headaches, and weight gain. A poor diet contributes to these symptoms.

Feelings and Emotions : Dislike a feminine energy cycle.

Diet	Vitamin & Minerals (Daily)	Essential Oils (Always dilute)	Herbs	Alternative Therapy	Avoid
Ayurvedic	Evening Primrose: 500 mg.	Clary Sage: VPK-	Raspberry Leaf: PK-V+	Acupuncture	Salt
diet for	2 x day	Rose: VPK=	Unicorn Root: VPK+	Chiropractic	Caffeine
body type	Calcium/Magnesium:	Cyperus: VPK-	Black Haw: PK-V+	treatments	Chocolate
	1000 mg.	Valerian: VK-P+	Dong Quai: VK-Po	Polarity	Cola
Whole grains	A: 10,000 IU	Jasmine: KP-V+	Milk Thistle: PKV+	Massage	Sugar
	E mixed tocopherals:	Sandalwood: PV-Ko	Licorice: PV-K+	Shiastsu	Honey
Legumes	400 IU 2 x day	Gardenia: PK-V+	Aloe Vera Gel: VPK-		Maple syrup
		Cinnamon: VK-P+	Turmeric: VK-Po		Dried fruit

Fruits	Zinc: 15 mg.	Black Pepper: K-PV+	Dill: PK-VO	Fruit juices
	Linseed oil: 2 Tbs.	Ginger: VK-P+	Fennel: VPK=	Dairy
Brewer's yeast	Bioflavonoids: 500 mg.	Calamus: VK-P+	Crampbark: KV-P+	Fats
	2 x day	Clove: VK-P+	Rosemary: VK-P+	Cabbage
Acidophilus	B-Complex : 100 mg.	Myrrh: VK-P+	Chamomile: PK-Vo	Brussel sprouts
	C: 2,000 mg.	Ylang Ylang: PV-K+	Comfrey: VP-K+	Cauliflower
Protein	B5-Pantothenic Acid:	Lavender: PK-Vo	False Unicorn: VK-P+	Tobacco
	2,500 mg.		Saffron: VPK=	Aspartame
Green leafy	Bromelin : 200 mg.	Chamomile:	Coriander. PKV-	
vegetables		PV-K+ (excess)	Brahmi: VPK-	
		Lemon Balm: KP-Vo	Dandelion: PK-V+	
			Shatavari: PV-K+	
			Ashwagandha: VK-P+	
			Jatamasi: VK-P+	
			Asafoetida: VK-P+	

Herbal Brew

Vata		Pitta		Kapha	
Shatavari	2 oz.	Raspberry Leaves	2 oz.	Raspberry Leaves	2 oz.
Licorice	1 oz.	Mint	1 oz.	Rosemary	1 oz.

Ginger	1 oz.	Fennel	1 oz.	Ginger	2 oz.
Comfrey	½ oz.	Coriander	1 oz.	Shatavari	1 oz.
Rosemary	½ oz.	Chamomile	1 oz.	Coriander	2 oz.
Vitex	1 oz.	Dandelion	2 oz.		
Ashwagandha	2 oz.	Shatavari	2 oz.		

Drink tea 2 weeks before menstruation 4 times per day. Also drink tea 1 day after menstruation ends.

Massage Formula

Chamomile	5 drops
Lemon Balm	5 drops
Clary Sage	5 drops
Ylang Ylang	2 drops
Vegetable oil	4 oz.

Self-Care

Exercise

Aromatherapy

Yoga

Women support groups

Wearing gemstones: pearl, moonstone, garnet, ruby

Apply warm sesame oil to head and lower abdomen

Kapha: Hot baths with essential oils that help eliminate water retention and are stimulating. **Use :** 10 drops Juniper, 10 drops Cypress, and 5 drops Orange.

Pitta : Refreshing cool baths which help relax and sweat: Use 5 drops Rose, 10 drops Clary Sage, and 10 drops Geranium.

Vata : Hot baths with essential oils to relax, calm the mind and assist with digestion. Use 10-15 drops Sandalwood, 5 drops Jatamasi, and 5 drops Ginger.

Wild Yam Cream (Progesterone cream)

SCIATICA

Sciatica may be either neuralgia or neuritis affecting the large sciatic nerve running down the back of the thigh. This sciatica nerve extends from the lower back down the leg to the heel of the foot. The chief symptom is pain and spasms along the line of the never at the back of the thigh usually caused by bulging lumbar discs rubbing against the sciatic nerve. Pain can also be felt on the side of the leg and the Achilles heel. Possible causes of sciatica are trauma or inflammation of the nerve itself, sprained joints in the lower back, rupture of a disc between the spinal bones, or a vertebra out of alignment causing neuritis.

Feelings and Emotions : Fear of going forward in life.

Cell Salts : Kali Sulph, Potassium Sulfate

Diet	Vitamin & Minerals (Daily)	Essential Oils (Always dilute)	Herbs	Alternative Therapy	Avoid
Anti-Vata Diet	B-Complex: 200 mg.	Chamomile: VPK-	Alfalfa: PK-V+	Acupuncture	Tomatoes
(if appropriate)	A: 50,000 IU (until clear)	Eucalyptus: VK-P+	Castor Oil: VP-Ko	Chiropractic	Rice
	E: 200 IU	Rosemary: VK-P+	Garlic: KV-P+	Massage	Potatoes
Ayurvedic diet	B5: 1500 mg.	Valerian: VK-P+	Ginger: VK-P+	Shiatsu	Eggplant

for body type	C: 3000 mg.	Wintergreen: PK-Vo	Kava Kava: VKP	Physical Therapy	Cauliflower
	Calcium: 400 mg.	Lavender: PK-Vo	Passion Flower: PK-V+	Myotherapy	Cold drafts
	Magnesium: 400 mg.	Skullcap: PK-Vo			
	Multi-Minerals	Valerian: VK-P+			

Note : Vata body types are susceptible to sciatica

Herbal Brew

Vata		Pitta		Kapha	
Chamomile	2 oz.	Passion Flower	2 oz.	Alfalfa	2 oz.
Ginger	1 oz.	Kava Kava	2 oz.	Kava Kava	1 oz.
Scullcap	2 oz.	Peppermint	1 oz.	Ginger	2 oz.
Valerian	1 oz.	Scullcap	1 oz.	Scullcap	1 oz.

Self-Care

Warm compresses with lavender and valerian
Muscle strengthening (i.e. swimming, walking)
Inversion therapy
Rest
Yoga Mudras

Yoga Postures:

Backbends	Knee to chest
Half wheel	Plough

SHINGLES (HERPES ZOSTER)

This is an infection that irritates the never endings in the skin and is characterized by blister and crust formations. It is accompanied by severe pain which may last up to several weeks. The most common site for the infection is across the chest and abdomen. Herpes Zoster, or shingles, received its name from a Greek word signifying a surcingle, or girdle, because it spreads in a zone-like manner around half the body. This virus lies dormant until injury or stress weakens the body.

Feelings and Emotions : Wanting control, wanting things your own way.

Cell Salts : Silica Q Oxide

Diet	Vitamin & Minerals (Daily)	Essential Oils (Always dilute)	Herbs	Alternative Therapy	Avoid
Ayurvedic diet	B-Complex: 200 mg.	Bergamot: VK-P+	Aloe Vera: VPK=	Acupuncture	Arginine rich
diets for body	2 x day	Camphor: VK-P+	Astralagus: VPK+	Chiropractic	Chocolate
type	B1: 200-300 mg.	Chamomile: VPK-	Chamomile: PK-Vo	Reiki	Coffee
Red grapes	B12: 300 mcg.	Clove: VK-P+	Eucalyptus: VK-P+	Therapeutic Touch	Colas
	B6: 200 mg.	Eucalyptus: VK-P+	Comfrey Root: VP-K+		Fatigue
Potatoes	Beta-carotene:	Tea Tree: VPK=	Echinacea: PK-V+		Nuts
	100,000 IU	Geranium: PK-V+	Goldenseal: PK-V+		Rice
Brewer's yeast	(until clear)	Lavender: PK-Vo	Neem: PK-V+		Skin drying out
	C: 2000 mg.	Clary Sage: VPK-	Shatavari: PV-K+		Stress
	Calcium: 500 mg.	Frankincense: VK-P+	Slippery Elm: PV-K+		Sun exposure
	Chlorophyll: 3 Tbs.	Rose: VPK=	Uva-Ursi: PK-V+		Tea

3 x day	Neem: PK-V+	Burdock: PK-V+
D: 600 IU	Lemon: VP-Ko	
Iron: 100 mg.	Myrrh: VK-P+	
L-Lysine: 750-1000 mg.	Peppermint: PK-Vo	
Thymus extract:	Thyme: VK-P+	
	Ylang Ylang: PV-K+	
2-3 tabs 3 x day		
E: 400 IU		
Zinc: 50-60 mg.		
Bioflavonoids: 1 gm.		

Herbal Brew

Vata		Pitta		Kapha	
Shatavari	2 oz.	Shatavari	2 oz.	Shatavari	2 oz.
Slippery Elm	1 oz.	Burdock	1 oz.	Uva Ursi	1 oz.
Comfrey	1 oz.	Astralagus	1 oz.	Burdock	1 oz.
Chamomile	1 oz.	Red Clover	1 oz.	Red Clover	1 oz.

Self-Care

Compress over the area twice per day with equal amounts of : Rose, Geranium, Levender, Chamomile.

SHOCK

Due to trauma, accident, or receiving alarming news. More common in Vata as they are easily frightened and put into fear, fainting, and affecting the nervous system. Not able to cope. May experience convulsions.

Feelings and Emotions : Not feeling centered. Not able to handle the challenges of life.

Diet	Vitamin & Minerals (Daily)	Essential Oils (Always dilute)	Herbs	Alternative Therapy	Avoid
Ayurvedic diet	B-Complex: 300 mg.	Lemon: PV-Ko	Calamus: VK-P+	Breathing therapy	Sugar
for body type	Multi-mineral	Lavender: PK-Vo	Mistletoe: VK-P+	Counseling	Animal proteins
	B6: 200 mg.	Sandalwood: PV-Ko	Horse Nettle: PK-V+	Therapeutic Touch	
Green	B15: 300 mg.	Basil: VK-P+	Astralagus: VPK+	Reiki	
vegetables	C: 1,000 mg.	Myrrh: VK-P+	Ashwagandha: VK-P+	Chakra Anointment	
	D: 500 IU	Shatavari: PV-K+	Bach Flower Rescue	Bach Flower Rescue	
High minerals	E: 100 IU	Chamomile: VK-P+	Arjuna: PK-V+	Remedy	
	L-tyrosine: 100 mg.	Rosemary: VK-P+	Lady's Slipper : VK-Po	Shirodhara	
Berries	Digestive Enzyme:	Peppermint: PK-Vo	Chamomile: PK-Vo		
	3-x day before meals	Hyssop: VK-P+			
Bee Pollen	Pituitary Extract:	Myrtle: PK-V+			
	2 x day				
	Bioflavinoids:				
	2000 mg.				

Herbal Brew

Vata		Pitta		Kapha	
Lobelia	2 tsp.	Chamomile	1 tsp.	Chamomile	1 tsp.
Valerian	1 tsp.	Scullcap	1 tsp.	Fennel	1 tbs.
Fennel	1 tsp.	Mint	1 tsp.	Brahmi	1 tsp.

Self-Care

Keep the person warm

Lay them down

Rescue Remedy

Anoint all chakras with essential oils

Wrap the body tight with a white sheet.

Breathwork

SINUS OR NASAL PROBLEMS

Congestion and inflammation of the nasal passages and upper respiratory system, clogging the inside passage of teh nasal cavity and the cheek behind the bridge of the nose. This could be caused by injuries, allergies, environmental irritants, and food allergies. Vata experiences sinus pain and headaches, Pitta experiences inflammation, and Kapha loses their sense of smell and has thick mucous drainage. When the mucous becomes green or yellow it has turned into an infection. This can lead to sore throat, laryngitis, or lung infection.

Feelings and Emotions : Feeling stuck, held back, confused, blocked. Afraid to act.

Diet	Vitamin & Minerals (Daily)	Essential Oils (Always dilute)	Herbs	Alternative Therapy	Avoid
Ayurvedic diet	A: 3,000-10,000 mg.	Eucalyptus: VK-P+	Horehound: PK-V+	Emetic Therapy	Dairy
for body type	Bioflavinoids: 300 mg.	Rosemary: VK-P+	Echinacea: PK-V+	Rebirthing	Sugar
	B-Complex: 200 mg./	Myrtle: PK-V+	Fenugreek: VK-P+	Pancha Karma	Fried Foods
Mucousless diet	2 x day	Lavender: PK-Vo	Lobelia: K-PV+	Ayurvedic	Poor food
	B6: 200 mg.	Sandalwood: VP-Ko	Goldenseal: PK-V+	consultation	combining
Cleansing foods	Pantothenic Acid:	Calamus: VK-P+	Garlic: KV-P+	Acupuncture	
	200 mg.	Sage: VK-P+	Onions: KV-P+		
Greens	3 x per day	Inula: KV-P+	Marshmallow: VP-K+		
	Germanium: 100 mg.	Camphor: KV-P+	Mullein: PK-V+		
	C (ascorbate) : 3,000 + mg.	Angelica: VPK-P+	Rosehips: V-KPo+ (in excess)		
		Basil: VK-P+	Basil: VK-P+		
			Angelica: VK-Po		
			Chrysanthemum: PK-V+		
			Ginger: VK-P+		
			Astralagus: VP-K+		
			Sitoplad Churna: VKP		
			Pippali: KV-P+		
			Elecampagne: VK-P+		
			Trikatu: VK-P+		

Herbal Brew

Vata		Pitta		Kapha	
Ginger	1 oz.	Mullein	1 oz.	Calamus	1 oz.
Marshmallow	1 oz.	Marshmallow	1 oz.	Ginger	½ oz.
Rosehips	1 oz.	Mint	1 oz.	Mullein	1 oz.
Astralagus	½ oz.	Horehound	1 oz.	Basil	1 oz.

Self-Care

Yoga	Compresses	Vapour rub on sinus areas
Inhalation of essential oils	Upper cervical & facial massage	Nasya Nosedrops

SORE THROAT

An infection of the throat when the adenoids become inflamed. Vata experiences dryness, Pitta has inflammaton, and Kapha experiences swelling of the throat.

Feelings and Emotions : Holding back communication. Fear of speaking truthfully.

Diet	Vitamin & Minerals (Daily)	Essential Oils (Always dilute)	Herbs	Alternative Therapy	Avoid
Ayurvedic diet for body type	C: 1000 mg. every 2 hours (until clear)	Sandalwood: VP-Ko	Echinacea: PK-V+	Therapeutic Touch	Sugar
	A: 25,000 IU	Lemongrass: PK-Vo	Amalaki: PV-Ko	Reiki	Dairy
		Ginger: VK-P+	Sage: VK-P+	Lymphatic	Fried foods

Drink large	Beta-Carotene: 1000 IU	Cardamom: VK-P+	Garlic: VK-P+	drainage	Alcohol
amounts of	Zinc: 50 mg.	Goldenseal: KP-V+	Sitopaladi: VP-K+		Poor food
water	Bioflavenoids: 1 gm. per day	Forsynthia: VPK+	Zedoaria: PK-V+		combining
	Thymus extract: 500 mg.	Talisadi: VPK-	Bibhitaki: PK-Vo		
Fresh squeezed	2 x day	Cinnamon: VK-P+	Korean Ginseng: V-PKo		
orange juice		Black Pepper: VK-P+	Honeysuckle: VPK+		
		Chamomile: VPK-	Siberian Ginseng: V-PKc		
Hot water with		Clary Sage: VPK-	Rosehips: V-PKo		
lemons		Eucalyptus: VK-P+	Licorice: VP-K+		
		Lavender: PK-Vo	Haritaki: VK-Po		
		Tea Tree: VPK=			
		Lemon: VP-Ko			
		Cajeput: VK-P+			
		Bergamot: VK-P+			
		Niaouli: PK-V+			
		Geranium: PK-V+			
		Thyme: VK-P+			
		Peppermint: PK-Vo			
		Pine: VK-P+			

Herbal Brew

Vata		Pitta		Kapha	
Ginger	1 oz.	Mullein	1 oz.	Sage	1 oz.
Cinnamon	½ oz.	Honeysuckle	2 oz.	Ginger	2 oz.
Cardamon	½ oz.	Chamomile	2 oz.	Bibhitaki	1 oz.
Lemon Peel	½ oz.	Liquorice	2 oz.	Basil	1 oz.
Haritaki	½ oz.	Fennel	2 oz.	Lemongrass	2 oz.
Liquorice	1 oz.	Lemongrass	1 oz.	Haritaki	1 oz.
Amla	½ oz.				
Anise	1 oz.				
Pitta Gargle		**Vata Gargle**		**Kapha Throat Spray**	
Water	2 oz.	Salt	½ tsp.	Tea tree oil	1 drop
Sandalwood	2 drops	Warm water	4 oz.	Cajeput	2 drops
Cajeput or tea tree	2 drops	Mix well.		Sandalwood	2 drops
				Water	4 oz.
Gargle 4-6 times per day, or every two hours or every 2 hours.				*Put in spray bottle. Spray onto throat every hour.*	

General caution : Always seek professional advice and treatment for children under 5 suffering from tonsillitis.

STRESS

Stress is a built-in system designed to prompt the "fight or flight" response. During the course of day, we experience many prolonged stresses, and we often tend to squelch the "fight or flight" response. After years of failing to respond, we inadvertently damage the body's immune system which, in turn, results in ill health. Side effects can manifest as ulcers, arthritis, cancer, high blood pressure, coronary heart disease, and a host of other conditions.

Alarm + Resistance + Exhaustion = Stress

Feelings and Emotions : Victim, Life is getting me. Caught in the illusion.

Diet	Vitamin & Minerals (Daily)	Essential Oils (Always dilute)	Herbs	Alternative Therapy	Avoid
Ayurvedic diet	B-Complex: 200 mg.	Lavender: PK-Vo	Echinacea: PK-V+	Massage	Smoking
for body type	B5 - Pantothenic Acid:	Lemongrass: PK-Vo	Goldenseal: PK-V+	Biofeedback	Cadmium
	2,500 mg.	Basil: VK-P+	Panax Ginseng: PKVo	Acupucture	Salt
Whole grains	A - (Beta carotene): 25,000 IU	Pine : VK-P+	Licorice: VP-K+	Polarity	Mental fatigue
	Bioflavinoids: 1000 mg.	Savory: VK-Vo	Valerian: VK-P+	Reiki	Physical fatigure
Legumes	C: 500 mg. every	Geranium: PK-V+	Skullcap: PK-Vo	Shirodhara	Sugar
	2 hours for 1 week	Cypress: VKP+	Lady's Slipper: VK-Po		Gaining weight
Cauliflower	Iron: 50 mg.	Hyssop: VK-P+	Cayenne: VK-P+		Tea
	Zinc: 100 mg.	Juniper: VK-P+	Black Cohosh Root: PK-V+		Coffee
Salmon	Calcium: 800 mg.	(in excess)	Guduchi: PKV+		Dairy
	Potassium: 3-5 gms.	Chamomile: VPK-	Ashwagandha: VK-P+		Anti-depressants

	L-Carnitine: 200 mg.	Sandalwood: VP-Ko	Chrysanthemum: PK-V+	Sleeping pills
	L-Tyrosine: 100 mg.	Ylang Ylang: PV-K+	Chamomile: PK-Vo	Protein
Sweet Potatoes	Folic Acid: 200 mcg.	Orange Blossom: VK-P+	Passion Flower: PK-V+	
	Phosphorus: 200 mg.	Vetiver: V-PK+		
Tomatoes	PABA: 200 mg.	Kava Kava: VPK-		
	Chromium: 200 mcg.			
Ghee	Copper: 100 mg.			

Herbal Brew

Vata		Pitta		Kapha	
Ashwagandha	2 oz.	Chamomile	2 oz.	Chrysanthemum	2 oz.
Liquorice	1 oz.	Chrysanthemum	2 oz.	Guduchi	1 oz.
Lady's Slipper	1 oz.	Shatavari	1 oz.	Skullcap	1 oz.
Shatavari	2 oz.	Liquorice	1 oz.	Chamomile	2 oz.
Chamomile	1 oz.	Passion Flower	1 oz.		

Self-Care

Meditation	Foot rubs	Whirlpool	Tai Chi
Steam	Exercise	Sports	Rest
Walking	Prayer, devotion	Yoga	Visualization
Laughter	Dancing	Aromatherpay bath with essential oils	
Chanting			

STOMACH ACHE

Cramping Pain is a sign that the stomach and intestines are sore and irritated. This is normally due to poor digestion, excessive nervous tension, food poisoning or infection. Stomach ache may occur on its own or lead to vomiting and diarrhoea. Garlic and marigold are antiviral and will help clear digestive infections. Relaxing herbs, such as German chamomile and cramp bark, relieve stomach spasm. For maximum benefit, they are mixed with carminative herbs to help relieve wind.

General Cautions : Seek professional advice if stomach pain is severe or recurrent. All species of mint (*Mentha spp.*) are unsuitable for children under 5.

(a) Stomach Spasm

Relaxing herbs : German chamomile (*Chamomilla recutita*), Lemon balm (*Melissa officinalis*), Cramp bark (*Vibumum opulus*).

Carminative herbs Anisa (*Pimpinella anisum*), Fennel (*Foeniculum vulgare*), Mint (*Mentha* spp), Angelica (*Angelica archangelica*).

Remedy : Mix 3 parts of a relaxing herb to 1 part of a carminative herb and make an infusion. For the carminative herbs, use fennel seeds, aniseed, mint leaves or angelica root. Drink up to 5 cups a day.

(b) Digestive infections

Herb : Garlic (*Allium sativum*)

Remedy : Eat 1-2 fresh cloves a day.

Herb : Marigold (*Calendula officinalis*)

Remedy : Infuse 2 tsp of herb in 750 ml of water and drink up to 5 cups a day.

Herbs : Yarrow (*Achillea millefolium*), Peppermint (*Mentha piperita*), Catmint (*Nepeta cataria*)

Remedy : Mix equal parts of each herb. Make an infusion of 2 tsp of mixture to 1 cup of water. Drink 2 cups a day.

Caution : Do not take yarrow in pregnancy.

ULCERS

Ulcers are an inflammation of the mucous lining of the stomach or the duodenum. They are associated with pain and burning in that area of the body. In advanced stages, bleeding occurs and when perforated, they can be life threatening. Ulcers are caused by excess acid from the small intestine which accumulates in the stomach and burns through the lining. It can sometimes be triggered by nervous sensitivity.

Feelings and Emotions: Stress and irritability.

Cell Salts: Nat Sulph, Sodium Sulfate

Diet	Vitamin & Minerals (Daily)	Essential Oils (Always dilute)	Herbs	Alternative Therapy	Avoid
Ayurvedic diet	A: 25,000-50,000 IU	Coriander: VPK-	Amalaki: PV-Ko	Biofeedback	Stress
for body type	B-Complex: 100 mg.	Mint: PK-Vo	Aloe Vera: VPK =	Reiki	Smoking
	C: 2,000 mg.	Chamomile: VPK-	Shatavari: VP-K +	Therapeutic touch	Caffeine
Bland diet	(in calcium	Fennel: VPK =	Liquorice: VP-K +	Polarity	Acid fruits
	ascorbate form)	Rose: VPK =	Marshmallow: VP-K +	Color therapy: blue,	Spicy foods
Milk	E: 600-1200 IU	Lavender: PK-Vo	Comfrey: VP-K +	green, indigo	Sour foods
	Calcium: 800 mg.		Barberry: PK-V +	Music/sound	Alcohol
Acidophilus	Iron: 50 mg.		Gentian: PK-V +	therapy	Spices,
	U: 300 mg.		Chiretta: PKV +	Cranial Sacral	including salt
Fruits			Katuka: PKV +	Homeopathics	Pickles
			Sudarshan: PVK		Vinegar

Vegetables	Mahasudarshan: PKV	Nightshade
	Coptis: PKV	Vegetables:
Pureed protein	Dry Ginger: KV-P +	tomato
	Noni Juice: VPK-	peppers
	Slippery Elm: VP-K +	
Cabbage juice	Goldenseal: PK-V +	potatoes
	Trikatu: VK-P +	
	Triphalla: VPK-	Cold food
3 x per day	Guggul: KV-P+	Raw food
Unsalted Millet		
Potato Juice		

Herbal Brew

Vata		Pitta		Kapha	
Slippery Elm	2 oz.	Mint	2 oz.	Marshmallow	1 oz.
Coriander	1 oz.	Shatavari	1 oz.	Coriander	2 oz.
Shatavari	2 oz.	Comfrey	1 oz.	Fennel	2 oz.
Liquorice	2 oz.	Slippery Elm	1 oz.	Mint	2 oz.
		Coriander	2 oz.	Shatavari	1 oz.
				Amalaki	1 oz.

Self-Care

Cool Compresses on the stomach with cooling essential oils

Visualization

VAGINITIS

There are three different types of vaginitis: infectious, hormonal and irritant. Infectious vaginitis may be sexually transmitted or may be a disturbance to the ecology of a healthy vagina. Examples of infectious vaginitis is simplex, chlamydia, gonorrhoea, trichomonas, or *Candida albicans*. Hormonal vaginitis is usually a problem in post-menopausal women and those whose ovaries have been removed. Another indication of hormonal vaginitis is increased vaginal discharge. Irritant vaginitis is directly related to certain medications, an injury, or foreign bodies in the vagina which irritate the delicate membranes. Vata generally experiences itching, Pitta usually has hormonal involvement, and Kapha tends to have heavy mucous discharge.

Feelings and Emotions : Irritation by male energy.

Diet	Vitamin & Minerals (Daily)	Essential Oils (Always dilute)	Herbs	Alternative Therapy	Avoid
Ayurvedic diet	A: 10,000 IU (until clear)	Anise: VK-P+	Alfalfa: PK-V+	Reiki	Alcohol
for body type	Aloe vera Gel: 1 Tbs.	Bergamot: VK-P+	Red Clover: PK-V+	Therapeutic	Antibiotics
	2 x day	Dhavana: PKV-	Don Quai: VK-Po	touch	Bad hygiene
Acidophilus	B-Complex: 100 mg.	Fennel: VPK=	Echinacea: PK-V+		Coffee
½ tsp.	Beta-carotene: 2,000 IU	Lavender: Pk-Vo	Garlic: VK-P+		Elevated vaginal pH
2 x day	Bioflavenoids: 2,000 mg.	Myrrh: VK-P+	Ginseng: V-PKo		Fats
	C: 2,500 mg.	Rose: VPK=	Goldenseal: PK-V+		Nylon tights

Raw garlic	Chlorophyll: 2-x day	Tea Tree: VPK=	Liquorice: VP-K+	Oral contraceptives
	Zinc: 15 mg.		Raspberry Leaves: PK-V+	Refined foods
Yogurt	E: 400 Iu		Shatávari: PV-K+	Sexual activity
	L-lysine: 2,000 mg.		Witch Hazel: PK+	Steroids
			Yarrow: PK-V+	Sugar
			Yellow Dock: PK-V+	Excessive douching

Vaginitis Herbal Brew

Vata		Pitta		Kapha	
Shatavari	2 oz.	Red Clover	2 oz.	Alfalfa	1 oz.
Ginseng	1 oz.	Rose	2 oz.	Red Clover	2 oz.
Rose	2 oz.	Yarrow	1 oz.	Yarrow	2 oz.
Liquorice	1 oz.	Liquorice	1 oz.	Witch Hazel	1 oz.
				Raspberry Leaves	2 oz.

VARICOSE VEINS

Varicose veins is a weakening in the wall of the veins, causing the lining to stretch and the pooling of blood in that area. Causes include poor circulation, lack of exercise, and long periods of either sitting or standing. This condition can be hereditary.

Feelings and Emotions : Stuck, Afraid to move.

Diet	Vitamin & Minerals (Daily)	Essential Oils (Always dilute)	Herbs	Alternative Therapy	Avoid
Molasses	C: 5000 mg.	Geranium: KP-V+	Ginger: VK-P+	Steam	Long periods of
	Bioflavinoids: 200 mg.	Lavender: KP-Vo	Juniper: VK-P+	Body wraps	standing or sitting
Greens	B-Complex: 200 mg.	Cypres: VKP+	Triphalla: VKPo	Lymphatic	Crossed legs
	D: 1500 mg.	Juniper: VK-P+	Cardamon: VK-P+	drainage	Dairy
Ayurvedic diet	Magnesium: 100 mg	(in excess)	Burdock: KP-V+	Massage	Red meats
for body type	E: 600 IU	Ginger: VK-P+	Aloe vera Gel: VKP=		Congesting foods
	Zinc: 60 mg.	Cardamon: VK-P+	Cinnamon: VK-P+		
Peaches	K: 150 mg.	Orange: VK-P+	Rosehips: V-KP+		
		Lemon: VP-Ko	Parsley: VK-P+		
Fresh spices		Parsley: KV-P+	Grape leaves: PVK		
		Lemongrass: PK-Vo	Uva Ursi: PK-V+		
All berries			Stone Root: PK-V+		
			Buckhorn: PK-V+		
			Butcher Broom: VPK-		

Herbal Brew

Vata		Pitta		Kapha	
Ginger	1 oz.	Burdock	1 oz.	Burdock	1 oz.
Cardamon	2 oz.	Colistonia	2 oz.	Colistonia	2 oz.
Lemon Peel	1 oz.	Parsley	1 oz.	Ginger	1 oz.
Cinnamon	1 oz.	Butchers Broom	2 oz.	Uva Ursi	1 oz.
Rosehips	2 oz.	Witch Hazel	1 oz.	Juniper	2 oz.
				Orange	1 oz.

Morning	Night
2 Tbs. of Aloe vera juice with lemon and lime juice.	Take 6 tablets of triphalla (500 mg.)

Self-Care

Elevate legs	Wear loose clothing	Sitz baths
Walking on cool water	Clay packs	Steam
Body wraps	Lymphatic drainage	Basti oil enema

Massage Formula

Cypress	5 drops	Lemongrass	5 drops
Juniper	5 drops	Vegetable oil	2 oz.

General caution : Do not massage or rub varicose veins.

VOMITING

The expulsion of the stomach contents by way of the mouth, caused by irritation, food poisoning, the flue, viruses, or nerves.

Feelings and Emotions : I am nauseated by my life; I am sick of it.

Cell Salt : Natrium Sulfate

Diet	Vitamin & Minerals (Daily)	Essential Oils (Always dilute)	Herbs	Alternative Therapy	Avoid
Cilantro juice (3x/dayu)	B-Complex: 150 mg. (yeast-free)	Anise: VK-P+	Poplar Bark: PK-V+	Ayurvedic consultation	Mucus forming foods
	C: 3,000 mg.	Fennel: VKP-	Spearmint: PK-Vo	Therapeutic touch	Poor food combining
Ayurveda diet for bodytype		Ginger: VK-P+	Peach Leaves: PK-V+		
Food combining		Mint: PK-Vo	Sweet Basil: VK-P+		
		Nutmeg: VK-P+	Fennel: VKP-		
		Cardamon: VK – P +	Cinnamon: VK-P+		
			Clove: VK -P+		
			Ginger: VK-P+		
			Nutmeg: VK-P+		
			Peppermint: VK-Vo		
			Raspberry Leaves: VK-P+		

Herbal Brew

VATA		PITTA		KAPHA	
Ginger	1oz.	Mint	1oz.	Raspberry leaves	1oz.
Nutmeg	1/2 oz.	Coriander	1/2 oz.	Ginger	1oz.
Cardamon	1oz.	Peach Leaves	1/2 oz.	Spearmint	1/2 oz.

Self-Care

Meditation

Relaxation techniques

Breathwork

Compress over stomach

Nosedrops

Aromatherapy inhalation after vomiting and in-between

Induce vomiting

General Cautions : Seek professional advice if nausea is severe or is recurrent All types or species of mint (*Mentha* spp.) are unsuitable for children under 5.

Bibliography

Agarwal, V.S. 1986. Economic Plants of India. Kailash Prakashan, Calcutta.

Agarwal, V.S. 1997. Drug Plants of India. 2 Vols. Kalyani Publishers, Ludihana.

Ainsile, W.L. 1813. Materia Medica of Hindoostan. Longman Rees Orme Browne , London.

Airy Shaw, H.K. 1973. A Dictionary of the Flowering Plants and Ferns. 8th Edition. Cambridge University Press, Cambridge.

Ambasta, S.P. 1986. The Useful Plants of India. Publication & Information Directorate, C.S.I.R., New Delhi.

Anonymous. 1951. Rastantra Sar Sangrah and Sidha Prayog Sangrah. Vol. I & II. Krishna Gopal Ayurved Bhawan, Ajmer.

Antol, M.N. 1996. Healing. Avery Publishing Group, New York.

Asolkar, L.V., Kakkar, K.K. and Chakre, O.J. 1992. Second Supplement to Glossary of Indian Medicinal Plants with Active Principles. Part I (A-K). Publication and Information Directorate, C.S.I.R., New Delhi.

Azmi, A. A. 1995. Basic Concepts of Unani Medicine: A Critical Study. Jamia Hamdard, New Delhi.

Badhwar, R. L. and Fernandez, R.R. 1968. Edible Wild Plants of the Himalayas. The Manager of Publications, Delhi.

Behl, P.N., Arora, R.B, Srivastava, G. and Malhotra, S.C. 1993. Herbs Useful in Dermatological Therapy. C.B.S. Publishers and Distributers, Delhi.

Bennet, S.S.R. 1987. Name Changes in Flowering Plants of India and Adjacent Regions. Triseas Publishers, Dehradun.

Bentley, R. and Trimen, H. 1880. Medicinal Plants: Being Descriptions with Original Figures of the Principal Plants Employed in Medicine and an Account of the Characters, Properties and Uses of their Parts and Products of Medicinal Value. Part I-IV. J. & A. Churchill, London.

Bhandari, C. R. 1993. Vanoushdhi Chandrodaya. Part I-X. Chowkhamba Sanskrit Sansthan, Varanasi. Originally printed by Gyan Mandir, Bhanpura, Indore Estate during 1938- 44.

Bhattacharjee, S.K. 1998. Handbook of Medicinal Plants. Pointer Publication, Jaipur (India).

Bose, K. C. 1932. Pharmacopoeia Indica. The Book Company Limited, Calcutta.

Campion, K. 1988. The Family Medical Herbal. Leopord Books, London.

Chatterjee, A. and Pakrashi, S.C. 1991-2001. The Treatise on Indian Medicinal Plants. V 1: 1991;V 2: 1992; V 3: 1994; V 4: 1995; V 5: 1997; V 6: 2001. Publications and Information Directorate, C.S.I.R., New Delhi.

Chevallier, A. 1996. The Encylopaedia of Medicinal Plants. Dorling Kindersley, London.

Chopra R.N., Chopra, I.C. and Verma, B.S. 1969. Supplement to Glossary of Indian Medicinal Plants. Publications and Information Directorate, C.S.I.R., New Delhi.

Chopra, R.N., Chopra, I.C., Handa, K.L. and Kapur, L.D. 1958. Chopra's Indigenous Drugs of India. 2nd Edition. U.N. Dhur and Sons Private Limited, Calcutta.

Chopra R.N., Nayar S.L. and Chopra I.C. 1956. Glossary of Indian Medicinal Plants. Publications and Information Directorate, C.S.I.R., New Delhi.

Chunekar, K.C. 1988. Bhavaprakasa Nighantu. Chaukhamba Bharti Academy, Varanasi.

Dash, B. andJunius, M. 1 987. A Handbook of Ayurveda. Concept Publishing Company, New Delhi.

Dastur, J.F. 1962. Medicinal Plants of India and Pakistan. 2nd Edition. D.B. Taraporevala Sons & Co. Private Ltd., Bombay.

Dastur, J.F. 1983. Everybody's Guide to Ayurvedic Medicine. D.B. Taraporevala Sons & Co. Private Ltd., Bombay.

Dey, A.C. 1980. Indian Medicinal Plants used in Ayurvedic Preparations. Bishen Singh Mahendra Pal Singh, Dehradun.

Dey, K. L. 1896. The Indigenous Drugs of India. 2nd Edition. Assisted by William Nair. Thacker Spink and Company, Calcutta.

Dhiman, A.K. 1998. Triphala : An Ayurvedic Formulation. *Sachitra Ayurved.* 50 (11): 767-68.

Dhiman, A. K. 1999. Notes on Ethnomedicnal uses of Important Fabaceous Plants in India. *Aryavaidyan.* 13: 22-29.

Dhiman, A.K. and Kaushik, P. 2000. Medicinal Uses of Some Spice Plants as in Ancient Literature. In A.K. De edited 'Recent Trends in Spices & Medicinal Plants Research', Calcutta. Associated Publishing Company, New Delhi. pp. 19-26.

Dhiman, A.K. 2003. Sacred Plants and their Medicinal Uses. Daya Publishing House, New Delhi.

Dhiman, A.K. 2004. Medicinal Plants of Uttaranchal State. Chowkhamba Sanskrit Series Office, Varanasi. (In Press)

Dhiman, A.K. 2004. Wild Medicinal Plants of India. Bishen Singh Mahendra Pal Singh, Dehradun. (In Press).

Drury, H. 1873. The Useful Plants of India. 2nd Edition. William H. Alien and Company, London.

Dutt, U.C. The Materia Medica of Hindoos. 2nd Edition. Thacker Spink & Co., Calcutta.

Dymock, W., Warden, C.J.S. and Hooper, D. 1890-93. Pharmacographia Indica. 3 Vols. Thacker, Spink and Co., Calcutta.

Garg, S. 1992. Substitute and Adulterant Plants. Periodical Experts Book Agency, Delhi.

Hooker, J.D. 1875-1897. The Flora of British India. Vol. I-VII. L. Reeve & Co. Ltd., Kent, England.

Jain, S.K. 1968. Medicinal Plants. National Book Trust, India, New Delhi.

Jain, S.K. and De Filipps, R. A. 1991. Medicinal Plants of India. 2 Vols. Reference Publication Inc., Algaonac, Machigan.

Kaushik, P. and Dhiman, A.K. 2000. Medicinal Plants and Raw Drugs of India. Bishen Singh Mahendra Pal Singh, Dehradun.

Khory, R. N. and Katrak, N. N. 1903. Materia Medica of India and their Therapeutics. Reprinted in 1981 by Neeraj Publishing House, Delhi.

Kirtikar, K.R. and Basu, B.D.1935. Indian Medicinal Plants. 2nd Edition. Vol. I-IV. Revised by E. Blatter, J.F. Caius and K.S. Mahaskar. Lalit Mohan Basu, Allahabad.

Miller, L. 2002. Ayurvedic Remedies for the Whole Family. Motilal Banarsidass Publishers Pvt. Ltd., Delhi.

Mowrey, D.B. 1993. Herbal Tonic Therapies. Wing Books, New York.

Nadkarni, K.M. 1914. Indian Plants and Drugs with their Medicinal properties and Uses. Popular Book Depot, Bombay.

Nadkarni, K.M. 1954. Indian Materia Medica. 2 Vols. 3rd Edition. Revised by A.K. Nadkarni. Popular Prakashan Pvt. Ltd., Bombay.

Ody, P. 1993. The Complete Medicinal Herbal. Dorling Kindersley, London.

Pandey, G. 1992. Medicinal Flowers. Sri Satguru Publication, Delhi.

Roberts, E. 1931. Vegetable Materia Medica of India. Reprinted in 1984 by Bishen Singh Mahendra Pal Singh, Dehradun.

Sanyal, D. P. 1924. Vegetable Drugs of India. 13 Radha Nath Bose Lane, Calcutta.

Shah, N.D.C.L. 1924-37. Bharat Bhaisajaya Ratnakar. 5 Vols. Unjha Ayurvedic Pharmacy, Ahemdabad.

Sharma, P.V. 1975-81. Dravyaguna Vijnana. (Vol. 1-1975; Vol. 2-1978; VoL-1979; Vol. 4-1977; Vol.5-1981). Chaukhambha Bharti Academy, Varaṇasi.

Sharma, P.V. 1996. Classical uses of Medicinal Plants. Chaukhambha Vishwabharti, Varanasi.

Sharma, D.P. 1965. Banoushdhi Shatak. Shree Baidyanath Ayurved Bhawan Pvt. Ltd., Calcutta.

Shastri, A. D. 1954. Shushrut Samhita. Chowkhamba Sanskrit Series Office, Benaras.

Shastri, K.N. 1994. Charak Samhita. Vol. I - II. 4th edition. Chaukhambha Sanskrit Sansthan, Varanasi.

Singh, R. S. 1983. Vanoushdhi Nirdeshika. Uttar Pradesh Hindi Sansthan, Lucknow.

Singh, T.B. 1948. Vanaushadhi - Darshika. Kashi Hindi Vishwavidyalaya, Varanasi.

Singh, T. D. 1949. Unani Dravyaguna Vigyan. Nirnay Sagar Press, Bombay.

Singh, T, D. 1985. Unani Chikitsa Sar. Shree Baidya Ayurved Bhawan Pvt. Ltd., Calcutta.

Sivarajan, V.V. and Balachandran, I. 1994. Ayurvedic Drugs and their Plant Sources. Oxford & IBH Publishing Company

Pvt. Ltd., New Delhi.

Swamy, B. 1936. Sandhigdh Nirnay Vanoushdhi Shastra. Pt. I-IX. 143, Harrison Road, Calcutta.

Thakur, R.S., Puri, H.S. and Husain, A. 1989. Major Medicinal Plant of India. Central Institute of Medicinal and Aromatic Plants, Lucknow.

Uniyal, M.R. 1977. Uttrakhand Vanousdhi Darshika. Central Council of Research in Indian Medicine and Homeopathy, Delhi.

Uniyal, M.R. 1989. Medicinal Flora of Garhwal Himalayas. Shree Baidyanath Ayurved Bhawan, Nagpur.

Uphof, J.C.T. 1959. Dictionary of Economic Plants. H.R. Engelmann (J. Cramer), Weinheim (Bergstrasse).

Vaidya, H.D.1990-97. Chikitsa Chandrodaya. Part I-VII (Pt. I-1994; Pt. II -1991; Pt. III -1990; Pt. IV -1995; Pt. V -1990; Pt. VI -1993 & Pt. VII -1997). Revised and enlarged by Chameli Devi, Vaidya and Shakuntia Devi. Haridas and Company Pvt. Ltd., Mathura.

Vaish, R. L. 1947. Abhinava Butidarpana. 2 Vols. Chowkhamba Sanskrit Series Office, Benaras.

Vaishya, S.L. 1953. Shaligram Nighantu. Khemraj Shree Krishan Dass, Bombay.

Vaishya, S.L. 1996. Bangsen : Hindi Tika. Khemraj Shree Krishan Dass, Bombay.

Vidyalankar, A.D. 1991. Ayurved Ka Itihas. Uttar Pradesh Hindi Sansthan, Lucknow.

Wahid, A. and Siddiqui, A. H. 1961. A Survey of Drugs. Institute of the History of Medicine and Medical Research, New Delhi.

Waring, E.J. 1868. Pharmacopoeia of India. W.H. Alien, London.

Waring, E.J. 1897. Remarks on the Uses of Some of the Bazar

Medicines and Common Medical Plants of India and Ceylon. J & A Chruchill, London,

Warrier, P.K, Nambiar, V.P.K. and Ramankutty, C. 1993-1996. Indian Medicinal Plants: A Compendium of 500 Species. Vol.1: 1993; Vol. II: 1994; Vol. III: 1994; Vol. IV: 1995 and Vol. V: 1996. Orient Longman, Madras.

Watt, G. 1889-96. A Dictionary of the Economic Products of India. 6 Volumes. W.H. Alien, London.

Wren, R.C. 1956. Potter's New Cyclopaedia of Botanical Drugs and Preparations. Enlarged by R.W. Wren. Sir Isaac Pitmen & Sons Ltd. London.

Appendix I

HERB CHART

Herbs are listed according to their common names. Taste is according to the six Ayurvedic tastes; sweet, sout, salty, pungent, bitter, astringent. Energy is heating or cooling. PD effect is *Vipaka* or post digestive effect (sweet, sour or pungent). Action on *dosha:* V is Vata, P is Pitta, K is Kapha, + is increases, - is decreases, 0 is neutral or mixed in effect. VPK = is balancing to all three doshas. Therepeutic properties are according to western herbalism. Herbs starred (*) are those also contained in the main text.

HERB	TASTE	ENERGY	PD-EFFECT	DOSHA	ACTIONS
AGRIMONY *Agrimonia eupatoria* *Rosaceae*	astringent, bitter	cooling	pungent	PK-V+	astringent, diuretic, vulnerary
AJWAN *Apium graveolens* *Apiaceae*	pungent	heating	pungent	KV-P+	stimulant, diaphoretic, antispasmodic
ALFALFA *Medicago sativa* *Fabaceae*	astringent, sweet	cooling	pungent	PK-V+	alterative, diuretic, antipyretic
ALLSPICE *Pimento officinalis* *Myrtaceae*	pungent	heating	pungent	VK-P+	stimulant, carminative

HERB	TASTE	ENERGY	PD-EFFECT	DOSHA	ACTIONS
ALMOND *Amygdalus communis* *Rosaceae*	sweet	heating	pungent	V-KP+	demulcent, expectorant, tonic
*ALOE *Aloe spp.* *Liliaceae*	bitter, astringent, pungent, sweet	cooling	sweet	VPK-	alterative, bitter tonic, rejuvenative, purgative
ANGELICA *Angelica archangelica* *Apiaceae*	pungent, sweet	heating	sweet	VK-P +	diaphoretic, carminative, emmenagogue
ANGELICA (Tang kuei) *Angelica spp.* *Apiaceae*	pungent, sweet	heating	sweet	VK-Po	tonic, emmenagogue, rejuvenative, diaphoretic
ANISE *Pimpinella anisum* *Apiaceae*	pungent	heating	pungent	VK-P+	carminative, stimulant, galactagogue
APRICOT SEED *Prunus armeniaca* *Asteraceae*	bitter, sweet	heating	pungent	KV-P+	antispasmodic, expectorant, laxative
ARNICA *Arnica montana* *Asteraceae*	pungent	heating	pungent	KV-P +	stimulant, vulnerary, tonic

HERB	TASTE	ENERGY	PD-EFFECT	DOSHA	ACTIONS
ASAFOETIDA *Ferula asafoetida* *Apiaceae*	pungent	heating	pungent	VK-P+	stimulant, carminative, antispasmodic, anthelmintic
ASPARAGUS *Asparagus officinalis* *Liliaceae*	sweet	cooling	sweet	PK-Vo	diuretic, laxative, tonic
*ASHWAGANDHA *Withania somnifera* *Solanaceae*	bitter, astringent	heating	sweet	VK-P+	tonic, rejuvenative, aphrodisiac, nervine
ATIBALA *Abutilon indicum* *Malvaceae*	sweet	cooling	sweet	PK-Vo	tonic, demulcent, diuretic, laxative
*BALA *Sida cordifolia* *Malvaceae*	sweet	cooling	sweet	VP-Ko	tonic, nervine, demulcent, rejuvenative
BALMONY *Chelone glabra* *Scrophulariaceae*	bitter	cooling	pungent	PK-V+	bitter tonic, anthelmintic, laxative

HERB	TASTE	ENERGY	PD-EFFECT	DOSHA	ACTIONS
*BARBERRY *Berberis aristata* *Berberidaceae*	bitter, astringent	heating	pungent	PK-V+	bitter tonic, alterative, antipyretic
BARLEY *Hordeum distichon* *Poaceae*	sweet	cooling	sweet	PK-V+	diuretic, demulcent, tonic
BASIL *Ocinum spp.* *Lamiaceae*	pungent	heating	pungent	VK-P+	diaphoretic, febrifuge, nervine
*BAYBERRY *Myrica spp.* *Myricaceae*	pungent, astringent	heating	pungent	KV-P+	diaphoretic, expectorant, astringent, emetic
BAY LEAVES *Laurus nobilis* *Lauraceae*	pungent	heating	pungent	VK-P+	carminative, stimulant, expectorant
BETONY WOOD *Stachys betonica* *Lamiaceae*	pungent, bitter	cooling	pungent	PK-V+	nervine, carminative, diuretic

HERB	TASTE	ENERGY	PD-EFFECT	DOSHA	ACTIONS
*BHRINGARAJ *Eclipta alba, etc.* *Asteraceae*	bitter, astringent, sweet	cooling	sweet	VPK=	tonic, alterative. nervine nervine, haemostatic
*BIBHITAKA *Terminalia belirica* *Combretaceae*	astringent	heating	sweet	KP-Vo	tonic, astringent, expectorant, laxative
BIRCH *Betula alba* *Betulaceae*	bitter, pungent	cooling	pungent	PK-V+	diaphoretic, diuretic, astringent,
BISTORT *Polygonum bistorta* *Polygonaceae*	astringent	cooling	pungent	PK-V+	astringent, diuretic, alterative
BITTER ROOT *Apocynum androsaemifolium* *Apocynaceae*	bitter, astringent	cooling	pungent	PK-V+	cathartic, emetic, diuretic
BLACKBERRY *Rubus fructicosus, etc.* *Rosaceae*	astringent	cooling	sweet	PK-V+	astringent, alterative, haemostatic

HERB	TASTE	ENERGY	PD-EFFECT	DOSHA	ACTIONS
BLACK COHOSH *Cimicufuga spp.* *Ranunculaceae*	bitter, pungent	cooling	pungent	PK-V+	alterative, emmenagogue, antiseptic
*BLACK PEPPER *Piper nigrum* *Piperaceae*	pungent	heating	pungent	KV-P+	stimulant, expectorant, carminative
BLESSED THISTLE *Carbenia benedicta* *Asteraceae*	bitter	cooling	pungent	PK-V+	emmenagogue, bitter tonic, galactagogue
BLUE COHOSH *Caulophyllum thalictroides* *Berberidaceae*	bitter, sweet	heating	pungent	KV- P+	emmenagogue, parturient, antispasmodic
BLUE FLAG *Iris versicolor* *Iridaceae*	bitter	cooling	pungent	PK-V+	alterative, antipyretic, laxative
BONESET *Eupatorium perfoliatum* *Compositae*	bitter, pungent	cooling	pungent	PK-V+	diaphoretic, antipyretic, laxative

HERB	TASTE	ENERGY	PD-EFFECT	DOSHA	ACTIONS
BORAGE *Borago officinalis* *Boraginaceae*	astringent, sweet	colling	pungent	PK-V+	diuretic, diaphoretic, demulcent
*BRAMHI *Centella asiatica* *Apiaceae*	bitter	cooling	sweet	PKV=	nervine, rejuvenative, alterative, diuretic
BUCHU *Barosma betulina* *Boraginaceae*	pungent, bitter	cooling	pungent	PK-V+	diuretic, diaphoretic, demulcent
BUCKBEAN *Menyanthes trifoliata* *Gentianaceae*	bitter	cooling	pungent	PK-V+	diuretic, antipyretic laxative
BURDOCK *Arctium lappa* *Compositeae*	bitter, pungent	cooling	pungent	PK-V+	alterative, diaphoretic, diuretic, astringent
BUTTERNUT *Juglans cinerea* *Juglandacae*	bitter, astringent	cooling	pungent	PK-V+	purgative, anthelmintic, astringent

HERB	TASTE	ENERGY	PD-EFFECT	DOSHA	ACTIONS
*CALAMUS *Acorus calamus* *Araceae*	pungent, bitter	heating	pungent	VK-P+	stimulant, decongestant, nervine, rejuvenative
CALENDULA *Calendula officinalis* *Asteraceae*	bitter, pungent	cooling	pungent	PK-V+	vulnerary, alterative antispasmodic
CALUMBA *Jateorhiza calumba* *Menispermaceae*	bitter	cooling	pungent	PK-V+	bitter tonic, antipyretic, antiemetic
*CAMPHOR *Cinnamomum camphora* *Lauraceae*	pungent, bitter	heating	pungent	KV-P+	diaphoretic, stimulant. decongestant, analgesic
CARAWAY *Carum carvi* *Apiaceae*	pungent	heating	pungent	KV-P+	carminative, stimulant
*CARDAMOM *Elettaria cardamomum* *Zingiberaceae*	pungent, sweet	heating	pungent	VK-P+	stimulant, carminative, expectorant

HERB	TASTE	ENERGY	PD-EFFECT	DOSHA	ACTIONS
CASCARA SAGRADA *Rhamnus purshianus* *Rhamnaceae*	bitter	cooling	pungent	PK-V+	laxative, astringent, bitter tonic
*CASTOR *Ricinus communis* *Euphorbiaceae*	pungent, sweet	heating	pungent	V- PK+	carthartic, demulcent, analgesic, nervine
CATNIP *Nepeta cataria* *Lamiaceae*	pungent	cooling	pungent	PK-Vo	diaphoretic, carminative nervine
CATTAIL *Typha spp.* *Typhaceae*	sweet, astringent	cooling	sweet	P-VK+	astringent, haemostatic, vulnerary
*CAYENNE *Capsicum annum* *Solanaceae*	pungent	heating	pungent	KV-P+	stimulant, carminative, alterative, haemostatic
CENTAURY AMERICAN *Sabbatia angularis* *Gentianaceae*	bitter	cooling	pungent	PK-V+	febrifuge, bitter tonic

HERB	TASTE	ENERGY	PD-EFFECT	DOSHA	ACTIONS
CENTAURY EUROPEAN *Erythraea centaurium* *Gentianaceae*	bitter, pungent	cooling	pungent	PK-V+	bitter tonic, antipyretic,
CHAMOMILE *Matricaria chamomilla(Ger)* *Anthemis nobilis (Roman)* *Asteraceae*	bitter, pungent	cooling	pungent	PK-Vo	diaphoretic, carminative nervine
CHAPARRAL Larrea divaricata Zygopyllaceae	bitter	cooling	pungent	PK-V+	atterative, diuretic, bitter tonic
CHIA SEEDS *Salvia polystachya* *Lamiaceae*	pungent, sweet	heating	sweet	KV-P+	expectorant, demulcent, diaphoretic
CHICKWEED *Stellaria media* *Caryophyllaceae*	bitter, sweet	cooling	sweet	PK-V+	alterative, demulcent, laxative, vulnerary
CHICORY *Cichorium intybus* *Asteraceae*	bitter	cooling	pungent	PK-V+	alterative, diuretic, antipyretic

HERB	TASTE	ENERGY	PD-EFFECT	DOSHA	ACTIONS
*CINNAMON *Cinnamomum Zeylanicum, etc. Lauraceae*	pungent, sweet astringent	heating	sweet	VK-P+	stimulant, diaphoretic, alterative
CHRYSANTHEMUM *Chrysanthemum indicum Asteraceae*	bitter, sweet	cooling	pungent	PK-V+	diaphoretic, antipyretic, alterative
CLEAVERS *Galium aparine Rubiaceae*	astringent, bitter	cooling	pungent	PK-V+	diuretic, alterative, vulnerary
CLOVES *Eugenia caryophyllata Myrtaceae*	pungent	heating	pungent	VK-P+	stimulant, carminative, aphrodisiac, expectorant
COCONUT *Cocus nucifera Palmaceae*	sweet	cooling	sweet	PV-K+	refrigerant, diuretic, tonic
COLTSFOOT *Tussilago farfara Asteraceae*	pungent, astringent, sweet	cooling	pungent	PK-Vo	demulcent, expectorant, astringent, antispasmodic

HERB	TASTE	ENERGY	PD-EFFECT	DOSHA	ACTIONS
COMFREY *Symphytum officinale* *Boraginaceae*	sweet, astringent	cooling	sweet	PV-K+	nutritive tonic, demulcent, emollient, vulnerary
*CORIANDER *Coriandrum sativum* *Apiaceae*	bitter, pungent	cooling	pungent	PKV =	alterative, diaphoretic, diuretic, carminative
CORN SILK *Zea mays* *Poaceae*	sweet	cooling	pungent	PK-V+	diuretic, demulcent, alterative
COTTON ROOT *Gossypium herbaceum* *Malvaceae*	sweet	heating	sweet	V-KP+	nutritive tonic, aphrodisiac, emmenagogue
CRAMPBARK *Viburnum opulus* *Caprifoliaceae*	bitter, astringent	heating	pungent	KV-P+	emmenagogue, astringent, antispasmodic
CRANESBILL *Geranium maculatum* *Geraniaceae*	astringent	cooling	pungent	PK-V+	astringent, haemostatic, vulnerary

HERB	TASTE	ENERGY	PD-EFFECT	DOSHA	ACTIONS
CUBEBS *Piper cubeba* *Piperaceae*	pungent	heating	pungent	VK-P+	stimulant, carminative, expectorant
CULVER'S ROOT *Leptandra virginica* *Scrophulariaceae*	bitter	cooling	pungent	PK-V+	cathartic, febrifuge, bitter tonic
*CUMIN *Cuminum cyminum* *Apiaceae*	pungent, bitter	cooling	pungent	PKV =	carminative, alterative, stimulant
DAMIANA *Turnera aphrodisiaca* *Turneraceae*	pungent, bitter	heating	pungent	K-VoP+	stimulant, aphrodisiac
*DANDELION *Taraxacum officinale* *Asteraceae*	bitter, sweet	cooling	pungent	PK-V+	alterative, diuretic, laxative
DATES *Phoenix dacytlifera* *Palmaceae*	sweet	cooling	sweet	VP-K+	demulcent, tonic, aphrodisiac

HERB	TASTE	ENERGY	PD-EFFECT	DOSHA	ACTIONS
DILL *Anethum graveolens* *Apiaceae*	pungnet, bitter	cooling	pungent	PK-Vo	carminative, alterative, expectorant
ECHINACEA *Echinacea augustifolia* *Asteraceae*	bitter, pungent	cooling	pungent	PK-V+	alterative, antibiotic, diaphoretic
ELDER FLOWERS *Sambucus spp.* *Caprifoliaceae*	bitter, pungent	cooling	pungent	KP-Vo	diaphoretic, diuretic, alterative
ELECAMPANE *Inula spp.* *Asteraceae*	pungent, bitter	heating	pungnet	VK-P+	expectorant, antispasmodic, rejuvenative
ELEUTHRO *Eleuthro senticosus* *Araliaceae*	pungent, sweet	heating	sweet	VK-P+	tonic, antispasmodic, antirheumatic
EPHEDRA *Ephedra vulgaris* *Gnetaceae*	pungent	heating	pungent	K-VP+	diaphoretic, diuretic, anti-cough, stimulant

HERB	TASTE	ENERGY	PD-EFFECT	DOSHA	ACTIONS
*EUCALYPTUS *Eucalyptus citriodora* *Myrtaceae*	bitter	cooling	pungent	KV-P+	diaphoretic decongestant, stimulant
EYEBRIGHT *Euphrasia officinalis* *Scrophulariaceae*	bitter	cooling	pungent	PK-V+	antipyretic, alterative, astringent
FALSE UNICORN *Helonias dioica* *Liliaceae*	bitter, sweet	heating	sweet	VK-P+	emmenagogue, aphrodisiac, diuretic
*FENNEL *Foeniculum vulgare* *Apiaceae*	sweet, pungent	cooling	sweet	VPK=	carminative, diuretic, antispasmodic
*FENUGREEK *Trigonella foenum-graeceum* *Fabaceae*	bitter, pungent sweet	heating	pungent	VK-P+	stimulant, tonic, expectorant, rejuvenative
*FLAXSEED *Linum usitatissimum* *Linaceae*	sweet, astringent	heating	pungent	V-KoP+	laxative, demulcent, nutritive tonic

HERB	TASTE	ENERGY	PD-EFFECT	DOSHA	ACTIONS
FO-TI *Polygonum multiflorum* *Polygonaceae*	sweet, bitter, astringent	cooling	sweet	PV-K+	tonic, rejuvenative, aphrodisiac, astringent
FRANKINCENSE *Boswellia thurifera* *Burseraceae*	bitter, pungent astringent, sweet	heating	pungent	KV-P+	alterative, analgesic, rejuvenative
GALANGAL *Alpinia officinarum* *Zingiberaceae*	pungent	heating	pungent	VK-P+	stimulant, diaphoretic, antirheumatic
*GARLIC *Allium sativum* *Liliaceae*	all but sour	heating	pungent	VK-P+	stimulant, carminative, antirheumatic
*GENTIAN *Gentiana kurroo* *Gentianaceae*	bitter	cooling	pungent	PK-V+	bitter tonic, antipyretic, alterative
*GINGER *Zingiber officinale* *Zingiberaceae*	pungent, sweet	heating	sweet	VK-P+	stimulant, diaphoretic, expectorant, carminative

HERB	TASTE	ENERGY	PD-EFFECT	DOSHA	ACTIONS
GINSENG *Panax ginseng* *Araliaceae*	pungent, bitter *sweet*	heating	sweet	V-KPo	tonic, stimulant, rejuvenative
*GOKSHURA *Tribulus terrestris* *Zygophyllaceae*	sweet, bitter	cooling	sweet	PK-Vo	diuretic, tonic, aphrodisiac
GOLD THREAD *Coptis spp.* *Ranunculaceae*	bitter	cooling	pungent	PK-V+	bitter tonic, antipyretic, alterative
GOLDEN SEAL *Hydrastis canadensis* *Ranunculaceae*	bitter, astringent	cooling	pungent	PK-V+	bitter tonic, antipyretic antibiotic
GRAVEL ROOT *Eupatorium purpureum* *Asteraceae*	bitter, pungent	cooling	pungent	PK-V+	diuretic, lithotriptic, nervine
GRINDELIA *Grindelia spp.* *Asteraceae*	pungent	heating	pungent	KV-P+	expectorant, diaphoretic antispasmodic

HERB	TASTE	ENERGY	PD-EFFECT	DOSHA	ACTIONS
GROUNDIVY *Glechoma hederacea* *miaceae*	pungent, astringent	heating	pungent	KV-P+	diaphoretic, astringent, carminative
*GUGGUL *Commiphora wightii* *Burseraceae*	bitter, pungent astringent, sweet	heating	pungent	KV-P+	rejuvenative, alterative, antispasmodic, expectorant
GUM ARABIC *Acacia senegal* *Fabaceae*	sweet	cooling	sweet	PV-K+	demulcent, emollient, tonic
*HARITAKI *Terminalia chebula* *Combretaceae*	all but salty	heating	sweet	VK-Po	rejuvenative, nervine, astringent, laxative
HAWTHORN *Crataegus oxycantha* *Rosaceae*	sour, sweet	heating	sour	V-KoP+	stimulant, antispasmodic, diuretic
HENNA *Lawsonia spp.* *Lythraceae*	bitter, astringent	cooling	pungent	PK-V+	antipyretic, alterative, nervine

HERB	TASTE	ENERGY	PD-EFFECT	DOSHA	ACTIONS
HIBISCUS *Hibiscus rosa-sinensis* *Malvaceae*	astringent, sweet	cooling	sweet	PK-V+	alterative, hemostatic, refrigerant, emmenagogue
HOPS *Humulus lupulus* *Articaceae*	bitter, pungent	cooling	pungent	PK-V+	nervine, bitter tonic, diuretic
HOREHOUND *Marrubium vulgare* *Lamiaceae*	bitter, pungent	cooling	pungent	KP-V+	expectorant, antispasmodic, diaphoretic
HORSERADISH *Cochlearia armoracia* *Brassicaceae*	pungent	heating	pungent	KV-P+	stimulant, diuretic, carminative
HORSETAIL *Equisetum spp.* *Equisetaceae*	bitter, sweet	heating	pungent	KV-P+	diuretic, diaphoretic, alterative
HYSSOP *Hyssopus officinalis* *Lamiaceae*	pungent, bitter	heating	pungent	KV-P+	diaphoretic, diuretic, carminative, anthelmintic

HERB	TASTE	ENERGY	PD-EFFECT	DOSHA	ACTIONS
INDIGO *Indigofera tinctoria* *Fabaceae*	bitter	cooling	pungent	PK-V+	alterative, antibiotic, laxative
*JASMINE *Jasminum grandiflorum* *Oleaceae*	bitter	cooling	pungent	PK-V+	alterative, refrigerant. emmenagogue, nervine
JUNIPER BERRIES *Juniperus spp.* *Cupressaceae*	pungent, bitter, sweet	heating	pungent	KV-P+	diuretic, diaphoretic, carminative, analgesic
KUDZU *Pueraria tuberosa* *Fabaceae*	sweet	cooling	sweet	PV-K+	tonic, diaphoretic, diuretic
LADY'S SLIPPER *Cypripedium pubescens* *Orchidaceae*	pungent, sweet, bitter	heating	sweet	VK-Po	nervine, antispasmodic, tonic
LAVENDER *Lavandula spp.* *Lamiaceae*	pungent	cooling	pungent	PK-Vo	carminative, diuretic, antispasmodic

HERB	TASTE	ENERGY	PD-EFFECT	DOSHA	ACTIONS
LEMON *Citrus limonum* *Rutaceae*	sour	cooling	sour	PV-Ko	expectorant, carminative, astringent
LEMON BALM *Melissa officinalis* *Labiatae*	pungent, sweet	cooling	pungent	KP-Vo	diaphoretic, carminative nervine
*LEMON GRASS *Cymbopogon citratus* *Poaceae*	pungent, bitter	cooling	pungent	PK-Vo	diuretic, diaphoretic: refrigerant
LILY *Lilium spp.* *Liliceae*	sweet	cooling	sweet	VP-K+	demulcent, nutritire tonic, nervine
LIME *Citrus acida* *Rutaceae*	sour, bitter	cooling	sour	PV-K+	refrigerant, carminative. expectorant
*LIQUORICE *Glycyrrhiza glabra* *Fabaceae*	sweet, bitter	cooling	sweet	VP-K+	demulcent, expectorant. tonic, laxative

HERB	TASTE	ENERGY	PD-EFFECT	DOSHA	ACTIONS
LOBELIA *Lobelia inflata* *Lobeliaceae*	pungent	heating	pungent	K-PV+	antispasmodic, emetic, expectorant, diaphoretic
*LOTUS *Nelumbo nucifera* *Nymphaeaceae*	sweet, astringent	cooling	sweet	PV-K+	nutritive tonic, astringent, nervine
MACE *Myristica fragrans* *Myristicaceae*	pungent, sweet	heating	pungent	VK-P+	antispasmodic, emetic, expectorant, diaphoretic
*MAHABALA *Sida rhombifoha* *Malvaceae*	sweet, bitter	cooling	sweet	PV – Ko	tonic, demulcent, rejuvenative, diuretic
MALVA *Malva spp.* *Malvaceae*	sweet, astringent	cooling	sweet	PV-K+	demulcent, emollient, astringent
MANDRAKE, AMERICAN *Podophyllum peltatum* *Berberidaceae*	bitter	cooling	pungent	PK-P+	cathartic, alterative, toxic

HERB	TASTE	ENERGY	PD-EFFECT	DOSHA	ACTIONS
MANJISHTA *Rubta cordifolia* *Rubiaceae*	bitter, sweet	cooling	pungent	PK – V +	alterative, hemostatic. emmenagogue. diuretic
MARJORAM *Origanum marjorana* *Lamiaceae*	pungent	heating	pungent	VK-P+	stimulant, antispasmodic, diaphoretic
MARSHMALLOW *Althea officinalis* *Malvaceae*	sweet	cooling	sweet	PV-K+	tonic, demulcent. diuretic, laxative
MISTLETOE *Viscum album* *Loranthaceae*	bitter, sweet	heating	pungent	VK-P+	nervine, antispasmodic. emmenagogue
MORMON TEA *Ephedra spp.* *Gnetaceae*	pungent	heating	pungent	K-VP+	diuretic, alterative
MOTHERWORT *Leonurus cardiaca* *Labiatae*	bitter, pungent	cooling	pungent	PK-V+	emmenagogue. diaphoretic, diuretic.

HERB	TASTE	ENERGY	PD-EFFECT	DOSHA	ACTIONS
MUGWORT *Artemesia vulgaris* *Asteraceae*	pungent, bitter	heating	pungent	VK-P+	antispasmodic, diaphoretic, emmenagogue
MULLEIN *Verbascum thapsus* *Scrophulariaceae*	bitter, astringent, sweet	cooling	pungent	PK-V+	expectorant, astringent, vulnerary, sedative
MUSTA *Cyperus rotundus* *Cyperaceae*	pungent, bitter	cooling	pungent	PK – Vo	carminative, astringent, alterative, emmenagogue
MUSTARD *Brassica campestris* *Brassicaceae*	pungent	heating	pungent	KV-P+	stimulant, expectorant, carminative
MYRRH *Commiphora myrrha* *Burseraceae*	bitter, pungent	heating	pungent	KV-P+	alterative, analgesic, emmenagogue, rejuvenative
NEEM *Azadiracta indica* *Meliaceae*	bitter	cooling	pungent	PK-V+	bitter tonic, antipyretic, alterative

HERB	TASTE	ENERGY	PD-EFFECT	DOSHA	ACTIONS
NETTLE *Urtica urens* *Urticaceae*	astringent	cooling	pungent	PK-V+	alterative, astringent, haemostatic
*NUTMEG *Myristica fragrans* *Myristicaceae*	pungent	heating	pungent	VK-P+	astringent, carminative, sedative, nervine
OAT STRAW *Avena sativa* *Poaceae*	sweet	cooling	sweet	VP-K+	nervine, antispasmodic, tonic
ONION *Allium cepa* *Liliaceae*	pungent, sweet	heating	sweet	VK-P+	diaphoretic, tonic, aphrodisiac
ORANGE PEEL *Citrus aurantium* *Rutaceae*	pungent, bitter	heating	pungent	VK-P+	carminative, expectorant, stimulant
OREGANO *Origanum vulgare* *Lamiaceae*	pungent	heating	pungent	VK-P+	stimulant, carminative, diaphoretic

HERB	TASTE	ENERGY	PD-EFFECT	DOSHA	ACTIONS
OREGON GRAPE *Mahonia repens* *Berberidaceae*	bitter	heating	pungent	PK-V+	alterative, antipyretic, laxative
OSHA *Ligusticum porteri* *Apiaceae*	pungent, bitter	heating	pungent	KV-P+	stimulant, antibacterial, expectorant
PAPRIKA *Capsicum annuum* *Solanaceae*	pungent	heating	pungent	KV-P+	stimulant, carminative
PARSLEY *Petroselinum spp.* *Apiaceae*	pungent	heating	pungent	KV-P+	diuretic, emmenagogue, carminative
PASSION FLOWER *Passiflora incarnata* *Passifloraceae*	bitter	cooling	pungent	PK-V+	nervine, sedative, diuretic, anodyne
PAU D'ARCO *Tabebuia avellanedae* *Bignoneaceae*	bitter	cooling	pungent	PK-V+	alterative, antipyretic, antibiotic

HERB	TASTE	ENERGY	PD-EFFECT	DOSHA	ACTIONS
PENNYROYAL *Mentha pulegium* *Lamiaceae*	pungent	heating	pungent	VK-P+	diaphoretic, carminative, emmenagogue
PEONY *Paeonia officinalis* *Ranunculaceae*	bitter, astringent	cooling	sweet	PK-Vo	alterative, emmenagogue, nervine
*PEPPERMINT *Mentha piperita* *Lamiaceae*	pungent	cooling	pungent	PK-Vo	diaphoretic, carminative nervine tonic
PERUVIAN BARK *Cinchona succirubra* *Rubiaceae*	bitter	cooling	pungent	PK-V+	bitter tonic, antipyretic
PIPPALI *Piper longum* *Piperaceae*	pungent	heating	sweet	VK – P +	stimulant, expectorant, aphrodisiac
PIPSISSEWA *Chimaphila umbellata* *Ericaceae*	bitter	cooling	pungent	PK-V+	diuretic, astringent. alterative

HERB	TASTE	ENERGY	PD-EFFECT	DOSHA	ACTIONS
PLANTAIN *Plantago major* *Plantaginaceae*	astringent, bitter	cooling	pungent	PK-V+	astringent, alterative, diuretic, vulnerary
PLEURISY ROOT *Asclepias tuberosa* *Asclepiadaceae*	bitter, pungent	cooling	pungent	PK-V+	diaphoretic, expectorant febrifuge
POKEROOT *Phytolacca spp.* *Phytolaccaceae*	bitter	cooling	pungent	PK-V+	alterative, emetic, cathartic
*POMEGRANATE *Punica granatum* *Punicaceae*	astringent, bitter, sweet	cooling	sweet	PK-Vo	astringent, alterative, anthelmintic, tonic
POPPY SEEDS *Papaver spp.* *Papaveraceae*	pungent, astringent, sweet	heating	sweet	VK-P+	stimulant, carminative, sedative
PRICKLY ASH *Xanthoxylum spp.* *Rutaceae*	pungent, bitter	heating	pungent	VK-P+	stimulant, carminative, anthelmintic

HERB	TASTE	ENERGY	PD-EFFECT	DOSHA	ACTIONS
PRIMROSE *Primula vulgaris* *Primulaceae*	bitter	cooling	pungent	PK-V+	nervine, demulcent expectorant
*PSYLLIUM *Plantago psyllium* *Plantaginaceae*	sweet, astringent	cooling	sweet	PV-K+	laxative, demulcent, astringent
PUMPKIN SEEDS *Cucurbita pepo* *Cucurbitaceae*	sweet	heating	sweet	V-PK+	anthelmintic, diuretic
*PUNARNAVA *Boerhaavia diffusa* *Nyctaginaceae*	bitter	cooling	pungent	PK-V +	diuretic, diaphoretic, laxative, rejuvenative
PURPLE LOOSESTRIFE *Lythrum salicaria* *Lythraceae*	astringent, sweet	cooling	pungent	PK-V+	alterative, astringent, demulcent
RASPBERRY *Rubus spp.* *Rosaceae*	astringent, sweet	cooling	sweet	PK-V+	astringent, alterative, emmenagogue

HERB	TASTE	ENERGY	PD-EFFECT	DOSHA	ACTIONS
RED CLOVER *Trifolium pratense* *Fabaceae*	bitter, sweet	cooling	pungent	PK-V+	alterative, diuretic, expectorant
RED ROOT *Ceanothus spp.* *Polygonaceae*	astringent	cooling	pungent	PK-V+	astringent, expectorant. sedative
REHMANNIA *Rehmannia glutinosa* *Scrophulariaceae*	sweet, bitter	cooling	sweet	PV-K +	nutritive tonic, rejuvenative, aphrodisiac
*RHUBARB *Rheum emodi* *Polygonaceae*	bitter	cooling	pungent	PK-V+	purgative, alterative, antipyretic
ROSE FLOWERS *Rosa spp.* *Rosaceae*	bitter, pungent, astringent, sweet	cooling	sweet	VPK=	alterative, emmenagogue, nervine
ROSEMARY *Rosmarinus officinalis* *Lamiaceae*	pungent, bitter	heating	pungent	KV-P+	diaphoretic, carminative stimulant, emmenagogue

HERB	TASTE	ENERGY	PD-EFFECT	DOSHA	ACTIONS
RUE *Ruta graveolens* *Rutaceae*	bitter, pungent	heating	pungent	KV-P+	nervine, emmenagogue anthelmintic
SAFFLOWER *Carthamus tinctorius* *Asteraceae*	pungent	heating	pungent	VK-P+	alterative, emmenagogue, carminative
*SAFFRON *Crocus sativus* *Iridaceae*	pungent, bitter, sweet	cooling	sweet	VPK=	alterative, emmenagogue, rejuvenative, carminative
SAGE *Salvia officinalis* *Lamiaceae*	pungent, bitter, astringent	heating	pungent	KV-P+	diaphoretic, expectorant, nervine, astringent
*SANDALWOOD *Santalum album* *Santalaceae*	bitter, sweet, astringent	cooling	sweet	PV-Ko	alterative, hemostatic, antipyretic, nervine
SARSAPARILLA *Smilax spp* *Liliaceae*	bitter, sweet	cooling	sweet	PV-Ko	alterative, diuretic, antispasmodic

HERB	TASTE	ENERGY	PD-EFFECT	DOSHA	ACTIONS
SASSAFRAS *Sassafras officinale* *Lauraceae*	pungent	heating	pungent	KV-P+	alterative, diaphoretic, stimulant
SAVORY *Satureia hortensis* *Lamiaceae*	pungent	heating	pungent	KV-P+	stimulant, carminative, astringent
SAW PALMETTO *Serenoa serrulata* *Palmaceae*	sweet, pungent	heating	sweet	V-PK+	tonic, rejuvenative, aphrodisiac, expectorant
SELF-HEAL *Prunella vulgaris* *Lamiaceae*	bitter, astringent	cooling	pungent	PK-V+	alterative, antipyretic, vulnerary
SENNA *Cassia acutifolia* *Fabaceae*	bitter	cooling	pungent	PK-V+	purgative, antipyretic, alterative
SESAME SEEDS *Sesamum indicum* *Pedaliaceae*	sweet	heating	sweet	V-PK+	nutritive tonic, demulcent, rejuvenative

HERB	TASTE	ENERGY	PD-EFFECT	DOSHA	ACTIONS
*SHATAVARI *Asparagus racemosus* *Liliaceae*	sweet, bitter	cooling	sweet	PV-K +	nutritive tonic, demulcent, emmenagogue, rejuvenative
SHEPHERD'S PURSE *Capsella bursapastoris* *Brassicaceae*	astringent, bitter	cooling	pungent	PK-V+	astringent, haemostatic. alterative
SKULLCAP *Scucttellaria spp.* *Lamiaceae*	bitter	cooling	pungent	PK-Vo	nervine, antispasmodic.
SKUNK CABBAGE *Symplocarpus foetidus* *Araceae*	pungent	heating	pungent	KV-P+	nervine, antispasmodic. expectorant
SLIPPERY ELM *Ulmus fulva* *Urticaceae*	sweet	cooling	sweet	PV-K+	nutritive tonic, demulcent, emollient
SOLOMON'S SEAL *Polygonatum spp.* *Liliaceae*	sweet, bitter	cooling	sweet	PV-K+	nutritive tonic, demulcent, astringent. rejuvenative

HERB	TASTE	ENERGY	PD-EFFECT	DOSHA	ACTIONS
SPEARMINT *Mentha spicata* *Lamiaceae*	pungent	cooling	pungent	KP-Vo	diaphoretic, diuretic, carminative
SPIKENARD *Aralia racemosa* *Araliaceae*	sweet, pungent	heating	sweet	KV-P+	demulcent, expectorant, tonic, alterative
SQUAW VINE *Mitchella repens* *Rubiaceae*	astringent, bitter	cooling	pungent	PK-V+	emmenagogue, astringent, diuretic, alterative
ST. JOHN'S WORT *Hypericum perforatum* *Hypericaceae*	bitter, pungent	cooling	pungent	PK-V+	antispasmodic, expectorant, astringent
STAR ANISE *Illicium verum* *Magnoliaceae*	pungent	heating	pungent	VK-P+	stimulant, carminative
STILLINGIA *Stillingia sylvatica* *Euphorbiaceae*	pungent	heating	pungent	KV-P+	alterative, diaphoretic, expectorant, tonic

HERB	TASTE	ENERGY	PD-EFFECT	DOSHA	ACTIONS
STONEROOT *Gollinsonia canadesis* *Lamiaceae*	bitter	cooling	pungent	PK-V+	diuretic, diaphoretic. astringent
STRAWBERRY LEAVES *Fragaria spp.* *Rosaceae*	astringent, sweet	cooling	sweet	PK-V+	alterative, astringent, diuretic
SUGAR CANE *Saccharum officinarum* *Poaceae*	sweet	cooling	sweet	PV-K+	nutritive tonic, demulcent, laxative
SUMACH *Rhus glabra, etc.* *Anacardiaceae*	astringent	cooling	pungent	PK-V+	astringent, alterative, refrigerant
TAMARIND *Tamarindus indica* *Fabaceae*	sour, sweet	heating	sour	VK-P+	stimulant, carminative, laxative
TANSY *Tanacetum vulgare* *Asteraceae*	bitter, pungent	cooling	pungent	PK-Vo	emmenagogue, diaphoretic, bitter tonic

HERB	TASTE	ENERGY	PD-EFFECT	DOSHA	ACTIONS
TARRAGON *Artemesia dracunculus* *Asteraceae*	bitter, pungent	heating	pungent	KV-P+	emmenagogue, diuretic, carminative
THYME *Thymus vulgaris* *Lamiaceae*	pungent	heating	pungent	VK-P+	antispasmodic, carminative, antispasmodic
TORMENTIL *Potentilla tormentilla* *Rosaceae*	astringent, bitter	cooling	pungent	PK-V+	astringent, hemostatic, antiseptic
*TURMERIC *Curcuma longa* *Zingiberaceae*	pungent, bitter,	heating	pungent	KV-Po	stimulant, alterative, antibacterial, vulnerary
UVA URSI *Arctostaphylos uva-ursi* *Ericaceae*	astringent, bitter	cooling	pungent	PK-V+	diuretic, astringent. antiseptic
*VALERIAN *Valeriana jatamansii* *Valerianaceae*	pungent	heating	pungent	VK-V+	nervine, antispasmodic. carminative, sedative

HERB	TASTE	ENERGY	PD-EFFECT	DOSHA	ACTIONS
VAMSHA ROCHANA *Bambusa arundinacea* *Poaceae*	sweet, astringent	cooling	sweet	PV-K +	demulcent, expectorant, tonic
VERVAIN *Verbena spp.* *Verbenaceae*	bitter	cooling	pungent	PK-V+	antipyretic, astringent
*VETIVERT *Vetiveria zizanioides* *Poaceae*	bitter, sweet	cooling	pungent	PK-V+	antipyretic, astringent refrigerant
VIDARI-KANDA *Ipomoea digitata* *Convolvulaceae*	sweet	cooling	sweet	VP-Ko	nutritive tonic, aphrodisiac, diuretic
VIOLET *Viola spp.* *Violaceae*	bitter, pungent	cooling	pungent	PK-V+	alterative, antiseptic, expectorant
WAHOO *Euonymus atropurpureus* *Celastraceae*	bitter	cooling	pungent	PK-V+	purgative, antipyretic, diuretic

HERB	TASTE	ENERGY	PD-EFFECT	DOSHA	ACTIONS
WALNUT *Juglans nigra* *Juglandaceae*	sweet	heating	sweet	V-PK+	demulcent, tonic, laxative
WATERCRESS *Rorippa nasturtium* *Brassicaceae*	pungent	heating	pungent	KV-P+	diuretic, expectorant, stimulant
WHITE OAK *Quercus alba* *Fagaceae*	astringent	cooling	pungent	PK-V+	astringent, haemostatic, antiseptic
WHITE PINE *Pinus alba* *Pinaceae*	pungent	heating	pungent	KV-P+	expectorant, diaphoretic carminative
WHITE POND LILY *Nymphaea odorata* *Nymphaeaceae*	sweet, astringent, bitter	cooling	sweet	PV-K+	demulcent, astringent, tonic
WHITE POPLAR *Populus tremuloides* *Salicaceae*	bitter	cooling	pungent	PK-V+	bitter tonic, antipyretic, diuretic

HERB	TASTE	ENERGY	PD-EFFECT	DOSHA	ACTIONS
WILD CARROT *Daucus carota* *Apiaceae*	pungent	heating	pungent	KV-P+	diuretic, stimulant, carminative, emmenagogue
WILD CHERRY BARK *Prunus spp.* *Rosaceae*	bitter, astringent	cooling	sweet	PK-Vo	antispasmodic, expectorant, alterative
WILD GINGER *Asarum Canadense* *Aristolochiaceae*	pungent	cooling	pungent	PK-V+	astringent, hemostatic, decongestant
WILD YAM *Dioscorea spp.* *Dioscoreaceae*	sweet, bitter	cooling	sweet	VP-Ko	antispasmodic, diaphoretic, tonic, rejuvenative
WILLOW BARK *Salix spp.* *Salicaceae*	bitter	cooling	pungent	PK-V+	bitter tonic, antipyretic, anodyne
WINTERGREEN *Gaultheria procumbens* *Ericaceae*	pungent	cooling	pungent	PK-Vo	carminative, astringent, analgesic

HERB	TASTE	ENERGY	PD-EFFECT	DOSHA	ACTIONS
WITCH HAZEL *Hamamelis virginiana* *Hamamelidaceae*	astringent, bitter, pungent	cooling	pungent	PK-V+	astringent, stimulant, vulnerary
WORMSEED *Chenopodium anthelminticum* *Chenopodiaceae*	pungent, bitter astringent	heating	pungent	KV-P+	anthelmintic, stimulant, antispasmodic
WORMWOOD *Artemisia absinthium* *Asteraceae*	bitter, pungent,	cooling	pungent	PK-Vo	anthelmintic, carminative, antispasmodic
YARROW *Achillea millefolium* *Asteraceae*	bitter, pungent astringent	cooling	pungent	PK-V+	diaphoretic, astringent, alterative
YELLOW DOCK *Rumex crispus* *Polygonaceae*	bitter, astringent	cooling	pungent	PK-V+	alterative, astringent, laxative

HERB	TASTE	ENERGY	PD-EFFECT	DOSHA	ACTIONS
YERBA SANTA *Eriodictyon glutinosum* *Hydrophyllaceae*	pungent	heating	pungent	KV-P+	expectorant, antispasmodic carminative
YERBA MATE *Ilex paraguariensis* *Aquifoliaceae*	pungent	heating	pungent	K-Vo P+	stimulant, diuretic

Appendix II

AYURVEDIC VITAMIN CHART

VITAMIN A

Stress, Depleted or Low Immune

Utilized in the Body	Helps in night vision. increases hair growth, strengthens all bone tissues, and balances all tissue linings
Deficiencies	Allergies, split ends of hair shafts, loss of smell, dry skin, susceptibility to frequent colds, tooth decay
Functions	Builds and strengthens immune system to fight infections; assists with aging process; prevents senility
Synthetic	Acetate or palmitate
Toxicity	300,000 IU
R.D.A.	5,000 IU with no special health problems; therapeutic dosage up to 100,000 IU with specific problems (i.e., acure infection, candidiasis).
Far Soluble	Animal sources
Water Soluble	Vegetable sources
Depleted By	Stress; overwork
VATA	Milk, Yogurt, Carrots, Spinach, Sweet Potatoes, Yams, Mangos, Soaked Seaweed
PITTA	Milk, Cottage Cheese, Kale, Collard Greens, Turmeric, Lemongrass, Mangos, Cabbage, Raspberry Leaf, Dandelion, Mints, Cilantro, Spirulina, Dark Leafy Greens

KAPHA	Buttermilk, Milk, Lemongrass, Parsley, Spinach, Mangos, Nettle, Mints, Dry Seaweed. Paprika, Sage, Cayenne, Chickweed, Kelp, Turmeric
Sources of Beta Carotene	Beta-carotene is a vegetable sourced precursor (can be made into) which must be converted by the liver into vitamin A at a ratio of 2 to 1 (i.e., 20,000 IU beta-carotene = 10,000 IU of vitamin A)

Note : The dosages of Vitamin A mentioned above regarding illnesses are often significantly higher than the maintenance does. The elevated amounts are not recommended for more than one month unless prescribed by a physician who understands vitamins. There have been a few reported cases of toxicity with long term use.

B-VITAMINS

B-vitamins work together as a complex and are often sold together in varying amounts or in equivalents (50 mg each). If you take an isolated B vitamin, it can create a deficiency of other B's so always take a balanced B-complex tablet also (i.e., B-1000 mg and B-complex 100 mg).

Depleted By	Smoking or second hand smokc, medication, antibiotic.

VITAMIN B-1 – THIAMINE

Metabolism

Utilized in the Body	Brain, ears, eyes, heart, muscle tissue, liver.
Deficiencies	Gastrointestinal problems, anger, irritability, muscle tone, numbness, nervousness of hands and feet, stabilizes appetite
Functions	Builds blood, assists with strengthening all

	tissue: circulation: assists digestion: nerves: stabilizes appetite
Synthetic	Thiamine hydrochloride: Thiamine mononitrate
R.D.A.	1.4 mg. Therapeutic dosage up to 240 mg
Toxicity	No known oral toxicity
Water Soluble	
Depleted By	Alcohol, coffee, sugar
VITA	Asparagus, Citrus, Garlic, Black Strap Molasses, Seaweed, Catnip, Watercress, Rice Bran
PITTA	Cauliflower, Kale, Barley Grass, Seaweed, Asparagus, Dandelion, Red Clover, Raspberry Leaf, Catnip
KAPHA	Cauliflower, Kale, Citrus, Spirulina, Garlic, Ghee,. Asparagus, Brewer's Yeast, Dandelion, Red Clover, Raspberry Leaf, Watercress, Rice Bran, Yeast

VITAMIN B-2 – RIBOFLAVIN

Emotional Balance, Blood

Utilized in the Body	Brain, nervous system, intestinal tract, epithelia tissue, spleen, liver
Deficiencies	Red bulging eyes, canker sores, nausea, weak digestion, sore cracked tongue, early gray hair, wrinkles
Functions	Metabolizes fat; assists functioning of antibodies and red blood cells; assists normal breathing patterns
Synthetic	Riboflavin
Toxicity	None Known
R.D.A	1.6 mg. Therapeutic Dosage: Up to 900 mg

Water Soluble	
Depleted By	Hot flashes, crying jags, antibiotics, tranquilizers
VATA	Raspberry Leaves, Catnip, Hops, Dulse, Currants, Watercress, Rosehips, Ginseng, Mushrooms, Organ Meats, Black Strap Molasses, Parsley, Dulse, Fenugreek, Rice Bran
PITTA	Brussel Sprouts, Red Clover, Raspberry Leaves, Alfalfa, Yarrow, Sago Palm, Steamed Onions, Legumes, Dandelions, Yellow Dock, Rice Bran
KAPHA	Nettles, Red Clover, Peppermint, Rosehips, Beans, Beet Greens, Asparagus, Legumes, Parsley, Dandelions, Fenugreek, Yellow Dock, Yeast

VITAMIN B-3 – NICACIN, NIACINAMIDE, NICOTIC ACID

Anxiety, Depression, Cholesterol, Heart pressure

Utillzed in the Body	Brain, gastrointestenal, nervous system, liver, skin, circulation, cholesterol, disorders, muscle weakness
Deficiencies	Skin problems, depression, nervous disorders, headaches, cold feet and hands, liver disorder, muscle weakness
Functions	Balances cholesterol levels; metabolies carbohydrates; balances hormones and hormorne production; dilation of blood flow and lymph movement
Syntheric	Nicotinic Acid, Niacin, Niacinamide
R.D.A.	1.6 mg.

Therapeutic Dosage: Up to 300 mg.

Toxicity	200 mg. in some people

Water Soluble	
Depleted By	Fatigue,digestion abnormalities
VATA	Rice Bran, Burdock Root, Hops, Slippery Elm, Asparagus, Organ Meats, Eggs, Avocados
PITTA	Slippery Elm, Spirulina, Echinacea, Cabbage, Red Clover, Liquorice, Nettles, Rice Syrup, Milk, Rice Bran, Potatoes, Burdock Root, Hops, Raspberry Leaf, Sunflower Seeds, Organ Meat, Lean Meat, Eggs, Avocado, Sunflower Seeds, Lean Meats, Peanuts
KAPHA	Spirulina, Bee Pollen, Nettles, Parsley, Potatoes, Burdock Root, Hops, Raspberry Leaf, Prunes

Note : Niacin in amounts greater than 100 mg will cause skin flushing. This property has been used in detox programs in combination with extended sauna (2-3 hours) at lowered temperatures (150 degrees) to promote elimination of toxins via the skin. Increasing amounts must be taken each day to elicit this response as body tolerance increases.

VITAMIN B-4 – CHOLINE

Utilized in the body	Brain, hair, gallbladder, kidneys, liver thymus, liver/bile production, endocrine system, urinary tract, balances cholesterol
Deficiencies	Ulcers, heart disorders, high blood pressure, kidney problems, stomach ulcers, intestinal bleeding, liver/gall bladder disorders, poor assimilation of fats
Functions	Works together with inositol: a basic constituent of lecithin; cell growth: emulsifies fat (cholesterol)
Synthetic :	Choline bitartrade or Biotin
Toxicity :	None known
R.D.A.	None established. Therapeutic dosage: Up to 1.500

Water Soluble

Depleted By	Alcohol, fried foods
VATA	Egg Yolk, Organ Meats, Wheat Bran, Wheat Germ, Liver
PITTA	Soybeans, Green Leafy Vegetables, Lecithin
KAPHA	Brewer's Yeast, Soybeans, Green Leafy Vegetable

VITAMIN B-5 – PANTOTHENIC ACID

Muscle Spasms, Allergies, Adrenal Insufficiency & Assists Body in Producing Cortisone

Utilized in the body	Fat metabolism, aids in breaking down proteins, adrenal support, brain tissue, digestive system, musculokeletal system, epithelia tissue, endocrine system, particularly the adrenal glands
Deficiencies	Constipation, duodenal ulcers, eczema, hypoglycemia, kidney disorders, hair loss, infection, sensitivity to gluten, auto accident injuries, muscle spasms, allergies, adrenal insufficiency, pain, muscle spasms, cramps, skin disorders, frequent colds
Function	Assists in producing cortisone; assists muscle healing antibody production; assimilation of vitamins; stops muscle spasms
Synthetic	Calcium pantothenate
Toxicity	10,000 - 20,000 mg
R. D. A.	10 mg

Therapeutic Dosage: Up to 1.000 mg.

Water Soluble

Depleted By	Stress, overwork, not enough self-care, muscle injury, accident, shock trauma

VATA	Rice Bran, Organ Meats, Egg Yolk, Liver, Molasses, Royal Jelly, Wheat Bran, Wheat Germ
PITTA	Green vegetables, Legumes, Soybeans, Peanuts, Whole Grains
KAPHA	Green Vegetables, Legumes, Soybeans, Royal Jelly, Brewers Yeast, Whole Grains
	Highest source is yeast and rice bran syrup

VITAMIN B-6 – PYRIDOXINE

Immune System, Skin, Herpes Sores, Cancer Preventative

Utilized in the Body	Circulation, muscles, nerves, skin, immune system
Deficiencies	Anemia, skin problems, kidney/bladder disorders, nervousness, nausea, vomiting, arthritis, depression, menstrual cramps, dizziness, frequent infections, anger, fear
Functions	Alleviates nause; antibody formation; digestion; weight control; assists in balancing sodium and potassium; cancer preventative; increases immune function; improves complexion; prevention of cancer
Synthetic	Pyridoxine hydrochloride
R. D. A.	2 - 100 mg

Therapeutic Dosage: Up to 1.800 mg

Toxicity	None Known

Water Soluble

Depleted By	Constipation, fasting, oral contraceptives, radiation , heart problems
VATA	Fish, Turnip. Cooked Spinach. Green Pepper. Organ Meats. Black Strap Molasses-unrefined. Wheat Germ. Carrots. Banana. Avocado

PITTA	Broccoli, Kale, Bananas, Leafy Greens, Peanuts
KAPHA	Fish, Spinach, Green Pepper, Leafy Green Vegetables

VITAMIN B-7 BIOTIN
(Also known as Vitamin H)

Utilized in the Body	Brain, hair, skin, muscular tissue, bone tissue
Deficiencies	Glandular disorders, dry hair, dry skin, dandruff, split ends, weak tissue, insomnia, early gray hair
Functions	Aids in recovery from fatigue; assists cell oxidation; metabolism of proteins, fats and sugar; nerves; antiseptic; assists antibody formation; assists assimilation of vitamins
Synthetic	Biotin
Toxicity	No oral toxicity
R.D.A.	30 -30 mg

Therapeutic Dosage: Up to 450 mcg

Water Soluble

Depleted By	Shock, trauma
VATA	Liver, Sardines, Whole Grains, Beef, Fruits, Nuts, Eggs
PITTA	Unpolished Rice, Legumes, Whole Grains, Fruits, Milk
KAPHA	Legumes, Whole Grains, Fruits, Basmati Rice

VITAMIN B - 8 – INOSITOL

Utilized in the Body	Brain, heart, kidneys, liver, muscle, hair, skin, bones, endocrine system, muscular system, assists choline and biotin

Deficiencies	Hypertension, constipation, eczema, eye disorders, hair loss, skin disorders, weak bones, cystitis
Functions	Calming effects; cholesterol reduction; prevents eczema; promotes hair growth; skin improvement; mental clarity and strength
Toxiciry	None known
R. D. A.	Unknown

Therapeutic Dosage: 100 - 1,000 mg

Water Soluble

Depleted By	Fried foods; excess fat
VATA	Black Strap Molasses - unrefined, Whole Grains, Nuts, Citrus, Organic Meats - Liver, Lecithin, Wheat Germ
PITTA	Milk, Whole Grains, Cabbage
KAPHA	Citrus, Whole Grains, Brewers Yeast, Raisins

VITAMIN B -9 – FOLIC ACID

Healthy Bones, Calm Nerves, Flexibility of Tissues, Adrenal Insufficiency

Utilized in the body	Endocrine, urinary tract, epithelia tissue blood, hair
Deficiencies	Canker sores, nervousness, anxiety, fatigue, depression, early gray hair, allergies, anaemia, edema, mental depression, overweight, infertility, muscle spasms
Functions	Relieves muscle spasms; production of hydrochloric acid; assists milk production; improved appetite; protein metabolism; formation of red blood cells; adrenal and pituitary enhancement; strong bones; pain reliever; division of body cells; hydrochloride

	acid production; red blood cell production
Synthetic	Pleroylglutamic Acid
Toxicity	None known
R. D. A.	4 mg

Therapeutic Dosage: Up to 4,000 mcg

Water Soluble

Depleted By	Stress; accident; overwork
VATA	Catnip, Comfrey, Dark Green Vegetables, Root Vegetables, Salmon, Sage, Mushrooms, Nuts, Asparagus, Cilantro
PITTA	Greens, Plantain, Chickweed, Peppermint, Kale, Broccoli, Milk, Nettles, Alfalfa, Asparagus, Legumes, Parsley
KAPHA	Nettles, Alfalfa, Parsley, Sage, Chickweed, Broccoli, Kale, Beet Greens, Dark Green Vegetables, Oysters, Root Vegetables, Catnip, Asparagus, Legumes

VITAMIN B - 12 – CYANOCOHALAMIN

Utilized in the body	All cells, nervous system, brain, circulation
Deficiencies	Anaemia, brain damage, poor appetite neuritis, chronic fatigue, general weakness, speech difficulties, irritability, stuttering, anaemia, hypoglycemia, fatigue
Functions	Increases appetite; blood cell formation; relieves depression; promotes longevity; memory; increases energy; promotes growth in children; pituitary function; balances nervous system; relaxes tissue
Synthetic	Cannot be synthetically made
Toxicity	None

R. D. A.	6 mcg

Therapeutic Dosage: 10 - 1,000 mcg

Water Soluble

Depleted By	Stress; poor diet
VATA	Cheese Lamb, Banana, Comfrey, Catnip, Concord Grapes, Cheese, Eggs, Seaweeds Liver, Wheat Germ
PITTA	Freshwater Fish, Milk, Banana, Alfalfa, Catnip, Miso, sunflower Seeds, Milk
KAPHA	Freshwater Fish, Kelp, Peanuts, Alfalfa, Miso

VITAMIN B-13 – CALCIUM ORATE

Utilized in the Body	All cell production
Deficiencies	Cancer, multiple sclerosis, aging, muscle weakness, early aging, degenerative disorders
Functions	Essential for biosynthesis of nucleic acid; cell rejuvenation; pregnancy; hormone production
Synthetic	Cannot be synthetically made
Toxicity	No known toxicity
R.D.A.	None established
Water Soluble	
VATA	Brown Rice, Apple Seeds, Grape Seeds, Nuts/seeds, Wheatgrass, Pink Lentils-well cooked, Root Vegetables, Yogurt Curdled Milk, Rejuvelac, Liquid Whey
PITTA	Sunflower Seeds, Apple Seeds, Grape Seeds, Legumes, Nuts/seeds-(diet/dosha specific), Wheatgrass, Liquid Whey
KAPHA	Brewer's Yeast. Pumpkin Seeds. Sesame Seeds. Apple Seeds. Grape Seeds. Lentils. Legumes. Nuts Seeds (diet/dosha specific)

VITAMIN B - 15 – CALCIUM PANGAMETE

Utilized in the Body	Kidneys, immune organs, nerves, urinary tract
Dediciendies	Heart disorders, glandular disorders
Functions	Aids in recovery from fatigue; cell oxygenation; fat, protein and sugar metabolism: endocrine system; lubrication of glands, cell regeneration
Synthetic	Pangamic acid
Toxicity	600 mg
R. D. A.	None established; possibly 50 mg

Therapeutic Dosage: 100 mg

Water Soluble

Depleted By	Fried foods; excess consumption of fat
VATA	Sesame Seeds, butter, Wheat, Brown Rice, Rice, Quince
PITTA	Rye,.Spelt, Sunflower seeds, Apricot Kernel
KAPHA	Pumpkin Seeds, Brewer's Yeast, Spelt, Almonds, Basmati Rice

VITAMIN B-17–LAETRILE (NITROSIDES)

Cancer Prevention

Utilized in the Body	Cell regeneration, hair, skin, endocrine, particularly the thyroid
Deficiencies	Cancer, immune disorders, viruses, autoimmune disorders
Functions	Controls cancer growth; prevention properties; reverses aging process; prevents cancer; strengthens organs; assists metabolism; balances endocrine system; protein assimilation; assists reproductive organs: cell regeneration

Synthetc Not available

Toxicity Over 1.0 gm may be toxic

R.D.A. Unknown.

Therapeutic Dosage: 25 - 1.0 gm. with meal

Water Soluble

Depleted By Stress, anxiety, fear

VATA Cheese, Lamb, Banana, Comfrey, Catnip, Concord Grapes, Cheese, Eggs, Seaweeds, Wheatgrass, Apricot, Peach, Almonds, Cranberries, Raspberries, Flaxseed, Plums

PITTA Freshwater Fish, Milk, Banana. Alfalfa, Catnip, Miso, Sunflower seeds, Garbanzo Beans, Mung Beans, Lima Beans. Wheatgrass, Raspberries

KATHA Kelp, Peanuts, Alfalfa. Miso, Miller, Flax, Blackberries, Cranberries, Mung Beans, Almonds

PABA – PARA AMINO BENZOIC ACID (B-COMPLEX)

Utilized in the Body Red blood cells

Deficiencies Tooth decay, muscle wasting constipation, low/high thyroid function, premature gray hair, aging, extreme tiredness, depression, miscarriage, intestinal disorders

Functions Sunscreens; hair pigmentation; healthy skin; intestinal functions; protein utilization; production of folic acid

Synthetic Not Known

Toxicity High doses over time can be toxic to the liver

R. D. A. None established

Therapeutic Dosage: 30 mg.

Water Soluble

Depleted By	Sulfur drugs; depression; constipation
VITA	Organ Meats, Wheatgerm Oil, Yogurt, Molasses, Rice Bran, Wheat
PITTA	Green Leafy Vegetables, Rice Bran, Legumes, Peanuts
KAPHA	Green Leafy Vegetables, Legumes, Yeast

VITAMIN C – ACEROLA, CITRUS, ASCORBATE ACID, SAGO PALM, AMLA

Strong Bones, Circulation, Night Sweats, Infections. Immune Builder, Adrenal Builder, Menopause

Utilized in the Body	Brain, heart, circulation, endocrine system, bones, ligaments, blood vessels
Deficiencies	Weak bones, mouth sores, anemia, weight loss, frequent infections, colds, flu, bleeding gums, thyroid disorders, poor digestion, bruising
Functions	Gum and teeth formation; smooth skin; collagen production; clear complexion; assists digestion and assimilation; strengthens immune system; prevents diarrhoea
Synthetic	Ascorbic acid, ascorbate
Toxicity	
R. D. A.	60 mg

Therapeutic Dosage: Up to 10,000 mg

Water Soluble

Depleted By	Aspirins, pain relievers, coffee, stress, smoking, baking soda, fevers, pain killers
VATA	Acerola, Tamarind, Lemon, Saffron, Strawberries, Rosehips, Comfrey, Primrose oil, Tomatoes, Guavas, Sweet Potatoes

PITTA	Yellow Dock, Dandelion, Raspberries, Red Clover, Alfalfa, Rosehips, Green Pepper, Saffron, Kale, Sago Palm, Cabbage, Primrose Oil, Cauliflower, Green Leafy Vegetables
KAPHA	Red Clover, Alfalfa, Yellow Dock, Raspberries, Rosehips, Spinach, Beet Greens, Parsley, Strawberries, Cayenne, Cabbage, Primrose Oil, Guava, Bell Peppers, Green leafy Vegetables

Note : Ascorbic acid is best for Vata and kapha. The ascorbate form is best for Pitta because, it is alkaline.

VITAMIN D – ERGOSTEROL

Strong Bones, Cancer Prevention, Balances Glucose

Utilized in the Body	Bones, never skin, teeth, thyroid
Deficiencies	Anaemia, constipation, diarrhoea, myopia, muscle weakness, poor absorption, tooth decay, soft bones
Functions	Assimilation of vitamin E and calcium in the intestinal tract; normal blood clotting
Synthetic	Calciferol of irradiated Ergosterol
Toxicity	25,000 IU may be toxic
R. D. A.	400 IU

Therapeutic Dosage: Up to 1,500 IU

Fat Soluble

Depleted By	Mineral oil
Best Source	Sunshine on the skin produces it in the body
VATA	Ghee, Eggs, Cod Liver Shrimp, Tuna, Mackerel, Sardines, Sunflower seeds, butter, Salmon, Fish Oils

PITTA	Trout, White Eggs, Ghee, Butter Sunflower Seeds, Alfalfa, Nettles, Raspberry Leaves, Red Clover, Fresh Water Tuna, Sprouted Seeds
KAPHA	Ghee, Trout, Sunlight, Alfalfa, Nettles, Raspberry Leaves, Red Clover, Sprouted Seeds

VITAMIN E – D- ALPHATOCOPHEROL; TOCOPHEROL ACETATE

Night Sweats, Cancer, Wrinkles, Arthritic Joints, Aging Process

Utilized in the Body	Heart, liver, lungs, adrenals, pituitary, all fatty tissue
Deficiencies	Baldness, prostate disorders, heart disorders, dry skin premature aging, miscarriage
Functions	Blood vessel dilator; reduces cholesterol; circulation; red blood cell production
Synthetic	D-Alpha tocopherol, Alpha tocopherol acetate
Toxicity	When taken for long periods of time in large amounts may produce toxicity
R. D. A.	10 IU

Therapeutic Dosage: Up to 1,000 IU

Fat Soluble

Depleted By	Stress, alcohol
VATA	Brown Rice, Oats, Shatavari, Cold Pressed Oils (diet/dosha specific), Organ Meats, Black Strap Molasses, Sweet potato, Watercress, Rosehips, Nuts (diet/dosha specific)
PITTA	Alfalfa, Rosehips Buckwheat, Sunflower Oil, Sweet Potato, Dandelion, Cold Pressed Oils (diet/dosha specific), soybean
KAPHA	Wheat, Corn, Rye, Almond Oil, Cold Pressed

	Oils (diet/dosha specific), Watercress, Dandelion, Soybeans, Greens

VITAMIN F – LINOLEIC, LINOLENIC AVACHIDONIC SEED, VEGETABLE & NUT OILS

Utilized in the Body	Adrenal, thyroid, cell production, skin, heart, arteries
Deficiencies	Allergies, dry skin, eczema, baldness, kidney disorders, cancer, nail problems, varicose veins
Functions	Normalizes blood pressure; blood coagulation; all glandular activity; healthy hair
Synthetic	None
Toxicity	None established
R. D. A.	10% of total calories. Men can take 5 times mores than women
Fat Soluble	
Depleted By	Radiation treatments
VATA	Ghee, Sunflower Seeds, Vegetable Oils (diet/dosha specific), Avocados, Flaxseed Oil
PITTY	Butter, Ghee, Sunflower Seeds, Vegetable Oils (diet/dosha specific), Peanuts, Castor oil
KAPHA	Ghee, Vegetable Oils (diet/dosha specific). Flaxseed Oil, Pumpkin Oils

VITAMIN K – ALFALFA

Utilized in the Body	Blood, circulation, liver
Deficiencies	Jaundice, bleeding ulcers, miscarriage, colitis, bruising, aging, varicose veins, miscarriage
Functions	Blood clotting; healthy liver; intestinal tract
Synthetic	Menadoine
Toxicity	1,000 mcg

R. D. A. 70 mcg

Fat Soluble

Therapeutic Dosage: 250 mcg

Depleted by Frozen foods, rancid fats, radiation, sulfate drugs & sulfates in foods

VATA Safflower Oil, Black Strap Molasses, Kelp, Green Leafy Vegetables (diet/dosha specific), Fish Oil Cherries, Pickles. Blackberries, Yogurt Molasses, Fermented Vegetables

PITTA Safflower Oil, Cauliflower, Alfalfa, Nettles, Green Leafy Vegetables (diet/dosha specific), All Berries

KAPHA Cauliflower, Alfalfa, Nettles, Kelp, Green Leafy Vegetables (dier/dosha specific), Safflower Oil

VITAMIN P – CITRIN, RUTIN, BIOFLAVONOIDS, HESPERIDIN

Varicose Veins, Circulation

Utilized in the Body Bones, blood, gums, teeth, ligaments, skin stomach

Deficiencies Asthma, bleeding gums, gum infections, liver disorders, hardening of the arteries, fevers, miscarriage, varicose veins, influenza, tremors, Alzheimer's, rheumatic fever

Functions Prevents bruising; strengthens immune system; blood vessel strengthening; habitual miscarriage; strengthens nervous system; memory enhancement; ulcer prevention

Synthetic None

Toxicity None Known

R. D. A. None established

Therapeutic Dosage: Up to 400 mg

Water Soluble

Depleted By	Excessive bleeding, poor diet, lack of exercise, pregnancy, gaining and losing weight, antibiotics, aspirin & pain relievers, sulfa, inhalation of petroleum fumes, genetics, stress
VATA	Apricots, Black Strap Molasses, Citrus, Amla Plum, Rosehips, Tomatoes, Black Currant, Grapefruit, Cherries
PITTA	Buckwheat, Greens, Bulgar, Broccoli, Papaya, Algae, Shepherd's Purse, Chervil, Flder Berries, Horsetail, Apricot, Sweet Pepper, Violet Leaf, Grapes
KAPHA	Buckwheat, Greens, Blue Green Algae, Rosehips, Pepper, Prune, Pepper, Lemon, Parsley, Violet Leaf, Tamarind, Horsetail, Citrus (diet/dosha specific)

VITAMIN T – SESAME SEED FACTOR

Utilized in the Body	Blood, skin, hair, bones, nails
Deficiencies	Senility, dry skin, bleeding, constipation, anaemia
Functions	Circulation, skin, moisturizer, hair growth, calcium, healthy skin, memory enhancement, blood platelet formation
Synthetic	None
Toxicity	None Known
R. D. A.	None established

Therapeutic Dosage: Achieved by including foods in diet

Fat Soluble

Depleted By	Deficient Diet
VATA	Sesame Seeds, Egg Yolk, Raw Seeds (diet/dosha specific), All Seeds

PITTA	Butter, Raw Seeds (diet/dosha specific), Sunflower Seeds
KAPHA	Raw Seeds (diet/dosha specific), Pumpkin Seeds, Almonds

VITAMIN U

Utilized in the Body	Stomach, Intestines
Deficiencies	Ulcers, Volitis, underweight
Functions	Assists digestion and assimilation; protects stomach lining
Synthetic	
Toxicity	Not known
R. D. A.	None established

Therapeutic Dosage: Achieved by including foods in diet

Fat Soluble

Depleted By	Stress, anger
VATA	Fermented Vegetables, Sauerkraut
PITTA	Raw Cabbage, Leafy Green Vegetables
KAPHA	Raw Cabbage, Sauerkraut, Leafy Green Vegetables

Appendix III

AYURVEDIC MINERAL CHART

CALCIUM

Utilized in the Body	Bones, teeth, hair, nails, circulation, blood, skin
Deficiencies	Heart palpitation, menstrual cramps, nervousness, numbness, tooth problems, tremors, muscles
Functions	Repairing of bones, regulates heartbeat, calming of nerves, relieves muscle spasms
Synthetic	Calcium lactate, calcium gluconate, dolomite, egg shell calcium, oyster calcium
Toxicity	No known toxicity
R. D. A.	100 mg

Therapeutic Dosage: 400 - 1,500 mg. In addition to what is in diet

Depleted By	Enemas, lack of exercise, coffee, sugar, alcohol, cortisone
VATA	Cheese, Apricots, Figs, Bran, Comfrey, Chamomile, Borage, Chicory, Kelp, Dulse, Sardines, Salmon, Walnuts, Sesame seeds, Almonds, Well Cooked Greens, Raisins
PITTA	Milk, Apricots, Figs, Cabbage, Alfalfa, Red Clover, Nettles, Shepherd's Purse, Horsetail, Plantain, Chamomile, Borage, Chicory, Dandelion, Kelp, Kale, Sun Flower Seeds, Oats, Navy Beans, Raisins, Greens
KAPHA	Greens, Apricots, Cabbage Bran, Alfalfa, Red Clover, Comfrey, Nettles, Shepherd's Purse,

	Horsetail, Coltsfoot, Plantain, Chamomile, Borage, Chicory. Dulse, Leafy Vegetables, Kale, Chard, Legumes, Almonds, Corn, Raisins, Sesame Seeds

CHLORINE

Utilized in the Body	Arterial walls, stomach, liver, gallbladder
Deficiencies	Low agni, hair loss, edema
Functions	Production of hydrochloric acid: production of enzymes; electrolyte balance, muscle contraction
Toxicity	14-28 grain is considered to be in excess
R. D. A.	500 mg
Depleted By	Drinking too many liquids with meals, salt free diet, excessive sweating
VATA	Salt, Cheese, Coconut, Beets, Radishes, Avocado, Kelp, Olives, Watercress, Celery, Turnips
PITTA	Goat and Cow Milk, Cream, Cheese, Coconut, Radishes, Asparagus, Celery
KAPHA	Celery, Asparagus, Turnips, Fish Beets, Radishes, Avocado

CHROMIUM

Utilized in the Body	Blood, arteries
Deficiencies	Diabetes, low blood sugar, pancreatic disorders
Functions	Regulates sugar levels, increases vitality
Toxicity	No known toxicity
R. D. A.	50 mcg

Therapeutic Dosage: Up to 300 mcg

Depleted By	Excess sugar; too much dairy; too much meat
VATA	Corn Oil, Clams, Whole Grain Cereals, Catnip, Sarsaparilla, Sugar Cane Juice, Shellfish
PITTA	Whole Grain Cereals, Barley Grass, Bee Pollen, Red Clover, Sarsaparilla, Freshwater Fish
KAPHA	Corn Oil, Brewer's Yeast, Barley Grass, Bee Pollen, Red Clover, Catnip, Meat, Corn

COBALT

Utilized in the Body	Blood, circulatory system
Deficiencies	Anaemia, low blood cells and enzymes
Toxicity	Excess may produce side effects
R. D. A.	6 mcg

Therapeutical Dosage: 5-8 mcg.

Depleted By	Long fasting, enemas
VATA	Organ Meats, Oysters, Clams, Green Leafy Vegetable, Fruits (diet/dosha specifict), Ginseng, Comfrey, Watercress, Ashwagandha
PITTA	Organ Meats, Polutry, Green Leafy Vegetables, Fruits (diet/dosha specific), Comfrey, Ginseng, Watercress, Blue-Green Algae, Ashwagandha
KAPHA	Oysters, Green Leafy Vegetables, Fruits-(diet/dosha specific), Garlic, Spirulina, Blue-Green Algae, Chlorella, Ashwagandha

COPPER

Utilized in the Body	Circulatory system, nervous system, brain
Deficiencies	Respiratory problems, canker sores, fatigue, weak blood
Functions	Mental clarity, coordination of thoughts, bone

	development, connective tissue, formation of red blood cells
Synthetic	Copper sulfate
Toxicity	20 times the RDA over time may be toxic
R D. A.	2 mg.

Therapeutic Dosage: 2-10 mg.

Depleted By	Hallucinogenic drugs, antibiotics
VATA	Organ Meats, Seafood, Nuts, Molasses, Watercress, Spinach, Chard, Almonds
PITTA	Legumes, Raisins, Spinach, Kale, Cabbage, Chickweed, Chard, Whole Grains
KAPHA	Legumes, Watercress, Garlic, Kale, Cabbage, Chickweed, Prunes

FLUORINE

Utilized in the Body	Bone, teeth, hair
Deficiencies	Split nails, hair loss, weak bones, tooth decay
Functions	Increases growth of hair, strengthens nails and bones
Toxicity	Fluoride is toxic
R. D. A.	1 mg.

Therapeutic Dosage: 1.5 - 4 mg

Depleted By	Excess sugar; carbonated sodas
VATA	Cheese, Egg Yolk, Carrots, Black Tea, Shellfish, Watercress
PITTA	Cauliflower, Cabbage, Raw Goat Milk, Brussel Sprouts, Sunflower Seeds
KAPHA	Cauliflower, Cabbage, Brussel Sprouts, Seafood, Watercress, Spinach, Garlic, Carrots

GERMANIUM

Utilized in the Body	Cell regenerator, endocrine system
Deficiencies	Autoimmune diseases
Functions	Builds immune system, rejuvenator, life extension
Toxicity	None known
R. D. A.	None established

Therapeutic Dosage: None Known

Depleted By	Processed foods; smoking; alcohol
VATA	Aloe, Comfrey, Watercress, Ashwagandha
PITTA	Aloe Vera, Comfrey, Chlorella, Ginseng
KAPHA	Garlic, Chlorella

IODINE

Utilized in the Body	Hair, nails, thyroid, brain, bones
Deficiencies	Cold hands and feet, anger, manic-depression, obesity, thyroid disorders
Functions	Mental development, enhances digestion stabilizes fat metabolism, improves circulation
Synthetic	Potassium oxide (added to table salt), Natural source is seaweeds
Toxicity	Over 1,800 mcg, can cause problems
R. D. A.	150 mcg

Therapeutics Dosage: Up to 1,000 mcg

Depleted By	Too much Protein
VATA	Seaweeds. Kelp. Seafood. Carrots. Tomatoes. Pineapple. Dulse. Mushrooms. Irish Moss. Citrus Fruit. Artichokes. Turnips. Watercress. Sea Salt

PITTA	Seaweeds, Pears, Onions, Parsley, Sarsaparilla, Dulse, Mushrooms, Artichokes, Turnips, Greens
KAPHA	Carrots, Pears, Onions, Pineapple, Parsley, Sarsaparilla, Turnips

IRON

Utilized in the Body	Circulation, bones, skin
Deficiencies	Anaemia, fatigue, pale skin, constipation, poor assimilation
Functions	Improves immune system, clear complexion, red blood cell formation and haemoglobin
Synthetic	Ferrous fumarate (best-gluconate, worst - sulfate)
Toxicity	1,000 mg
R. D. A.	10 mg (Men) - 18 mg (Women)

Therapeutic Dosage: 10-15 mg.

Depleted By	Black tea, High protein diet, bleeding in ulcers etc.
VATA	Organ Meats, Eggs, Shellfish, Poultry, Prunes, Blackstrap Molasses, Apricots, Comfrey, Sorrel; Watercress, Fennel, Bananas, Dulse
PITTA	Lentils, Shellfish, Organ Meats, Poultry, Apricots, Potato Peelings, Nettles, Dandelion, Alfalfa, Yellow Dock, Comfrey, Chickweed, Mullein, Fennel
KAPHA	Lentils, Shellfish, Poultry, Potato Peelings, Nettles, Dandelion, Alfalfa, Yellow Dock, Chickweed, Mullein, Sorrel, Watercress, Fennel, Prunes

LITHIUM

Utilized in the Body	Brain, muscular system, nervous system
Deficiencies	Manic-depression, nervousness, anxiety
Functions	Balances and transports sodium metabolism to nerves, brain and muscles
Toxicity	None
R. D. A.	None available
Depleted By	Alcohol, hallucinogenic drugs, bi-polar disorder
VATA	Cream, Yogurt, Milk, Kelp, Dulse, Seafood
PITTA	Kelp, Dulse, Seafood
KAPHA	Buttermilk, Kelp, Dulse, Seafood

MAGNESIUM

Utilized in the Body	Brain, endocrine system, arteries, nervous system, stomach
Deficiencies	Weak bones, infections, confusion, irritability, excessive anger, trembling
Functions	Balances acid/alkaline, regulates blood sugar, metabolism of calcium of calcium and vitamin C
Synthetic	Magnesium palmatate, Magnesium sulfate
Toxicity	Large doses over a period of time 400 mg
Therapeutic Dosage: 300 - 1,800 mg	
Depleted By	Chemical drugs, alcohol
VATA	Lemons, Peaches, Beet Tops, Nuts, Figs, Seafood, Molasses, Yellow Corn, Water-cress, Oatstraw, Carrots, Almonds, Raspberries, Brown Rice, Sesame Seeds
PITTA	Peaches, Beet Tops, Sunflower Seeds, Apples, Alfalfa, Green Vegetables, Nettles, Burdock, Horsetail, Sage, Raspberries, Clover

KAPHA	Lemons, Beet Tops, Apples, Almonds, Green Vegetables, Coconut, Apples, Watercress, Alfalfa, Oatstraw, Nettles, Burdock, Carrots, Horsetail, Almonds, Sage, Clover

MANGANESE

Utilized in the Body	Circulation; blood; brain; endocrine system, especially the pituitary and thyroid
Deficiencies	Stomach disorders, hot flashes, dizziness, loss of hearing
Functions	Production of enzymes, hormonal function, muscular system, nervous system
Synthetic	Manganese gluconate
Toxicity	5 - 7.5 mg
R.D.A.	4 - 6 mg.

Therapeutic Dosage: 2 - 50 mg.

Depleted By	Too much fat; constipation
VATA	Egg Yolks, Beets, Citrus, Rice Bran, Kelp, All Nuts, All Seeds, Pineapple, Wheat Germ
PITTA	Peas, Rice Bran, Green, Vegetables, Sunflower Seeds, Blueberries
KAPHA	Peas, Citrus, Green, Vegetables, Almonds, Kelp

MOLYBDENUM

Utilized in the Body	Circulation, blood, stomach
Deficiencies	Poor digestion and assimilation
Functions	Important for oxidation
Toxicity	In large amounts
R. D. A.	None established

Therapeutic Dosage: 150 mcg - 500 mcg

Depleted By	Alcohol, carbonated drinks

VATA	Whole Grain Cereals-(diet/dosha specific)
PITTA	Legumes, milk, Liver. Dark Green Vegetables
KAPHA	Legumes, Whole Grain Cereals-(diet/dosha specific),Brewer's Yeast. Millet

PHOSPHORUS

Utilized in the Body	Circulation, blood, heart, urinary tract, nerves, teeth
Deficiencies	Loss of appetite, breathing disorders, sudden weight loss or gain, low blood sugar
Functions	Cell regeneration, vitality, assists heart and muscle contractions, calcium metabolism, assists nerve and muscular activity, assimilation of vitamins
Synthetc	Calcium phosphate
Toxicity	None known
R. D. A.	1000 mg

Therapeutic Dosage: 1500 mg

Depleted By	Sugar, mental stress, high fat diet
VATA	Cheese, Meat, Whole Grains-(diet/dosha specific), Egg Yolk, Lentils-(well cooked), Caraway Seeds, Parsley, Comfrey, Watercress, Licorice, dried fruit-(well soaked), All Nuts
PITTA	Dried Fruits-(well soaked), Milk, Fish, Poultry, Whole Grains-(diet/dosha specific), Legumes-(diet/dosha specific), Peas, Comfrey, Nettles, Chickweed, Alfalfa, Marigold, Dandelion, Licorice
KAPHA	Almonds, Whole Grains-(diet/dosha specific), Legumes-(diet/dosha specific), Peas, Caraway Seeds, Parsley, Watercress, Nettles, Chickweed. Alfalfa, Marigold, Dandelion

POTASSIUM

Utilized in the Body	Blood, heart, urinary tract, muscle tissue, nerves skin
Deficiencies	Fatigue, constipation, insomnia, weak reflexes
Functions	Balances sodium, assists all body activities, nerve functions and tissue growth
Synthetic	Potassium gluconate, Potassium chloride
Toxicity	None known
R. D. A.	2,500 mg

Therapeutic dosage: Up to 6,000 mg

Depleted by	Excessive urination, excessive perspiration, salt
VATA	Sweet potatoes, Tomatoes, Watercress, Dried Soaked Fruits, Vegetables, Whole Grain Cereals-(diet/dosha specific), All Nuts, Seeds, Comfrey, Coltsfoot, Parsley, Kelp, Dulse
PITTA	Potatoes, Sweet Potatoes, Sunflower Seeds, Lean Meats, Dried Soaked Fruits, legumes-Well Soaked-(diet/dosha specific), Vegetables, Whole Grain Cereals-(diet/dosha specific), Alfalfa, Comfrey, Coltsfoot, Borage, Chicory, Eyebright, mint, Plantain
KAPHA	Potatoes, Lean Meats, Dried Fruits, Vegetables, Whole Grain Cereals-(dosha/diet specific), Alfalfa, Coltsfoot, Water Cress, Borage, Chicory, Eyebright, Mint, Plantain, Parsley.

SELENIUM

Utilized in the Body	Male reproductive system, blood circulation
Deficiencies	Premature aging, hair loss, brittle nails, fatigue
Functions	Slows the aging process, antioxidant, blood oxidation

Synthetic	Natural sources only
Toxicity	Nausea occurs with excessive dosage
R. D. A.	50 mcg

Therapeutic Dosage: Up to 150 mcg

Depleted By	Stress, smoking, lack of B-vitamins
VATA	Tuna Fish Herring, Brewer's Yeast, Wheat Germ and Bran, Whole Grains-(diet/dosha specific), Eggs, Wheat Germ, Kelp
PITTA	Milk, Herring, Broccoli, Whole Grains-(diet/dosha specific), Kelp
KAPHA	Brewer's Yeast, Broccoli, Whole Grains-(diet/dosha specific), Kelp

SILICON

Utilized in the Body	Bones. nail. hair. teeth. endocrine system, reproductive system
Deficiencies	Premature aging. weak bones
Function	Promotes hair growth. strengthens bone tissue and nails. complexion. enhances immune system
Toxicity	None known
R. D. A.	None known
Depleted By	Stress, smoking. alcohol. fear. lack of B vitamins
VATA	Steel Cut Oats. Beets. Kelp. Grapes. Sweet Onions-(well /cooked). Almonds. All Seeds Parsnips, Whole Grains-(diet/dosha specific), Tomatoes, Horsetail. Leeks. Strawberries. Flaxseed
PITTA	Peanuts, Strawberries. Apples. Sweet Onions. Grapes. Parsnips. Whole Grains-(diet/dosha specific). Spinach. Horsetail. Dandelion. Nettles. Leeks

KAPHA	Peanuts, Strawberries, Apples, Almonds, Parsnips, whole Grains-(dosha/diet specific), Spinach, Horsetail, Dandelion, Nettles, Leeks, Strawberries, Flaxseed

SODIUM

Utilized in the Body	Lymph movement, muscular, arterial balance, all glandular activities, blood
Deficiencies	Chronic pain, diarrhoea, sugar imbalance, gallbladder problem
Functions	Lymphatic system, production of bile, adrenaline production, pancreatic enzymes, preparation
Synthetic	Sodium chloride
Toxicity	Loss of potassium; high blood pressure
R. D. A.	500 mg

Therapeutic Dosage: 2.000 mg.

Depleted By	Too much sugar, meat and dairy
VATA	Watermelon, Celery, Kelp, Sea Salt, Asparagus, Okra, Pork, Carrots, Beets, Organ Meats
PITTA	Romaine Lettuce, Celery, Asparagus, Okra, Coconut, Beet Greens
KAPHA	Romaine Lettuce, Celery, Asparagus, Carrots, Coconut, Irish Moss, Beet Greens

SULPHUR

Utilized in the Body	Bone tissue (hair, nails, skeletal), nervous system
Deficiencies	Early aging
Functions	All body tissue formation, collagen production
Toxicity	Possible with inorganic source
R. D. A.	None established.

Therapeutic Dosage : 500 - 1,000 mg Considered adequate when protein needs are met

Depleted By	Not known
VATA	Lean Meats-(diet/dosha specific), Eggs, Ocean Fish, Horseradish, Shrimp, Parsley, Sage, Celery, Watercress, Coltsfoot
PITTA	Celery, Legumes-(diet/dosha specific), Freshwater Fish, Cabbage, Brussel Sprouts, Chestnuts, Nettles, Plantain, Kale, Coltsfoot, Mullein, Shepherd's Purse, Cabbage
KAPHA	Legumes-(diet/dosha specific), Celery, Meat-(diet/dosha specific), Freshwater Fish, Cabbage, Brussel Sprouts, Horse Radish, Shrimp, Kale, Coltsfoot, Mullein, Shepherd's Purse, Cabbage, Sage

VANADIUM

Utilized in the Body	Circulatory system, blood
Deficiencies	High blood pressure, heart disorders
Functions	Breaks down cholesterol
R. D. A.	None established
Depleted by	Not known
VATA	Herring, Sardines
PITTA	Sea vegetables
KAPHA	Sea vegetables

ZINC

Utilized in the Body	Blood, brain, prostate, reproductive system, skin
Deficiencies	Late blooming, low appetite, loss of taste, poor circulation, liver disorders, prostate disorders,

	reproductive disorders, infertility, insulin insufficiency
Functions	Heals cuts and burns, assists breakdown of pancreatic enzyme production, prostate functions, maturity and development of all organs
Toxicity	None
R. D. A.	15 mg

Therapeutic Dosage: Up to 50 mg

Depleted By	Air pollution, alcohol, pregnancy
VATA	Sunflower Seeds, Seafood, Organ Meats, Mushrooms, Watercress, Pumpkin Seeds
PITTA	Sunflower seeds, Mushrooms, Soybeans
KAPHA	Soybeans, Brewer's Yeast, Watercress, Pumpkin Seeds

TRACE MINERALS

Arsenic

VATA	Asparagus, Celery, Salmon
PITTA	Celery
KAPHA	Asparagus, Celery

Boron

VATA	All Sweet and Sour Fruits, Purslane
PITTA	Dandelion, Yellow Dock, Chickweed, Astringent Fruits
KAPHA	Chickweed, Bitter Herbs

Borium

VATA	Organic Fruit, Vegetables, Nuts, Purslane, Dandelion Roots
PITTA	Organic Fruit, Vegetables Chickweed,

	Purslane, Nettles, Dandelion Leaf, Yellow Dock
KAPHA	Organic Fruit, Vegetables, Chickweed, Nettles, Dandelion Leaf, Yellow Dock

Bromine

Utilized in the Body	Heart, circulation
Deficiencies	Heart disorders, kidney/bladder disorders and edema
Functions	Circulation and water balance
Depleted By	Excess alcohol and sugar
VATA	Melons, Cucumber, Seafood
PITTA	Melons, Cucumber, Alfalfa
KAPHA	Alfalfa, Turnips, Seafood

NICKEL

Utilized in the Body	Tissue repair, bones, heart, and circulation
Functions	Builds strong Bones, healthy tissue
Depleted By	Not known
VATA	All vegetables (diet/dosha specific), all herbs (diet/dosha specific), Fenugreek
PITTA	All vegetables (diet/dosha specific), All Herbs (diet/dosha specific), Alfalfa, Red Clover, Oat Straw, Fenugreek
KAPHA	All Vegetables (diet/dosha specific), All Herbs (diet/dosha specific), Alfalfa, Red Clover, Oat Straw, Fenugreek

Appendix IV

DIETS FOR TRIDOSHAS

DIET FOR REDUCING VATA IMBALANCE

Grains

Take	Avoid/Reduce
Basmati rice	Barley
Brown rice	Rye
Oats	Corn
Wheat	Granola
Couscous	Millet
Spelt	No dry cereals
Amaranth	Corn chips unless eaten
Buckwheat	with cheese

Vegetables

Take	Avoid/Reduce
Well cooked	Bean Sprouts
with butter,	Peas
lemon	Brussel sprouts
Beets	Cauliflower
Cucumber	Lettuce
Carrots	Fresh corn
Yams	Raw vegetables
Jerusalem	(these vegetables may be
artihokes	eaten in small quantities)
Mushrooms	-always cooked
All tubers	

Take	Avoid/Reduce
Okra	
Pickled veggies	
Celery	
Potato	
All squash	
Kale	
Turnip	
Spachetti and winter squash	
Asparagus	
Yucca	
Animal Foods	
Pork	Rabbit
Seafood	Beef
Turkey	
Chicken	
Duck	
Spices	
Anise	Chili
Bay	Tarragon
Juniperberry	Cayenne
Asafoetida	Caraway
Basil	Peppermint
Caraway	
Cardamon	
Cinnamon	
Black pepper	

Take	Avoid/Reduce
Clove	
Coriander	
Sage	
Cumin	
Fennel	
Garlic	
Ginger	
Onion	
Thyme	
Turmeric	
Fenugreek	
Nutmeg	
Allspice	
Horseradish	
Fruits	
Avocado	Apple
Banana	Cranberry
Cantaloupe	Dried fruits
Cherries	Melon
Coconut	Pear
Fresh figs	Pomegranate
Peaches	Jujube
Grapefruit	
Kiwi	
Dates	
Lime	
Lemon	

Take	Avoid/Reduce
Mandarine	
Mango	
Papaya	
Grapes	
Persimmons	
Sweet fruits	
Sweet berries	
Sweet oranges	
Sweet pineapple	
Sweet plums	

Dairy Products

• Take all dairy products unless there is an allergy, Especially, fermented like Keifer, cream cheese.

Beans

All beans should be avoided except for pulses, green beans and tofu, Make into a paste or dahl: chick peas, mung beans, pink lentils.

Oils

Take	Avoid/Reduce
All oils, although the best are sesame oil, ghee and mayonnaise	Canola Corn oil Mustard oil

Nuts and Seeds

Take	Avoid/Reduce
All nuts – best soaked	Peanuts – dry roasted
Peanuts in butter	Pumpkin

Take	Avoid/Reduce
Sweeteners	
Sugar cane products	Raw honey
Molasses	Carob
Stevia	
Rice syrup	
Sucanat	
Cooked honey	
Beverages	
Hot herbel teas	Cold drinks
I small glass wine – (no sulfates) with meals.	Coffee Black tea
Warm rice milk	All other alcohols
No carbonated drinks	

DIET FOR REDUCING PITTA IMBALANCE

Take	Avoid/Reduce
Grains	
Barley with spice	Brown rice
Buckwheat	Yellow corn
Quinoa	Yeasted breads
Oars	
Kumut	
Soda Breads and pancakes	
Wheat	
Rye	

Take	Avoid/Reduce
Millet	
White basmati rice	
Corn	
Vegetables	
Asparagus	Beets
Broccoli	Carrots
Alfalfa sprouts	Chard
Brussel sprouts	Chilis
Artichokes	Eggplant
Gabbage	Garlic
Green bell	Onions
Peppers	Hot peppers
Cauliflower	Mustard greens
Celery	Tomatoes
Eggplant	Parsley
Cucumber	Pickles
Green beans	Purpple peppers
Lettuce	Radish
Mushrooms	Spinach
Okra	
Peas	
Potatoes	
Pumpkin	
Turnips	
Sweet Potatoes	
Steamed sweet onions	
Turmips	

Take	Avoid/Reduce
Zucchini	
Lots of greens	
Animal Foods	
Chicken	Beef
Egg white	Egg yolk
Pork	Lamp
Turkey	Duck
Pheasant	
Freshwater fish	
Spices	
Chlantro	Clove
Milk curies	Fenugreek
Cinnamon	Ginger
Mint	Nutmeg
Cumin	Horseradish
Fennel	Oregano
Lotus seeds	Rosemary
Dill	Sage
Lemongrass	Salt
Lemon skin	Asofoetida
Braggs Aminos	Hing, All other spices, hot spices
Beverages	
Cold drnks	Alcohol
Soy milk	Coffee Tea
	Hot drinks

Take	Avoid/Reduce
Fruits	
Coconut	Grapefruit
Cherries	Lemon juice
Grapes	Limes
Melon	Olives
Pear	Papaya
Pomegranate	Peaches
Sweet fruits	Persimmon
Sweet oranges	Sour oranges
Sweet Pineappples	Sour Pineapple
Sweet plnms	Mango
Dairy Products	
Butter	Cheese (highly
Cottage cheese	fermented)
Cream cheese	Cultured
Ghee	buttermilk
Milk	Kefie
Rice dream	Salry cheeses
Soybean	Sour cream
Ice cream	Yogurt

Beans

Most beans are advisable, especially mung, tofu, aduki, black chickpeas, lima, soybeans, fava.

Oils

Sesame

Corn

Others

Take	Avoid/Reduce
Nuts	
Lotus seed	Peanuts
Sunflower	Almonds
Cashews	Pine nuts
(best to skip	Pumpkin
in the summer)	Sesame seeds
Sweeteners	
Maple syrup	Honey
Rice syrup	Molasses
Stevia	White sugar
Barley syrum	Chocolate
Best to Avoid/Reduce	
Fermented products	
Vinegars	
Red meat	
Salt	
Tobacco	

Note: *Avoid/Reduce means; When balanced, decrease consumption eat occassionally, When imbalaneed, avoid completey, If unclear as to your your body type, consult an ayurvedic practitioner*

DIET FOR REDUCING KAPHA IMBALANCE

Grains

Take well cooked (with spices)	Avoid/Reduce
Basmati rice	Millet
	Brown rice

Take well cooked (with spices)	Avoid/Reduce
Buckwheat	Wheat
Corn	White rice
Rye	Oats
Dry cereals	
Roasted grains	
Quinoa	
Couscous	
Barley	
Vegetables (75% of diet)	
Artichokes	Cucumber
Beets	Okra
Fresh corn	Sweet
Turnips	potatoes
Asparagus	Tomatoes
Bok choy	Zucchini
Bitter melon	Sweet and juicy veggies
Bell peppers	
Carrots	
Broccoli	
Cabbage	
Spinach	
Swiss chard	
Celery	
Eggplant	
Green salads	
Leafy greens	
Lettuce	

Take	Avoid/Reduce
Mushrooms	
Chili peppers	
Mustard greens	
Onions	
Sprouts	
Potatoes	
Squash	
Hot peppers	
Radish	
Animal Foods	
Freshwater fish	Beef
Rabbit	Chicken
Turkey (dark meat)	Duck
Venison	
Beverages	
Almond milk	Ice cold
Ginger tea	drinks
Coffee (1 cup per day)	Avoid
Cranberry juice	All Vinegars
Tea	
Carbonated drinks	
I small glass wine with meals	
Fruits (especially dry)	
Apple	Bananas
	Coconut
Cranberry	Dates

Take (especially dry)	Avoid/Reduce
Dried fruits	Figs
Lemons	Prunes
Grapefruit	Grapes
Pears	Kiwi
Persimmons	Melons
Pomegranate	Orange
Raisins	Pineapple
Papaya	Sweet fruits
Blueberries	
Strawberries	
Apricots	
Dairy Products	
Small amounts	Fermented,
unsalted ghee	aged dairy
soft chese,	
cottage cheese	
Beans	
All beans, especially aduki,	Tofu in extreme Kapha
fave, kidney,	chickpeas
lentils, lima	Hummus
Oils (Small Amounts)	
Beat cold pressed	All others
Canola	
Flax	
Corn	
Mustard	

Take	Avoid/Reduce
Almond	
Sunflower	
Soya	
Mayonnnaise	
Peanuts	
Sweeteners	
Small amounts of raw uncooked honey	All other sweeteners
Nuts and Seeds	
Best if sprouted	All others
Flax	Peanuts
Pumpkin	
Sunfower	
Spices	
All spices, especially ginger	Pickles
	Salt vinegar

***Note** : Avoid/Reduce means; When balanced, decrease consumption eat occassionally, When imbalaneed, avoid completey, If unclear as to your your body type, consult an ayurvedic practitioner.*

DIET FOR REDUCING VATA-KAPHA OR KAPHA-VATA IMBALANCE

(When Vata is obstructed, it is best to follow a Kapha diet)

Take	Avoid/Reduce
Grains (cooked well)	
Basmati rice	Barley
	Buckwheat
Oats	Corn
Wheat	Granola
Couscous	Miller
Spelt	Rye
Amaranth	No dry cereals
	Corn chips unless eaten with cheese
Vegetables - (well cooked)	
With butter, lemon	Bean sprouts
	Brussel sprouts
Beets	Raw vegetables
Cilantro	Caulifower
Carrorts	Lettuce
Yams	Rresh corn
Cucumber	(the above vegetables may be eaten in small quantities-always cooked)
Celery	
Jerusaleum Artichockes	
Mushrooms	
Okra	
Okara	

Take	Avoid/Reduce
Green beans	
Broccoli	
Pickled veggies	
Spinach	
Potato	
Acorn	
Turnips	
Asparagus	
Cooked Kale	
Turnips	
Asparafus	
Cooked greens	
Cooked eggplant	
Animal Foods	
Pork	Rabbit
Seafood	Beef
Turkey	
Chicken	
Duck	
Spices	
Anise	Chile
Bay	Cayenne
Asofoetida (Hing)	Peppermint
Bay	
Caraway	
Cardamon	
Cinnamon	

Take	Avoid/Reduce
Juniper	
Black pepper (small amounts)	
Clove	
Coriander	
Sage	
Cumin	
Fennel	
Garlic	
Ginger	
Onion	
Caraway	
Tarragon	
Turmeric	
Thyme	
Fenugreek	
Nutmeg	
Allspice	
Horseradish	
Fruits	
Avocado	Apple
Banana	Cranberry
Payaya	Dried fruits
Cantelope	Pear
Cherries	Pomegrante
Grapes	Jujube
Coconut	Melons
Fresh figs	

Take	Avoid/Reduce
Peaches	
Grapefruit	
Kiwi	
Dates	
Lemons	
Lime	
Mandarine	
Mango	
Persimmons	
Sweet berries	
Sweet plums	
Sweet fruits	
Sweet pineapples	
Add spices to fruits	

Dairy Products

All dairy products, unless there is an allergy, especially fermented like yogurt, buttermilk, keifer, cream cheese, soy, rice, almond cheeses.

Beans

All beans should be avoided except for pulses, beans and tofu.

Oils

Take	Avoid/Reduce
All oils, although,	Canola
the best are:	Corn oil
sesame, ghee	Mustard oil
Mayonnaise	

Nuts and Seeds

Take	Avoid/Reduce
All nuts-best	Peanuts-dry

Yes	Avoid/Reduce
soaked	roasted.
	Pumpkin
Sweetners	
Cooked honey	Raw honey
Molasses	Carob
Stevia	
Rice syrup	
Sucanat	
Beverages	
Hot herbal teas	Cold drinks
1 small glass wine	Coffee
(with no sulfates)	Black tea
with meals	All other
Warm rice milk	alcohols
	No carbonated drinks

Note : *Avoid/Reduce means; When balanced, decrease consumption eat occassionally, When imbalaneed, avoid completey, If unclear as to your body type, consult an ayurvedic practitioner*

DIET FOR REDUCING PITTA-VATA OR VATA-PITTA IMBALANCE

(When there is extreme imbalance or allergies, diet may have to be modified)

Grains

Take	Avoid/Reduce
(well cocked)	Barley
Basmati rice	Brown rice

Take	Avoid/Reduce
Spelt	Wheat
Oats	Buckwheat
Amaranth	Corn
Couscous	Granola
Rye	Millet
Quinoa	No dry cereals
	Corn chips unless eaten with cheese

Vegetables (well cooked with butter and lemon)

Take	Avoid/Reduce
Carrots	Bean sprouts
	Peas
Yams	Cabbage
Cucumber	Cauliflower
Okra	Lettuce
Jerusalem	Fresh corn
Artichokes	Eggplant
Mushrooms	Raw vegetables
Brococli	(these vegetables
Celery	may be eaten in
Sweet potato	small quantities,
Acorn squash and all squash	always cooked)
Kale	
Turnips	
Spaghetti and winter squash	
Asparagus	
Steamed onion	
All greens	
Dandelion	

Take	Avoid/Reduce
Fennel	
Animal Foods	
Seafood	Rabbit
Turkey	Beef
Chicken	
Duck	
Spices	
Anise	Chili
Bay	Juniper berries
Asofoetida (Hing)	Sage
Basil	Cayenne
Cilantro	Caraway
Cardamon	Clove
Cinnamon	Garlic
Black pepper (small amounts)	
Coriander	
Sage	
Cumin	
Fennel	
Fresh garlic	
Peppermint	
Onion	
Milk curries	
Sea salt	
Tarragon	
Thyme	

Take	Avoid/Reduce
Fenugreek	
Nutmeg	
Allspice	
Turmeric	
Fruits	
Avocado	Apple
Banana	Cranbery
Cantaloupe	Dried fruits
Melon	Pomegramate
Cherries	Jujube
Coconut	
Fresh figs	
Peaches	
Grapefruit	
Kiwi	
Dates	
Lime	
Lemon	
Mandarine	
Mango	
Papaya	
Grapes	
Persimmon	
Sweet berries	
Sweet fruits	
Sweet oranges	
Sweet pineapples	

Yes	Avoid/Reduce
Sweet plums	
Cooked apples	
Cooked pears	

Dairy Products

All dairy products are advisable unless there is an allergy.

Beans

All beans should be avoided except for pulses (dahl), beans with ghee and beans with tofu.

Nuts and Seeds (all nuts best soaked)

Yes	Avoid/Reduce
Sunfoower, sprouted	Peanuts dry
Peanuts in butter	Pumpkin roasted

Sweeteners

Yes	Avoid/Reduce
Sucanat	Raw honey
Fructose	Carob
Stevia	
Rice syrup	
Cooked honey	

Beverages

Yes	Avoid/Reduce
Herbal teas	Cold drinks
1 small glass	Coffee
wine (no	Black tea
sulfates) with meals	All other alcohols
Warm rice milk	No carbonated drinks

Note : *Avoid/Reduce means; When balanced, decrease consumption eat occassionally, When imbalaneed, avoid completey, If unclear as to your body type, consult an ayurvedic practitioner*

DIET FOR REDUCING PITTA-KAPHA OR KAPHA-PITTA IMBALANCE

Take	Avoid/Reduce
Grains (well cooked)	
	Millet
Barley	Brown rice
Basmati rice	Wheat
Buckwheat	White rice
Corn	
Rye	
Dry cereals	
Roasted grains	
Quinoa	
Couscous	
Vegetables (75% of diet)	
Artichokes	Cucumber
Asparagus	Okra
Bell peppers	Sweet Pota toes
Beets	Tomatoes
Turnips	Zucchini
Bitter melon	Sweet and juicy
Bok choy	vegetables
Fennel	Radish
Broccoli	Carrots

Take	Avoid/Reduce
All greens	Hot peppers
Swiss chard	
Cabbage	
Cauliflower	
Celery	
Egglant	
Spinach	
Green pepper	
Lettuce	
Green salads	
Leafy greens	
Mushrooms	
Mustard greens	
Dandelion	
Onions	
Sprouts	
Potatoes	
Squash	
Animal Foods	
Freshwater fish	Beef
Turkey	Seafood
Venison	Chicken
	Duck
	Lamb
	Pork
	Fatty foods
	Fried, greasy, meats

Yes	Avoid/Reduce
Spices	
Coriander	Pickles
Mint	Salt
Cardamon	Vinegar
Cilantro	
Turmeric	
Ginger	
Anise	
Fennel	
Cinnamon	
Milk curries	
Fruits (especially dry)	
Apple	Banana
Dried fruits	Dates
Lemon	Figs
Gapefruit	Prunes
Pear	Grapes
Persimmon	Kiwi
Pomegranate	Melons
Raisins	Oranges
Papaya	Pineapple
Strawberry	Sweet fruits
Apricot	
Blue berries	
Dairy Products	
Goatmilk (small amount, unsalted)	Fermented, aged dairy products

Take	Avoid/Reduce
Ghee Soft cheese Cottage cheese	
Beans	
All beans, especially aduki, fava, kidney, lentils, lima	Tofu in extreme Kapha Chickpeas Hummus
Oils (small amounts)	
Best cold pressed Canola Flax Corn Mustard Almond Sunflower Soy Maynnaise Peanut	All others
Sweeteners	
Small amount only - raw uncooked honey	All other sweeteners
Nuts and Seeds	
Best if sprouted Flax seed	All others Peanuts

Yes	Avoid/Reduce
Pumpkin seed	
Sunfolwer	
Beverages	
Almond milk	Ice cold drinks
Ginger tea	
Coffee (1 cup per day)	
Lemonade	
Tea	
Carbonated drinks	
Wine - l small glass with meals	

Note : *Avoid/Reduce means; When balanced, decrease consumption eat occassionally, When imbalaneed, avoid completey, If unclear as to your body type, consult an ayurvedic practitioner*

Appendix V

LIST OF PLANTS FROM WHICH IMPORTANT AYRUVEDIC PREPARATIONS ARE MADE

Acacia catechu: Khadirarist, Khadir sar, Khadiradi kwath, Khadirastak, Kadiradi vati, Kutajarista, Lavangadi vati, Chandanadi vati, Vrihtkhadiradi vati, Jarurkula and Marham kharishjadin.

Achyranthes aspera: Apamargkshar taila, Apamarg asav, Apamarg avaleh, Cystone, Kushta samul-far, Kustha shangraf and Kushta hartal warqi. Besides, Somal bhasm, Hartal bhasm and Vang bhasm also obtained with the help of apamarg.

Aegle marmelos : Bilvapanchak kwath, Bilvadichurna, Bilvadighrit, Bilva taila, Bilvadileh, Brhidgangadhar churna and Majun bawasir; also one of the ingredients of Dashmula.

Allium cepa: Majun piyaz:

Allium sativum: Lasunadivati, Lasunadhyaghirit, Rasonpinda, Rasonashtak, Majunseer and Rasonasura. Some companies are selling the oil of garlic in pear-shaped, capsules under the trade name 'Garlic' or 'Gasgo' for the gastric disorders.

Aloe barbadensis: Kumariasva, Kumarikavati, Kumaripak, Rajparvatni vati, Habb shabyar, Habb-ayariz, Habb sibra, Habbantkar and Suful dama.

Alstonia scholaris: Saptparnasatvadi vati, Saptchhadadi kwath and Malariasamhar vati. Besides, Grieve (1973), stated that the plant is also used in homoeopathy for its bitter, tonic and astringent properties.

Asparagus racemosus: Shatavari ghirit, Phalghirit, Shatmulyadi louh, Shatavari panak, Narayan taila, Dhatupaushtik churna, Shatavari churna, Suparipak, Lakshmivilas ras, Basant kusumakar ras, Phalkalyan ghirit, Saraswatrisht, Geriforte, Halwa-i-supari pak, Halwa-i-ghaikwar, Majun zanjibil, Majun shir bargadh wali and Majun musli pak.

Azadirachta indica: Nimbadi kwath, Nimbadi churna, Nimbarisht, Nimbharidrakhand, Amber mezhugu and Habbebawasir.

Bambusa arundinacea: Sitopaladi churna, Talishadi churna, Sudarshan churna, Chandraprabha vati and Kurs tabashir.

Bauhinia variegata: Kachnar guggulu, Kachnaradi kwath, Kachnar gudika, Hab mussafi khun, Sufuf kalan and Majun suparipak.

Boerhavaia diffusa: Punarnava mandur, Punarnava-kshar kwath, Punarnava ark, Punarnava ashtak, Punarnava asav, Punarnava churna, Calcury and Jawarish zaruni ambari ka naksha Kalan.

Bombax ceiba: Musli-pak, Shalmali ghrit, Pushyanug churna, Brihadgangadhar churna, Musli simbhal, Halwa-i-chakwar, Majun kalan and Sufuf habis.

Butea monosperma: Palashbijadi churna, Palashkshar ghirt, Palashadi kwath, Calcury (used against ureteric calculus), Majun zanzgbil and Majun supari pak.

Caesalpinia bonduc: Bijai churna, Karanjadi ghrit, Karanjadi churna and Visham javarghani vati.

Cannabis sativa: Madnanand modak, Jati-phaladi churna, Lai churna and Majunphalakser. Besides, In homeopathy, flowering tops of freshly harvested plants are used.

Capsicum annum: Visam jawaraghni vati and Lanka sura.

Cassia fistula: Aragvadhadi-kshar, Aragvadhadi taila, Aragvadhadi leh, Aragvadharishta, Aragvadhadisutravarti and Aragvadha kwatham.

Centella asiatica: Brahmi rasayana, Brhami taila, Brahmi sarbat, Brhami ghirt, Brahmi pak, Brahmi panak, Saraswatarisht, Saraswat ghrit, Brahmi halwa, Brahmi malhar and Majun brahmi.

Curcuma longa: Haridrakhanda, Chandraprabha vati, Laghu-vis-garva-taila, Pippalasav, Punarnava mandur, Sudarshan churna, Vidangadi lep, Geriforte, Majnoon-e-falsfa and Habs harkachur.

Cynodon dactylon: Durvadi kwath, Durvadi ghrit and Durvadi taila.

Cyperus rotundus: Mustakadi Kwath, Mustakarisht, Mustadi churna, Mustadileh, Shandgapaniya, Jawarish jalinush and Majun-murrawal-ul-anwah.

Datura metal:	Kanakasava, Dhaturdhum, Martyuanjaya ras, Dattuphal vasma, Dhatturadi pralep, Laghu-vis-garva taila, Dugdha vati, Jawrankush, Haba shafa and Roghan dhatura.
Datura stramonium:	Kankasav, Dhaturdhum, Martyuanjaya ras and Jawarankush.
Derris indica:	Karanjadi churna, Karanjadi ghrit, Karanjadi taila, Karanjadi yog, Vidangadi lep and Habb karanjaba,
Desmostachya bipinnata:	Trinpanchmul, Kusableha and Kusadya-ghrit.
Eclipta prostrata:	Bhringraj taila, Shadbindu taila, Bhringraj ghrit, Bhringrajadi churna, Tafroli, Hab miskeen nawaz, Roghan amala khas and Majun murrawah-ularwah.
Emblica officinalis:	Chavyanprash, Brahma rasayan, Dhartri louha, Triphala, Amalkyadi churna, Sudarshan churna, Sarvajawar louha, Agnitundi vati, Sanjivani vati, Phaltrikadi kwath, Punarnava mandur, Navayas louha, Rakta pittantak louha, Pippalayasav, Sringayadi churna, Karanjadi yog and Itriphan ustkhudus.
Ficus bengalensis:	Nyagrodhadi churna, Nyagrodhadi ghrita, Nyagrodhadi kwath and Majun bargad.
Ficus racemosa:	Udumbar sar.
Ficus religiosa:	Hartal bhasm and Sharbat peepar.
Fumaria indica:	Parpati kwath, Parpatadhyarist, Shadgapaniya, Sharbat murakkab

	musaffi khun, Sufuf chob mala and Sufuf burghina wala.
Gloriosa superba:	Kasisadi taila, Languli rasayan and Laghuvis garva taila.
Gmelina arborea:	Dashmularisht, Kutajarisht, Sriparnyadi kwath, Sriparni taila and Brihat panchmuladi kwath.
Holarrhena antidysenterica:	Kutajarista, Kutajavaleha, Kotari-ras, Bhuinimbadi churna, Brihat sudarshan churna, Pathadya, Pradoranilauha, Amritastak kwath, Sudarshan churna, Sarvajwar hara louha, Atsayakadi kwath, Majunregmahi, Majunsalab, Majun bawasir and Sufuf habis.
Justicia adhatoda:	Vasaka churna, Vasaka kwath, Vasakarista, Vasaka ghirta, Vasa avieha, Vasa kshar, Vasa chandanaditaila, Phalatrikadi kwath, Vasadi kwath, Kanakasav, Vunimbadi kwath, Chavyanprash, Geriforte, Shagat aijaz and Bakhor dama.
Madhuca longifolia:	Madhukasav, Kutajarishta, Kanakasav, Parthadyarishta and Madhukadi him.
Moringa oleifera:	Shobhanjandi lep, Syamadi churna, Sudarshan churna, Sarva-jwar-har louha and Shobhanjanadi kwath.
Oroxylum indicum:	Dashmula ghrit, Dashmula taila, Dashmularisht, Chavyanprash and Shyonak putpak.
Piper longum:	Gurpippali, Pippalikhand, Pippalasav, Pippalimuladi Kwath, Videngadi-louha, Chandraprabha vati, Gokshuradi kwath, Kukwadi churna, Khadirarista, Aragbadhyadi kwath, Arnlakayadi

	churna, Sudarshan churna, Sarvajwarhar-louha, Amritarista, Anandbhairav ras, Hingavastak churna, Lavanbhaskar churna, Rasonvati, Agnitundi vati, Sanjivani vati, Punarnava mandur, Nayas louha, Rakta pittantak louha, Talisadi churana, Sitopaladi churna, Trikatu churna, Kaphketu ras, Sringadi churna, Kanakasav, Karanjadi yog, Yograj guggulu, Narachras, Itriphal fauladi, Angaruya-i-kabir and Majun khadar.
Plumbago zeylanica:	Chittrakadi gutika, Chittrak haritaki, Chittrak ghrit, Chittrakadi churna, Devdaradi kwath, Arnlyadi churna, Sudarshan churna, Sarvajwar louha, Agnitundi vati, Punarnava mandur, Navayas louha, Pipplyasav, Yograj guggulu, Laghuvis-garva taila, Aryogyavardhini vati, Chandraprabha vati, Aquaruva-i-kabir, Hab ashkhar, Majun baladur and Majun raigmahi.
Punica granatum:	Dadima chatusham, Dadimastak, Dadimadi churna, Dadima ghirt, Dadimadi taila and Lavanbhaskar churna.
Rauvolfia serpentina:	Sarpgandhaadi churna, Sarpgandha yog, S arpgandha vati and Hala fisher.
Ricinus communis:	Erandpak, Erandmuladi kwath, Erandsaptak kwath, Rasnadi kwath, Rasna panchak kwath, Vishgarbh taila and Jimade sheeraeshutur.
Saccharum : spontaneum	Trinapanchmul kwath, Kusavleha and Kusadya ghrit

Sapindus mukorossi: Tiriyak afuyun.

Saraca asoca: Ashokarishta and Ashokaghrit.

Sida species: Baladikwath, Baladya ghrit, Baladya arista, Chandanbala lakshadi taila, Sudarshan churna and Kukuvadi churna.

Solanum ferox: Brihatyadi kwath, Brihatyadi gan, Sudarshan churna, Dashmularishta, Devdarvadi kwath, Dashmula taila, Chavyanprash and Satayadi kwath.

Solanum surattense: Dashmula ghrit, Dashmularishta, Dashmula taila, Dashmula kwath, Nidigdhikadi kwath, Bayaghri haritaki, Bayaghri taila, Kantkari ghrit, Kantkari avieha, Sudarshan churna, Sarva hara louh, Kanakasav, Devadarvadi kwath and Sringayadi churna.

Stereospermum chelonoides: Dashmula ghrit, Dashmula taila, Dashmularisht, Dashmuladi kwath and Chavyanprash.

Tamarindus indica: Juwarishae tamarae nindi, Sharbetae tamarae hindi, Astanga lavan and Tartaric acid.

Terminalia arjuna: Arjunarista, Arjunaghirt, Parthodhyarista, Arjunatwak churna, Kukubhadi churna, Hridayarnava ras and Arjun ksheerpak.

Terminalia chebula: Abhaya modak, Abhayarista, Agastiharitaki, Agnitundivati, Amrita haritaki, Arnlakyadi churna, Arogyavardhini vati, Aragbadhyadi kwath, Byaghri haritaki, Chittrak haritaki, Chandraprabha vati, Gokshuradi guggulu, Danti haritaki.

Haritaki khand, Haritakadi kwath, Khadirarista, Kukuvadi churna, Karanjadi yog, Laghu-vis-garva taila, Navayas louha, Pathyadi kwath, Pathyadi churna, Panchaskar churna, Phaltrikadi kwath, Punarnava mandur, Sanjivani vati, Sarvajwar louha, Sringayadi churna, Sudarshan churna, Dashmula haritki, Triphala, Vasadi kwath, Vidangadi lep, Itriphalsagir, Sharbat murrakale musaffi khun and Majun mochras.

Tinospora cordifolia: Gudachyadi Kwath, Guduchi louha, Guduchayadi churna, Amritarista, Kirattiktodi kwath, Sudarshan churna, Sanjivani vati, Amritastak kwath, Phalatrikadi kwath, Guduchi taila, Pippalimuladi kwath, Panchbhadra kwath, Rasnasaptak kwath, Yograj guggulu, Kaisur guggulu, Rasnapanchak kwath, Sansmani vati, Arkharabhara, Sat giloe and Arq maul laham mako kashiwala.

Tribulus terrestris: Dashmula kwath, Gokshuradi churna, Gokshuradi kwath, Gokshuradi guggulu, Gokshuradi avaleha, Abhayarista, Chavyanprash, Rasna saptak kwath, Haritakayadi kwath, Vrihatvarunadi kwath, Ark murkkab mussafikhoon, Sharbat bazuri motadil, Sharbat mudir, Lulab-al-asrar, Majun zangibil and Sufuf kalan.

Vitex negundo: Nirgundi kalpa, Nirgundi taila, Vishgarbha taila and Safuf fanjkisht.

Withania somnifera: Ashwagandhadi churna, Ashwagandha rasayan, Ashwagandha ghirt, Ashwagandharishta and Narayana taila.

Woodfordia fruticosa: Dhatkayadi churna, Dhatkayadi taila, Kutajarista, Laghugangadhar churna, Abhyayarista, Pippalayasav, Kanakasav, Khadirarista, Parthadyarista, Ashokarishta, Majun zangibil and Arq faulad.

Zingiber officinale: Amritarista, Adarkkhand, Panchsam churna, Samsharkar churna, Rasnadi kwath, Saubhagya shunthi, Shunti sura, Shunthi panak, Talishadi chura, Lavangadi churna, Hingvastak churna, Javarish zangibil, Majun izaraqui and Murraba adrak.

Zizyphus mauritiana: Sharbat zufah murrakab, Sharbat sadar, Sharbat unnab, Sharbat murakkab musaffikhun and Arq murkkab musaffikhun.

Appendix VI

COMMON GROUPS OF HERBS

The following are some common herbal formulas used in ayurveda, either by themselves or as part of greater formulas.

Groups	Constituents
Triphala The three fruits : laxative, rejuvenative	Haritaki, bibhitaka, amalaki
Trikatu The three spices : stimulant, digestive	Dry ginger, long pepper, black pepper
Trijata Carminative, anti-emetic	Cinnamon, cardamom, cinnamon leaf
Chaturjata Carminative, appetizer	Trijata and nagakeshar
Trimada Clears consiousness, opens channels, removes obstructions	Vidanga, cyperus, chitrak
Chaturbija The four seeds: carminative, stimulant	Fenugreek, watercress, kalajaji, yavani
Parichakola The five barks: astringent, anti-styptic, anti-diuretic, haemostatic	Long pepper (pippali), pippali ashwattha, plaksha, parisha
Panchapallava Astringent, anti-diarrhoeal, for diabetes	Mango, jambu, kapittha, citron, bilwa
Trinaparichamula Increase urination, for urinary tract stones	Kusha, kasa, nala, darbha, sugar cane

Panchatikta The five bitters: antipyretic, febrifuge, alterative	Vasa, guduchi, neem, kantakari, patola
Brihat Panchamula The greater five roots: alleviates Vata	Bilwa, patala, agnimantha, syonaka, sambhari
Laghu Panchamula The lesser five roots : alleviates Vata	Shalaparni, prishniparni, kantakari, gokshura, brihati
Dashamula The ten roots: alleviates Vata, good for basty (enema therapy)	Combines Brihat and Laghu Panchamula

Appendix VII

LIST OF AYURVEDIC PREPARATIONS

Kwatha	Decoction
Phanta	Hot infusion
Hima	Cold infusion
Swarasa	Fresh juice
Kalka	Crushed pulp of the plant
Ghana	Herbal decoction evaporated to solid
Arka	Liquid extracts
Avaleha	Herbal jellies
Asava and Arista	Fermentations or tinctures of herbs
Churna	Powders
Ghrita	Medicated ghee
Kshara	Extraction of alkalies from plants
Lavan	Salts
Guggul	Resins and balsams
Lepa	Pastes
Upanaha	Poultices
Malahara	Ointments
Panak	Crushed fruits and their preparations
Sattva	Active or concentrated herb principles
Taila	Medicated oils
Varti	Suppositories
Guti-vati	Tablets

Bhasma	Herbal oxide ashes
Sara	Resins
Kshira	Exudations
Anjana	Ointments
Dravak	A mixture of various ashes of plants, salts, and alkalies distilled to produce a liquid substance, like Shankhadrava
Druti	Solid Substances converted into liquids, like liqeuefied sulphur

—

Appendix VIII

GLOSSARY OF MEDICAL TERMS

Abcess	Collection of pus in a tissue
Abortifacient	Agent that cause abortion
Abortion	Giving birth to an embryo or fetus prior to stage of viablity
Adenitits	Inflammation of a gland
Alexteric	Defensive to infectious diseases
Amenorrhoea	Absence or abnormal cessation of the menses
Anaemia	Reduction of erythrocytes below normal number in the blood
Analgesic	Agent that relieves pain
Anasarca	Accumulation of fluid in subcutaneous tissues
Angina	A severe constricting pain, commonly used interm of angina pectoris
Anodyne	Agent capable of relieving pain
Anorexia	Loss of appetite
Anthelmintic	Agent that destroys expulsion of intestinal worms
Antidote	Counteracts poison
Antiemetic	Counteracting nausea and vomiting
Antiperiodic	Agents that prevents the regular occurrence of a disease or a symptoms
Antiphlogistic	Preventing or relieving inflammation
Antipyretic	Agent that reduces fever

Antiscorbutic	Effective in prevention of scurvy
Antispasmodic	Preventing spasms
Aperient	Mild purgative
Aphrodisiac	Arousing sexual desire
Aphthous	Relating to ulcer on mucous membrane with exudate
Ascites	Abnormal accumulation of serous fluid in peritonial cavity
Asthma	A condition marked by recurrent attacks of paroxysmal dyspnea with wheezing
Astringent	Agent that causes contraction, usually after local application
Atonic	Without normal tension
Bechic	Pertaining to cough
Beriberi	A disease due to deficiency of Vitamin B1
Billiousness	Complex system of nausea, abdominal discomfort, headache and constipation due to excessive bile secretion
Blindness	Loss of ability to see
Bronchitis	Inflammation of bronchi
Bruise	Superficial discolouration of the skin due to hematoma without rupture
Buboes	Inflammatory swelling of lymph-glands in the groin
Carbuncle	Deep infection of several contagious hair follicles with formation of connecting sinus which results in ulceration and formation of pus
Carminative	Relieving flatulence
Cataract	Opacity of crystalline lens of the eye
Catarrh	Inflammation of mucous membrane with discharge

Cathartic	Strong purgative
Cephalgia	Headache
Chilblain	A recurrent localized itching, swelling and painful erythema of finger
Cholagógue	Which stimulates gall bladder contraction and promotes the flow of bile into the intestine
Cholera	Acute infectious disease caused by *Vibrio cholerae*
Cirrhosis	Intestinal inflammation of an organ, particularly of liver
Colic	Spasmodic pain in the abdomen
Coma	Unconsciousness from which the patient cannot be roused even by powerful stimuli
Congestion	Abnormal accumulation of blood in part of the body
Conjunctivitis	Inflammation of the mucous membrane covering the anterior surface of the eye ball
Contraceptive	Agent for prevention of conception
Contusion	Bruise without rupture of blood vessels
Convulsion	Violent spasm
Coryza	Inflammation of the nasal mucous membrane with discharge
Cystitis	Inflammation of the urinary bladder
Debility	Weakness
Delirium	Mental disturbance of relatively short duration usually reflecting a toxic state marked by illusion and excitement
Demulcent	Soothing
Diarrhoea	Abnormal frequent evacuation of watery stools
Diphoretic	Agent that promotes sweating
Diphtheria	An acute disease, caused by *Corynebacterium*

	diphterieae and marked by formation of grey white pseudomembrane in nose and throat or larynx with fever and also respiratory obstruction
Diuretic	Agent that promotes the flow of urine
Dropsy	An abnormal accumulation of fluid in intercellular spaces of the body.
Dysentery	Inflammation of intestine with frequent stools with blood
Dysmenorrhoea	Painful menstruation
Dyspepsia	Impairment of power or function of digestion
Dyspnea	Difficult breathing
Dysuria	Discharge of urine with pain and difficulties
Eczema	Superficial inflammation of the skin marked by redness itching and minute papules and later by scaling, lichenification and often pigmentation
Edema	An abnormal accumulation of fluid in intercellular spaces of the body
Elephantiasis	Inflammation of fibrous tissues caused by filarial worms
Emaciation	Growing pain
Emetic	Agent that causes vomiting
Emmenagogue	Agent that promote menustral flow
Emollient	Agent that softens the skin and soothes irritation of the skin
Epilepsy	Syndromes characterized by paroxysmal transient disturbances of brain function that may be manifesed as episodic impairment or loss of consciousness psychic disturbances or perturbation of the autonomic nervous system

Epitaxis	Nose bleeding, usually due to rupture of small vessels over lying anterior part of the cartilaginous nasal septum
Erysipelas	A disease characterized by the inflammation and redness of the skin
Euphoria	Absence of pain or distress
Expectorant	Agent that increases bronchial secretion and facilitates its expulsion
Fatigue	A state of diminished capacity to respond effectively to stimulus reducing the efficiency
Febrifuge	A remedy for fever
Febrile	Feverish
Fistula	Abnormal passage, usually between two organ, especially near anus
Flatulence	Excessive gas formation in stomach intestine
Galactagogue	Agent that promotes the secretion and flow of milk
Glaucoma	Eye disease, characterized by an increase in ocular pressure causing visual defects
Gonorrhoea	A contagious inflammation of the genital mucous membrane transmitted chiefly by coitus and due to *Neisseraia gonorrhoae*
Haemeplegia	Paralysis of one side of body
Haemoptysis	Spitting of blood from the lungs or bronchial tubes
Haemorrhoids	Piles
Haemostasis	Arrest of bleeding
Helimintniasis	Vomiting of worms
Hemicrania	Unilateral headache
Herpes	Any inflammatory skin disease marked by formation of small vesicles in clusters

Hydrocele	A circumscribed collection of fluid, especially in tunica vaginallis of testis or along the spermatic cord
Hydrophobia	Fear of water caused by rabies
Hyperglycaemia	Abnormal high concentration of glucose in blood
Hypertension	Persistent high blood pressure
Hypotension	Low blood pressure
Hyptonic	Decreased tension
Hysteria	A term used widely in psychiatry; sudden onset of dream states, stupor and paralysis
Impetigo	Scabby eruption commonly occurring on the face caused by bacteria
Impotency	Lack of sexual power
Indigestion	Lack of failure of digestion, usually used to denote vague abdominal discomfort after meals
Indolent	Painless
Inflammation	Injury or destruction to protective tissues, signs are pain, heat, redness, swelling and loss of function etc.
Insomnia	Sleeplessness
Jaundice	Yellowness of skin, mucous membrane and excretion due to hyper biliruinemia and deposition of bile pigment
Lactagogue	Agent that promotes milk flow
Leprosy	Chronic communicable disease, caused by *Mycobacterium lepreae* characterized by production of mucous membranes and peripheral system
Leucoderma	Depigmentation of the skin

Lochia	Discharge from the reproductive tract occurring after childbirth
Lumbago	Pain in lumbar region
Mania	A phase of bipclar disorder and characterized by expansiveness, elation, agitation, hyperexcitablity, hyperactivity and increased speed of thought and ideas
Measles	Contagious viral infection, usually of childhood marked by an eruption of discrete , red papules which become flatten, confluent and brown
Melancholia	Depressed and unhappy emotional state with abnormal inhibition of mental and bodily activity
Menorrhagia	Excessive or prolonged menstruation
Nausea	An unpleasant sensation, vaguely referred to epigastrium and abdomen
Neuralgia	Nerve pain
Nyctalopia	Night blindness
Opthalmia	Inflammation of eye
Orchitis	Inflammation of testis
Otatgia	Ear-ache
Otitis	Inflammation of bone
Paralysis	Impairment or loss of motor function in a part due to lesion of the neural or muscular mechanism
Pityriasis	Skin disease marked with formation of fine and braining scales
Pleurisy	Inflammation of pleura, serous membrane investing the lungs
Pneumonia	Inflammation of lungs with exudation and consolidation
Prolapse	Descending of an organ from normal position

Prurigo	Skin diseases marked by intense itching
Pruritus	Itching
Psoriasis	Chronic or heriditary recurrent dermatitis marked by discrete vivid red macules, papules or plaques covered with silvery lamellated scales
Pubescent	Arriving at puberty stage
Puerperal	Post natal period
Purgative	Agent that causes bowel evacuation
Purulent	With pus formation
Rabies	Infectious viral disease of central nervous system results from rabid animal bite
Refrigerant	Agent that causes cooling effect
Rinderpest	Cattle plague
Rubefacient	Reddening of the skin
Scabies	Contagious skin disease, caused by itch mite; *Sarcoptes scabiei*
Sciatica	Neuralgic along the course of the sciatica nerve, most often with pain radiating into buttock and lower limb
Scorbutic	Relating to scurvy
Scrofula	Tuberculosis with glandular swellings
Scurvy	A disease caused due to vitamin C deficiency
Sedative	Agent that cause excitement
Sialagogue	Agents that enhance the flow of saliva
Spasmolytic	Agent that relieves spasm
Spermatorrhoea	Involuntary discharge of semen
Sprains	Rupturing of ligaments but they remain intact
Sprue	Chronic form of malabsorption syndrome
Stomatitis	Inflammation of the mucous membrane of the mouth

Strangury	Slow and painful discharge of urine
Sudorific	Agent that causes sweating
Suppuration	Formation of pus
Syphilis	An acute and chronic infectious disease caused by *Treponema pallidum* (Syn. *Spirocheta pallida*) and transmitted by direct contact, usually through sexual intercourse
Tetanus	An acute often fatal infectious disease caused by *Clostridium tetani* whose spores entered in body through wounds
Thermoplegia	Heatstroke or sunstroke
Tuberculosis	Infectious disease, caused by *Mycobacterium* and marked by tubercle formations and caseous necrosis in any organ tissue
Tumour	Swollen part of the body, one of the cardinal signs of inflammation
Ulcer	A wound with superficial loss of tissue
Urethritis	Inflammation of urethra
Urothrorrhoea	Abnormal discharge from urethra
Urticaria	An eruption of the skin characterized by transient appearance of slightly elevated reddish patches associated with severe itching
Vermicidal	Agent that is lethal to intestinal animal parasites
Vertigo	Dizziness
Vesicant	Producing blisters
Whitlow disease	Primary herpes, simplex infection of terminal segment of a finger with much tissue destruction

General Index